The Web of Poverty
Psychosocial Perspectives

HAWORTH Marriage & the Family
Terry S. Trepper, PhD
Senior Editor

Christiantown, USA by Richard Stellway

Marriage and Family Therapy: A Sociocognitive Approach by Nathan Hurvitz and Roger A. Straus

Culture and Family: Problems and Therapy by Wen-Shing Tseng and Jing Hsu

Adolescents and Their Families: An Introduction to Assessment and Intervention by Mark Worden

Parents Whose Parents Were Divorced by R. Thomas Berner

The Effect of Children on Parents by Anne-Marie Ambert

Multigenerational Family Therapy by David S. Freeman

101 Interventions in Family Therapy edited by Thorana S. Nelson and Terry S. Trepper

Therapy with Treatment Resistant Families: A Consultation-Crisis Intervention Model by William George McCown, Judith Johnson, and Associates

The Death of Intimacy: Barriers to Meaningful Interpersonal Relationships by Philip M. Brown

Developing Healthy Stepfamilies: Twenty Families Tell Their Stories by Patricia Kelley

Propagations: Thirty Years of Influence from the Mental Research Institute edited by John H. Weakland and Wendel A. Ray

Structured Exercises for Promoting Family and Group Strengths: A Handbook for Group Leaders, Trainers, Educators, Counselors, and Therapists edited by Ron McManus and Glen Jennings

Psychotherapy Abbreviation: A Practical Guide by Gene Pekarik

Making Families Work and What to Do When They Don't: Thirty Guides for Imperfect Parents of Imperfect Children by Bill Borcherdt

Family Therapy of Neurobehavioral Disorders: Integrating Neuropsychology and Family Therapy by Judith Johnson and William McCown

Parents, Children, and Adolescents: Interactive Relationships and Development in Context by Anne-Marie Ambert

Women Survivors of Childhood Sexual Abuse: Healing Through Group Work: Beyond Survival by Judy Chew

Tales from Family Therapy: Life-Changing Clinical Experiences edited by Frank N. Thomas and Thorana S. Nelson

The Practical Practice of Marriage and Family Therapy: Things My Training Supervisor Never Told Me by Mark Odell and Charles E. Campbell

The Therapist's Notebook: Homework, Handouts, and Activities for Use in Psychotherapy edited by Lorna L. Hecker and Sharon A. Deacon

The Web of Poverty: Psychosocial Perspectives by Anne-Marie Ambert

The Web of Poverty
Psychosocial Perspectives

Anne-Marie Ambert

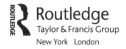

Routledge
Taylor & Francis Group
New York   London

First published in 1998 by The Haworth Press, Inc., 10 Alice Street, Binghamton, NY 13904-1580

This edition published 2014 by Routledge

711 Third Avenue, New York, NY 10017, USA
2 Park Square, Milton Park, Abingdon, Oxon OX14 4RN

Routledge is an imprint of the Taylor & Francis Group,an informa business

Cover design by Monica L. Seifert.

Library of Congress Cataloging-in-Publication Data

Ambert, Anne-Marie.
   The web of poverty : psychosocial perspectives / Anne-Marie Ambert.
      p.   cm.
   Includes bibliographical references and index.
   ISBN 0-7890-0232-9 (alk. paper).
   1. Poor–North America. 2. Poverty–North America. 3. Poverty–North America–Psychological aspects. 4. Inner cities–North America. I. Title.
HV4042.A5A53   1997
362.51097–dc21   97-14968
                                                                                       CIP

CONTENTS

Foreword   xi
        Terry S. Trepper

Acknowledgments   xiii

Introduction   1

Origins of This Volume   2
Volume Contents   3
Intended Audiences   4

Chapter 1. Poverty in the United States and Canada   7

Across the World   7
Poverty in North America   11
    Canada and the United States   11
    The Extent of Poverty   12
    Other Aspects of Poverty   13
The Gap Between Rich and Poor   14
Mobility Out of and Back into Poverty   16
The Reduction of Rural Poverty   19
Conclusion   20

Chapter 2. Systemic Causes of Poverty   23

Globalization of the Economy   23
Evolving Structure of the Economy   25
    Relative Loss of Manufacturing Jobs   25
    Expansion of the Service Sector   27
    Increase in Part-Time Employment   28
    Increase in Low-Paying Jobs   29
    Increase in Two-Wage-Earner Families   30
    Higher Educational Requirements   31
    Job Relocation   32
    Emphasis on Financial Profit   33
Unemployment   34
National Debt   36

Low Social Assistance Payments 36
Low-Skilled Immigration 38
Conclusion 39

Chapter 3. Personal Causes of Poverty 41

Single Parenting 42
   Single Parenting and Poverty 43
   Divorced Single Parenting 45
   Never-Married Parenting 46
   Effects on Children 48
Poverty in the Family of Origin 50
School Dropout and Lack of Education 51
Additional Factors: Delinquency and Ill Health 53
Conclusion 54

Chapter 4. Urban Neighborhoods in Poverty 57

The Canadian Exception 58
The Development of High-Poverty Neighborhoods 59
Depletion of Neighborhood Resources 62
Poor Neighborhoods and Negative Socialization of Children 64
Poor Neighborhoods as Risk Factors for Children 67
Homelessness 70
The Nonpoor in Disadvantaged Neighborhoods 71
Conclusion 72

Chapter 5. Schools and Education in Poor Districts 75

Schools in Impoverished Neighborhoods 75
Quality of School Personnel and Disadvantaged Families 78
Disadvantaged Students and Schools 80
Family Routine and Organization 81
Parental Resources and Involvement in Schooling 82
Low-Income Minority Students 85
Involuntary and Voluntary Minorities 87
Conclusion 90

Chapter 6. Disadvantaged Families   **91**

Family Size   92
Adolescent Single Parenting   93
    The Situation   93
    Consequences for Offspring   95
    Types of Single Adolescent Mothers   97
    Single Fathers: The Real Problem?   99
Family Conflict and Violence   100
    Marital Conflict and Spousal Abuse   100
    Child Abuse   101
    Child Neglect   102
    Abuse of Parents by Children   103
Parenting Skills and Poverty   104
Parental Dilemmas   106
Conclusion   107

Chapter 7. Women, Children, and the Elderly   **109**

Women   109
Mothers in Poverty   111
    Their Burden   111
    The Matter of "Proper" Childrearing Practices   112
    Mothers as Victims   114
Children   115
    The Extent of Child Poverty   115
    Consequences of Poverty for Children   117
    Negative Child Outcomes   118
Homeless Children   120
The Elderly   122
Elderly Women   124
Conclusion   125

Chapter 8. Visible Minorities, Discrimination,
and Segregation   **127**

Recent Roots of Inequalities   128
Racial and Ethnic Inequalities and Poverty   131
Segregation   133
Work Discrimination   135
Health Differentials   138

Reduced Life Expectancy   140
Conclusion   141

Chapter 9. Health and Illness Differentials   **143**

Health and Socioeconomic Status   143
Life Expectancy   145
    The Differentials   145
    Myths About Life Expectancy   147
Explanation for Differentials   149
Illness-Related Problems   150
Psychiatric Problems   152
Cognitive Problems   154
Is More Medical Care the Solution?   156
Conclusion   158

Chapter 10. Poverty and Delinquency   **159**

Aspects of Delinquency   159
Personal Pathways to Delinquency   160
Causes of Delinquency   162
Poverty and Delinquency   164
    Poverty and Social Control   164
    Poverty and Segregated Minorities   166
    Poverty and Dysfunctional Opportunity Structure   169
Poverty and the Media   171
Conclusion   173

Chapter 11. Poverty Undermines Genetic Potential   **175**

Genetics and Child Outcomes   176
    Outline of Behavior Genetics Principles 176
    Genotype-Environment Correlations   178
Genetically Influenced Chains of Events   180
Environmentally Influenced Chains of Events   181
Environmental Rather Than Personal Deficits   182
Poverty Creates Inferiority   186
The Absurdity of African-American Inferiority   187
Conclusion   189

Chapter 12. Conclusions, Implications, and Critiques   **191**

    A Subculture of Poverty?   193
    Ethnic Cultures and Subcultures of Poverty   194
    A New Meritocracy   196
    Social Pathologies   198
    A Subculture of Wealth: The "Overclass"   200
    Reducing the Concentration of Neighborhood Poverty   201
    The Global Perspective   204

Glossary   **207**

Reference Notes   **213**

Bibliography   **227**

Author Index   **281**

Subject Index   **293**

ABOUT THE AUTHOR

Anne-Marie Ambert (PhD, Cornell University) is Professor in the Department of Sociology at York University, Toronto, where she has taught for well over two decades. Prior to joining the faculty at York, Dr. Ambert was on the faculty of three different American universities. The author of seven books and the editor of two volumes, she has published widely in the areas of family, child development, and youth in journals such as *Criminologie, American Journal of Psychiatry, Canadian Review of Sociology and Anthropology, Social Science and Medicine,* and *Journal of Marriage and the Family.* Her current research interests reside in poverty as it relates to family life and human development. Dr. Ambert holds memberships in sociological, psychological, and child development associations.

Foreword

I came from a middle-class background, went to middle-class schools, and was taught and supervised by middle-class professors. While always considering myself "sensitive" to the problems of the poor, I certainly was not knowledgeable about those problems. One of the difficulties of not clearly understanding the causes and effects of poverty is that it leads to a naïve assumption that family problems have the same origin and treatment for *all* families regardless of economic status. I now wish I had read a book like *The Web of Poverty* years ago, as it would have lessened my naiveté about the interaction between poverty and mental health.

This book, written by one of Canada's premier family sociologists, Anne-Marie Ambert, is a comprehensive look at both the causes and effects of poverty. Her approach is highly systemic, examining in depth the multiple systems involved with the development of poverty, and those systems that are impacted by poverty. While most books on poverty less than subtly advocate one particular agenda or another, this text is clearly an unbiased scholarly endeavor. That makes this work unique and very important, both as a nonevaluative review for scholars and as a textbook for upper-division and graduate students.

This book should be of interest to family research scholars and students, since most all of the current sociological research and theory on poverty and the family is described and analyzed. This book should also be read by all clinicians, from each of the therapy disciplines, who may ever see a poor family in therapy. It will expand their view of social inequalities, and help them better see poverty as a cause of mental health problems. Finally, this book will also be of interest to general readers who may be interested in this critical problem of poverty and its effect on families.

I hope you enjoy this book as much as I have. It is very well written, extremely interesting, and a very important work on a major North American problem.

Terry S. Trepper, PhD
Executive Editor
Haworth Marriage and the Family
Professor of Psychology and Marriage and Family Therapy
Purdue University Calumet

Acknowledgments

The research necessary for this book and for the preceding one, *Parents, Children, and Adolescents,* took several years to gather. This enterprise would not have been possible without a grant from the Social Sciences and Humanities Research Council of Canada (grant #410-91-0046). I am grateful to Tonda March, former Managing Editor for the *Journal of Marriage and the Family,* for copyediting. I also benefited greatly from the patient editing of Peg Marr and Deb Johnston at Haworth. My daughter Stephanie has contributed to the preparation of my recent books throughout her adolescence. Now, as a social work student, she has been responsible for the entire technical production of the manuscript, from word processing, to bibliography, to indexing. The book would not have proceeded as rapidly without her help. Terry Trepper, Executive Editor, Haworth Marriage and the Family, and Bill Palmer, Vice President of The Haworth Press Book Division, have encouraged my ideas for books with their repeated confidence. It is worth mentioning that I have stayed with The Haworth Press because it is the most author-friendly publisher I have ever encountered.

Introduction

Poverty is the most urgent social problem facing North America. Poverty diminishes the effectiveness of a society and its institutions, and blunts the quality of life of families and their individual members. In the United States and Canada, the paradox of poverty amidst affluence is particularly troubling. This is the more so because the possibility of substantially reducing poverty exists, but the will of political and financial institutions is lacking. In this text, the causes of poverty are examined, but the focus is on consequences, particularly for families, children, and minorities. The approach combines both psychological and sociological perspectives.

The deleterious effects of poverty on individuals cannot be adequately grasped without consideration of the cultural and social contexts in which their lives unfold. The meaning of poverty in North America is quite different from that in Latin America and particularly in Africa. In many non-Western societies, poverty is endemic, historically rooted, and seemingly intractable. The reality of poverty is therefore different around the world in terms of its causes and contexts. It affects all human beings similarly on certain dimensions no matter where they live. However, on other dimensions, it affects citizens of various countries in different ways because of the types of cultures, social systems, and economies in which their lives are embedded. Thus, while many of the life risks attached to economic disadvantage, such as illness, malnutrition, and shortened life expectancy, are universal, others are culture specific. Here one can think of teenage pregnancy and delinquency in North America compared with child labor and lack of schooling in some parts of Asia and Africa.

A further complication attached to the study of poverty is that there is some overlap between consequences and personal causes. For instance, school dropout is a cause of future poverty for youngsters who do not pursue their education. In addition, it is a consequence of poverty for those youth born into families that are economically disadvantaged or who live in areas where job opportunities are scarce. Therefore, personal causes of poverty are also likely to be consequences, while systemic causes generally operate only at the broader causality level. A case in point is unemployment created by corporate downsizing. It operates only at the causality level and is not a consequence of poverty.

Yet another problematic aspect of the study of poverty arises when, by looking at aggregates—that is, the *average* for all poor people compared with others—we fail to take into account the *diversity* that exists among the disadvantaged (Furstenberg et al., 1994). Not only do poor individuals vary among themselves according to sociodemographic characteristics such as age, gender, race, and place of residence, but they also vary in the reasons for their poverty, the length of time during which they are poor, their psychological characteristics, individual resources, and coping skills. In this text, we try to reflect this diversity, although the lack of data in several of these domains makes such a task difficult to accomplish.

ORIGINS OF THIS VOLUME

This book was written as one of the possible extensions of a text on parent-child relations and human development, titled *Parents, Children, and Adolescents: Interactive Relationships and Development in Context* (Ambert, 1997a). It arose out of my frustration, due to space considerations, of not being able to discuss at greater length the context of poverty as it impacts family relationships, places adults and children at risk of suffering from numerous difficulties, and prevents parents—particularly mothers—from raising their children as effectively as more fortunate parents can. Thus, I had already gathered a great deal of research material on poverty but could not fit it within the scope of my earlier book without substantial digressions.

A second incentive to write this volume stemmed from the realization that books on poverty in general do not address the personal issues and data related to individuals' experiences with disadvantage, whether in terms of health, family, or human development. The other side of the coin is that texts on human development cannot address the global or systemic causes and consequences of poverty.

As a social psychologist and sociologist with extensive interest not only in family relationships and human development but also in social structure, the necessity to amalgamate the psychological and sociological aspects of poverty seemed obvious. It is my hope that I have achieved this goal so that this text is of use to a diverse group of scholars.

VOLUME CONTENTS

The book opens with an introduction to the global dimensions of poverty in North America, that is, the United States and Canada. It is followed by two chapters on the origins of poverty: societal or systemic causes (Chapter 2) and personal causes (Chapter 3), the latter including variables such as single parenting and low educational levels. The two chapters are closely interlinked in that the individual causes of poverty cannot exist on such a large scale as is currently the case without the promoting effect of societal factors. The remainder of the book focuses on the consequences of poverty.

Chapters 4 through 6 examine social units and institutions as they are affected by the multiple causes of economic disadvantage. Chapter 4 discusses the development of the concentration of poverty in neighborhoods and the dangers that are experienced by children and youth living in these areas. In Chapter 5, the emphasis is on schools located in poor districts, which are often racially segregated, and how these schools contribute to the creation and perpetuation of inferiority among their students. The focus of Chapter 6 is on families that are disadvantaged: their structure, domestic violence and abuse, the parenting role, and the dilemmas that impoverished parents face are discussed. A particular emphasis is placed on adolescent parenting, both as a consequence and as a cause of poverty.

With Chapter 7, we begin inquiring into the effects of poverty on specific categories of individuals, in this case, women (including women as mothers) children, and the elderly. Chapter 8 examines the plight of minority groups that are disproportionately poor, and the role of discrimination and segregation in causing and maintaining disadvantage. This chapter includes a discussion of both systemic and personal causes of poverty at the source of minority impoverishment. In Chapter 9, health and illness differentials stemming from poverty are examined. Chapter 10 introduces another consequence of poverty, that is, widespread delinquency. The focus of Chapter 11 is most unusual for a book on poverty: it is on the interaction of genes and environment. It tackles the question of what poverty does to individuals' genetic endowments. The chapter explains how poverty prevents the actualization of positive qualities and fosters negative outcomes in human development. The suggestion that the poor, and particularly blacks, may be genetically inferior is examined. The concluding chapter offers perspectives, critiques, and thought-provoking comments on the "subculture of poverty," the new meritocracy, and social pathologies, as well as on the "subculture of wealth" and the "overclass."

INTENDED AUDIENCES

Most of the books on poverty are written from an economic or macrosociological perspective, where large economic, historical, and social variables predominate. There are some books, albeit fewer, in other disciplines focusing on specific issues related to poverty such as ethnic/racial groups, children, or women. The various readerships do not generally meet because they are separated by disciplinary boundaries, access different scholarly journals, and are constrained by lack of time from exploring the research carried out in other fields. In the present volume, I have tried to include all the perspectives mentioned above in order to provide a certain level of cross-fertilization between disciplines and domains. As a result, this text is more interdisciplinary than many other books on poverty.

This volume aims to inform a double potential audience. The first includes scholars in one field or another who may wish to use the book to familiarize themselves with areas concerning poverty that fall outside their own disciplines. For example, most scholars who write on poverty have not had the opportunity to become acquainted with the literatures on family relations, child socialization, behavior genetics, education, urban sociology, or even delinquency. For their part, scholars who write on these same topics are generally not familiar with the various global perspectives on poverty that could pertain to their concerns.

The book was also written for a student audience as a text for advanced courses in social problems, social stratification, family studies, social work, and education, as well as for specialized courses in disciplines that are apparently unrelated, that is, economics, political science, and human development. Multidisciplinary references and endnotes will help students develop essay topics. In addition, a glossary of terms is included at the end of the book; concepts covered in the glossary are highlighted by boldface characters when they are first mentioned in the text. The volume is clearly written, with a minimum of jargon, and although it does include many basic statistics, tables have been intentionally left out. Instructors who adopt this work as a text will find several pedagogic features in an accompanying Instructor's Manual designed to facilitate their task.

Several areas of specialization are covered in different chapters, although the single largest focus of this book is on families and youth: seven of the twelve chapters discuss families and children. Therefore, for researchers and advanced students interested in these topics, the contents of Chapters 3 through 7, as well as Chapters 10 and 11, discuss these domains under various perspectives. For the more specialized topics of parenting, childrearing, and child development, a number of sections can be considered synchronously, given that they cover complementary aspects and viewpoints on the condition of impoverished parents, particularly mothers, and their children. These sections include, in Chapter 1, the section on mobility out of and back into poverty; in Chapter 3, the four subsections pertaining to single parenting; in Chapter 4, the section on poor neighborhoods and negative socialization of children, and the section on poor neighborhoods as risk factors for children; most of Chapter 5; in Chapter 6, the sections on adolescent parenting, parenting skills and poverty, and parental dilemmas; in Chapter 7, the sections on mothers in poverty, children, and homeless children; in Chapter 10, some aspects of the sections on delinquency and poverty; and much of Chapter 11.

Researchers and students interested in minorities and poverty can similarly find relevant and complementary sections in several chapters. These include several sections on the evolving structure of the economy, as well as on low-skilled immigration, in Chapter 2;

single parenting and school dropout in Chapter 3; much of Chapters 4 and 5; adolescent parenting in Chapter 6; several sections of Chapter 7; the entirety of Chapter 8; delinquency and poverty in Chapter 10; the last three sections of Chapter 11; and several sections of Chapter 12.

Last, but not least, for those interested in women's studies, it should be noted that many of the sections listed earlier under the topic of mothers and parents are relevant. To these should be added the subsection on two-wage-earner families in Chapter 2, the section on elderly women in Chapter 7, and, to a more limited extent, the section on psychiatric problems in Chapter 9.

Finally, an interesting and unusual aspect of this book is that it contains both U.S. and Canadian data. Research and governmental statistics from the two adjoining countries are presented and discussed. However, because there are more American than Canadian research publications, the bulk of the literature reviewed is American. Nevertheless, as is explained later, there are more similarities than differences between the two countries in the causes and consequences of poverty so that research results and government statistics obtained in one country generally apply to the other. Exceptions are noted where applicable. It is therefore hoped that this cross-border perspective produces a larger framework for the study of poverty than would otherwise be possible.

Chapter 1

Poverty in the United States and Canada

In this chapter, the extent and dimensions of poverty in the United States and Canada are described. We then discuss the widening gap between rich and poor, and families' mobility out of and back into poverty. The reduction of rural poverty in recent decades is documented. However, the extent of poverty among various ethnic and racial groups in the population is discussed in subsequent chapters. But, first, we begin by situating poverty within the context of continents characterized by endemic low income. This allows us to place the American and Canadian situation within a more global perspective.

ACROSS THE WORLD

Poverty is not as widespread in Western and industrialized countries as it is in Africa, Latin America, and parts of Asia. Many of the countries on these continents are paralyzed by seemingly intractable impoverishment that frequently cohabits with a multitude of social problems. Among these are government corruption, civil wars, abuses of human rights, lack of infrastructure, lower education levels (particularly among women), ill health, and elevated fertility rates, to mention only a few of the social ills that plague many economically disadvantaged countries. In contrast, poverty in North America is less widespread, more temporary for the majority of those affected, appears more tractable, and stems from different causes. However, the high level of deprivation that North America's two contiguous nations tolerate among their citizens is or should be an anomaly. The reasons for this anomaly reside in these countries' affluence, their level of economic development, their democratic institutions, and their ability to manage large-scale international crises. The fact that they are considered to have an enviable standard of living, are favored by prospective immigrants throughout the world, and are at the forefront of technological innovations makes this situation even more paradoxical.

Today, the African continent, particularly the sub-Saharan portion, contains the greatest concentration of what is referred to as low-income economies. These are countries with a per capita **GNP***** of $580 or less. They include Mozambique ($80), Ethiopia ($120), and Tanzania ($130).[1] The per capita GNP of middle-income countries, such as South Africa, and nations in South America/Northern Africa, and Eastern Europe is less than $6,000 per year. High-income economies, such as those in North America, enjoy a per capita GNP well above $6,000 a year.

What characterizes most sub-Saharan Africa is that it is the only part of the globe that, after a period of growth in the early 1960s, has recently slipped more deeply into the abyss of poverty. This has been occurring at a time when the rest of the world is progressing markedly at the economic and technological levels (Kingue, 1996). Causes of African impoverishment are external debt, decline in both industrial and agricultural output, and weak exports (Yansane, 1996). Because of the lack of resilience of the various African economies, they have been buffeted more than others by externally created disruptions, such as sharp rises in oil prices in the 1970s and 1980s (Simon, 1995). Other causal features of poverty are totalitarian and corrupt regimes that exploit and deprive the masses (Tshishimbi, Glick, and Thorbecke, 1994). Consequently, these nations exhibit a huge gap between the very rich and the very poor.

African poverty is regularly aggravated by droughts and famines, which are often created when violence disrupts villagers' lives and agricultural activities are then abandoned (Scheper-Hughes, 1987). Thus, civil wars constitute another cause of impoverishment. Some recur in the same country or last for a decade, while others seem to

---

*Glossary terms are set in boldface type upon first mention.

flare up briefly, devastating the economic infrastructure, displacing peasants whose lands then lie fallow, and creating entire generations of dislocated youth. These youths, who are often regimented as "boy soldiers" (Fyfe, 1989), are not only unschooled, hence untrained for any occupational sector, but are also seeped in a culture of lawlessness and violence.

Sub-Saharan Africa has the lowest rate of capital formation and foreign investment in the world, two ingredients necessary to create an economic revival. This situation arises because potential investors are deterred by political instability and inadequate infrastructures, as well as by the populations' lack of modern education and work habits compared with those of other developing nations. During the globalization of the economic and financial sectors, the growth of investment and trade has increased internationally.[2] This expansion has, however, largely bypassed the turbulence of sub-Saharan Africa and left it economically isolated (O'Connor, 1991).

The majority of Africans have known nothing but a simple, traditional life in terms of material possessions. However, many of these societies had seen better days in the 1960s, after colonialism, or even under colonialism. These countries all boast educated elites and a well-to-do class, but the middle class is comparatively small, and the bulk of the population is either indigent or ekes out a simple existence in villages and agricultural areas. Subsistence life in rural regions of Africa is not necessarily a matter of poverty in the perception of the peasants and villagers, as long as their lands are fertile, their communities are intact, and their children can attend school—conditions that are unfortunately eroding in too many countries. Material expectations are basic and feelings of relative deprivation are not as **prevalent** as they might be in cities or in more affluent societies, where the poor are deprived not only in absolute terms, but in comparative ones as well.

Rural poverty in areas that have not been socially disrupted exists mainly in the eye of Western beholders. The level of life satisfaction, self-fulfillment, family orientation, and community cohesiveness may be far superior to our own. But these contented villagers are becoming fewer because various forces in their countries, as well as external, cultural, and economic influences, are destroying their traditional ways of life, and slowly transforming them into indigent people clinging at the fringes of a materialist economy (e.g., Holm, 1995). However, even the reasonably contented African citizens do not generally receive adequate health care, and they are often malnourished or suffer from a variety of medical conditions that drastically reduce their life spans and sap their energies. Intestinal and blood parasites are a case in point. Moreover, because children receive only minimal schooling, modern avenues of employment are closed to them as adults.

Fertility rates in poor nations are generally high (Grant, 1992), and the population growth that results places additional pressure on an already burdened economy. Elevated fertility prevails because of traditional values, the economic usefulness of children in peasant societies, infant mortality, low education (particularly among women),[3] and the absence of reliable birth control methods. As global market economies advance into these societies, a plentiful and inexpensive labor force may attract some foreign investment, but the demographic profile maintains wages at an extremely low level. In addition, the intrusion of global markets disrupts traditional economic life so that families can no longer fall back on the agricultural resources they have left behind in order to "improve" their life conditions by moving to large cities (Korten, 1995).

Rural poverty in Africa, Latin America, and many Asiatic countries often leads to internal migrations of individuals to cities in search of work or the fulfillment of dreams. These migrants, bereft of marketable skills and material resources, settle into shantytowns that are generally devoid of even the most rudimentary sanitary facilities, and where competition for scarce resources makes life precarious (Scheper-Hughes, 1992). Child mortality is endemic, adult life expectancy is low, fertility begins at a younger age than in the general population, human growth is stunted,[4] schooling may be unavailable, and opportunities for employment (except for domestic service, working in small shops, or searching trash heaps for food or items to sell) are practically nonexistent. The result is that these new urban areas of absolute poverty, no longer buttressed by their residents' traditional communities, harbor a strong element of illegal activity that brings violence and personal insecurity—as is the case in the inner cities of American metropolitan areas.

POVERTY IN NORTH AMERICA

Canada and the United States

In both Canada and the United States, poverty is the result of an unequal distribution of wealth rather than an overall lack of riches (Ross, Shillington, and Lockhead, 1994). Nevertheless, this poverty impacts negatively on the fabric of the two societies as well as on their overall economies. Poverty is not a phenomenon that is compartmentalized strictly to the poor and their neighborhoods: it affects everyone, even the rich, albeit in different ways. Of Western societies, only the United States and Canada harbor a large and entrenched population of very disadvantaged citizens,[5] many of whom live in urban areas that are decaying, socially disorganized, and unsafe. The United States is the only Western country where residents do not benefit from universal health care, thus compounding the problems of the poor who cannot afford health insurance. When we speak of economic disadvantage in North America, welfare recipients come readily to mind. However, this is a misconception because, as amply documented later on, *only a minority of people who are poor are on social assistance. A majority of the poor and near poor are employed*—they work in low-paid jobs or part-time occupations. Even a substantial proportion of women on welfare are gainfully employed (Harris, 1993).

The United States and Canada share more economic similarities than differences. The two nations' poverty levels are equivalent, and along with the United Kingdom, both have the highest rates of child poverty, divorce, and single parenting among Western industrialized countries. Both countries trade extensively with each other. However, because the Canadian economy is dependent upon the American economy, unemployment in Canada is more prevalent, generally by four or five percentage points. A second major difference between the two nations is that Canada's cities have not (yet) been transformed into ghettos, so that there are not as many socially disorganized census tracts in Canada as in the United States. Canadian crime rates are substantially lower and cities safer. Other differences reside in the two countries' population sizes, the more varied ethnic composition of Canadian cities, the two nations' health care and welfare systems, taxation and salaries, as well as the American hegemony in terms of economy, mass media, and technology (Cheal, 1996). In addition, as pointed out earlier, more research exists on the American economy so that much of the literature surveyed in this text is American.

The Extent of Poverty

In the United States, in 1993, 15 percent of the population was poor, with a total of 39.3 million economically disadvantaged individuals.[6] In Canada, 16 percent or over 4 million persons were poor; 13.3 percent of families and 39.7 percent of individuals living by themselves were impoverished. In the United States, 23 percent of all children were poor, compared with 21 percent in Canada. Thus, the overall poverty rates are quite similar in both countries, despite differences in cutoff points. In the United States in 1995, the poverty threshold was $7,811 for one person and $15,662 for a family of four (Schiller, 1995). In Canada, an annual low-income cutoff is established on the basis of the number of persons in a household, the size of the community of residence (larger cities are more expensive to live in), and a percentage of the median income in that community. In 1990, this figure was $14,155 for one person and $24,389 for an urban family of three, substantially higher cutoff points than in the United States.

Nevertheless, these basic statistics do not tell the entire story because, in both countries, *at least 30 percent of the poor's income is below the poverty level by 50 percent—thus extreme indigence.* One also has to consider that today's poverty income provides only goods and services equivalent to the 1959 poverty level; the erosion of the buying power of the disadvantaged over the decades has been substantial (Devine and Wright, 1993). Consequently, in 1959, the standard of living of the poor was closer to the average than is currently the case, and an ever-widening gap between the disadvantaged and the relatively affluent has arisen (Mishel and Simon, 1988). Furthermore, the income of middle-class families has also eroded.[7]

A Roper survey conducted in April 1994 revealed that Americans needed $25,000 for a family of four "just to get by," and $40,000 "to live in relative comfort." There is therefore a substantial gap between what is officially defined as the poverty level and the subjective experience of what is necessary just to get by. As Devine and Wright (1993:3) point out, "One might even argue that in American society today, television sets and automobiles are necessities of life, even though the vast bulk of the world's population continues to exist with neither." Clearly, any definition of poverty has to take into consideration a society's level of development.

There is disagreement on the accuracy of estimates of poverty. Haveman and Buron (1993:64), among others, suggest that official statistics understate the incidence of poverty among minority groups, female-headed families, large families, and those headed by persons with insufficient schooling. For his part, Schiller (1995) points out that overestimation of poverty can result from official statistics that include only the family's *cash* income; in fact, a family of four may receive $2,000 in food stamps and another $2,000 in housing subsidies, as well as Medicaid. According to this line of reasoning, an American family of four with an income of $15,000 is designated as poor while, in reality, the in-kind transfers add another $4,000 to $5,000 a year to its receipts. Schiller (1995:42) estimates that when in-kind aid is included, the total of 39.3 million poor persons (or 15 percent) diminishes to 31.7 million poor or 12.2 percent of the total population. Then, if the rental value of a house owned by the family is added, 25.4 million people, or 9.8 percent of the population, are poor. Furthermore, there is repeated evidence that people tend to underreport their income by an average of $2,000 per person, and the average poor family spends nearly twice as much as it reports earning. This gap between expenditure and disclosed income continues to widen (Mayer and Jencks, 1993), perhaps again indicating that other revenues remain unreported. Obviously, such divergent statistics, some claiming an underestimation of poverty, others an overestimation, can be used to buttress the interests of various factions in governmental and financial sectors.

Other Aspects of Poverty

Another important aspect of poverty in North America is that it more often than not involves what is referred to as the "working poor," that is, families in which at least one member has been employed part of the year or the entire year. In 1990, 60 percent of disadvantaged households were so composed. In 18 percent of poor households, there were more than two workers. Additionally, 53 percent of single poor individuals, including single mothers, were employed at least part of the year.[8] Obviously, the poor *do* work, but their wages are too low and, in other cases, the jobs available to them are only part-time, thus carrying an insufficient income. Among two-parent poor families, 53.8 percent of their income comes from earnings and 12.6 percent from social assistance, compared with 24.9 and 42.7 percent, respectively, in one-parent poor families (Ross, Shillington, and Lockhead, 1994).

Other descriptive dimensions of poverty, based on the 1980 U.S. Census,[9] indicate that, compared with other families, the poor on average reside in more crowded households, live in older buildings, and fewer have central heating or air conditioners. Moreover, 43 percent own their houses compared with 70 percent for the middle class and 91 percent for the rich. The mean number of automobiles for low-income households is 0.733, whereas the average for the middle class is 1.457 and for the affluent, 2.157 (in 1980). The relatively low proportion of home ownership among the poor is one factor that in part prevents them from accumulating savings that could ease the hardships during periods of unemployment, compensate for low income in old age, and be transmitted to the next generation.

In 1991, in Canada, renters were paying a higher proportion of their income for shelter than were homeowners. Thirty-five percent of renters were spending a third or more of their income for housing, compared with 23 percent of homeowners with a mortgage and five percent of those with no mortgage.[10] In a study including welfare recipients from Quebec and Ontario, Deniger et al. (1995) found that 72 percent of their respondents were in debt. For a majority, the debt load was on the order of $1,000 to $5,000, substantial sums at that income level, and it covered mainly monthly expenses such as telephone, heating, and clothes. A majority reported limiting leisure activities with their children because of a lack of money.

THE GAP BETWEEN RICH AND POOR

As societies leave subsistence agriculture and develop a surplus, inequalities begin to arise until a level of development via industrialization and the democratization of education is reached that allows for a more equitable distribution of resources nationally.[11] Thus, in the first 70 years of this century, "economic development fed social development by diminishing inequality" (Nelson, 1995:14). In contrast, "today's economic development escalates inequality."[12] Therefore, unless policies are redirected, increases in the GNP and **GDP** will no longer necessarily lead to rewarding employment and appropriate wages for perhaps 50 percent of the population. Indeed, the share of the national income that reaches the poorest has been declining since 1973 (Harrison, Tilly, and Bluestone, 1986). In 1973, the share of the national income received by the bottom 20 percent of the population was 5.5 percent, whereas in 1993 it stood at only 4 percent. During that same period, the share of the top 20 percent accrued from 41.4 to 48.2 percent (Schor and Menaghan, 1995).[13]

These findings indicate that the gap between the rich and the poor and, for that matter, between the rich and the rest of the population, is widening (Nelson, 1995). In Canada, in 1990, the average after-tax income of the top 10 percent of families was $88,000 compared with $11,600 for the bottom 10 percent, or a ratio of 8 to 1. Without government transfer payments, the ratio would be 65 to 1.[14] The gap between the rich and the poor is narrower in countries such as Sweden and Norway, while it is wider in others such as Germany and Israel. In 1985, the ratio of highest to lowest income by quintile was an astonishing 19 to 1 for West Germany, 9 to 1 for the United States and the United Kingdom, 8.8 to 1 for Israel, 7.9 to 1 for Norway, 6.7 to 1 for Canada, and 5 to 1 for Sweden.[15] These ratios are much higher in poor countries and may well reach over 100 to 1.

In Western societies, the redistribution of income via transfer payments can translate into a substantial reduction of the difference between the rich and the poor. It also alleviates poverty, as is illustrated in the recent decrease of poverty among the elderly described in Chapter 7.[16] In 1985, total social programs, with the exception of health and education, accounted for 21 percent of the GDP for Denmark and France, 15 percent for West Germany, 10.7 percent for the United Kingdom, 10.3 percent for Canada, and 8.5 percent for the United States. In 1995, in both Canada and the United States, tax revenues constituted a smaller percentage of the GDP (35.7 percent and 30 percent, respectively) than in many other European countries—such as Sweden (over 55 percent), Denmark (50 percent), and France (over 42 percent)—whose social programs account for a larger share of the GDP. A country's ability to help low-income groups depends in part on its taxation policy and, currently, on the government deficit that has to be serviced out of taxation revenues.

MOBILITY OUT OF AND BACK INTO POVERTY

Four studies illustrate the movement of individuals in and out of welfare and poverty, as well as the recurrence of these phenomena in the lives of people. Harris (1996) reports that, in the Panel Study of Income Dynamics (PSID) for the years 1983 to 1988, 25 percent of mothers formerly on welfare returned to welfare within a year, 42 percent returned within two years, and close to 60 percent returned at least once during the six years of the study. They exit welfare through work, marriage, or family and personal events. However, *even after exit, 67 percent of these mothers remain poor* because of insufficient wages. Younger women return to welfare more often than older women. Women with higher incomes and who live in areas that are economically flourishing are more likely to remain off welfare. Overall, "work among poor women should be viewed as the *problem* rather than the solution" (Harris, 1996: 424) because they have little hope of advancement, they lose their Medicaid benefits when they resume paid employment, and they experience difficulties finding stable, quality day care for their children. Harris (1996) argues that current welfare reforms are unrealistic if they do not provide health and child care when women shift from welfare to work.

In Canada, it is estimated that one in three Canadians will be poor at some point in their working life (Economic Council of Canada, 1992:22). Each year, approximately as many Canadians leave the ranks of poverty as join them. There is therefore a great deal of mobility in and out of poverty, although many of those who enter already have experienced at least one poverty spell in the past. A **longitudinal study** conducted between 1982 and 1986 documented that the longer people remain out of poverty after leaving it, the lower their subsequent rate of reentry.[17] Thus, 21 percent of those who had escaped poverty in 1982 reentered it one year later, but only 12 percent returned to it three years later. The same study also found that 49 percent of people escaped poverty the year following their entry into it, but only 23 percent escaped after three years of poverty. The longer people remain in poverty, the more difficult it is to exit.

The Economic Council of Canada (1992:23) concludes that "it is reasonable to suspect that at least some poor people tend to become dependent on one social-security program or another and lose their ability and motivation to become self-reliant." The ECC also established that, from 1982 to 1986, 15 percent of those who were poor in a given year had two or three spells of poverty during the five-year period, and that nearly 40 percent of those who had escaped poverty in 1983 had reentered it within three years. In a complementary vein, Corcoran (1995) finds that less than 25 percent of black and 10 percent of white disadvantaged children remain poor by early adulthood. Of those who have been persistently poor as children, 46 percent of blacks and 24 percent of whites remain so as adults.

In the study by Deniger et al. (1995) comparing a number of Quebec and Ontario welfare recipients, the Quebec sample was obtained from neighborhoods characterized for several decades by a relatively high concentration of poverty. The Quebec respondents felt less stigmatized by their welfare status (68 percent vs. 87 percent), less useless (47 percent vs. 74 percent) , and less guilty for possible inconveniences that "your children have to cope with because you are on welfare" (44 percent vs. 75 percent) than the Ontario respondents. These results lead to the implication that residing in an area where many other low-income families live lessens the stigma of poverty. It may also reduce mobility out of poverty and out of welfare, a situation that is of utmost pertinence to American inner cities with high concentrations of poverty.

In both Quebec and Ontario samples, over 90 percent of the welfare recipients were women younger than age thirty. The researchers compared the respondents who had participated in an employability program with those who had not. The latter seemed to experience fewer negative feelings concerning stigma and self-esteem than the participants. They were also less aware of the need to upgrade their skills and of the obstacles they could encounter on the job market. The authors suggest that employability or workfare programs that do not result in credible jobs may have a negative effect on self-esteem and feelings of worthlessness. In contrast, motherhood gives meaning to women's lives.[18] As Deniger et al. (1995: 88) point out: "In a way it provided them with more opportunities for autonomy and affirmation than if they constantly had to deal with programs and obtaining work experience which, in any event, would be unlikely to integrate them reasonably well into society."

Some of the implications are that, for indigent and uneducated women, motherhood, at least when their children are small, provides a certain status, a source of gratification, and feelings of worthiness, even though poverty prevents them from giving their children as much as they wish to (Fernandez Kelly, 1995). Deniger et al. (1995:87) ask: "Does daily life at home with, in many cases, the care of children as the main occupation serve to a certain degree to protect these respondents from the personal and structural limits and obstacles to be found in the current socioeconomic situation?" Within this perspective, motherhood acts as a shelter, at least temporarily. However, we have seen that the longer the interval of poverty, the more difficult it becomes to move out of poverty—and the consequences may be long-lasting for the children involved (Ensminger, 1995). Therefore, these women may later on experience more difficulty adjusting to the world of employment than same-age women who are also poor but do hold jobs, or participate in workfare, even if only temporarily (Butler, 1996).

One can well wonder whether, for mothers who are not employed, the feelings of worthiness will last into the children's adolescence. "It is at this step that . . . the need to develop other skills, to be more than a parent and, as a result, to want to change one's strategy for succeeding in life" may develop (Deniger et al., 1995:90). However, inadequate schooling and lack of work experience may slow these women's reentry into the labor market. But, then, even if employed, they are likely to remain poor (Edin and Lein, 1997). This situation applies particularly to adolescent mothers who remain on social assistance much longer than older women (Bane and Ellwood, 1986). Therefore, adolescent mothers and their children are at far greater risk than older mothers of initiating a cycle of dependence that will be transmitted to a great proportion of their children (Gottschalk, 1992).

THE REDUCTION OF RURAL POVERTY

Farm poverty in North America has decreased substantially from 50 percent in 1959 to 11 percent in 1990; it now accounts for only 1.6 percent of all poverty in the United States compared with 20 percent in 1959 (Devine and Wright, 1993:63). This reduction in farm poverty is both the result of a decline in the farm population from 15 million in 1957 to less than 5 million in 1990, and a result of the restructuration of farming to adapt to the competitive nature of the general economy (Flora et al., 1992). Farming efficiency has increased dramatically and requires less labor, explaining in part the reduction in the farm population. But what is also reflected is that small family holdings have frequently been replaced by larger ones, either owned by more affluent families or by large agribusinesses.

Apart from technologization and rising cost of energy, some of the processes that precipitated the farm crisis of the 1970s and 1980s were heavy debt load resulting from the devaluation of farm lands, and the practice of borrowing to purchase the latest models of heavy machinery. Small landowners and marginal farmers were forced to sell out at reduced prices, and many farms were repossessed by banks and other creditors—thus diminishing farm poverty by default. In other instances, fathers pushed their adult sons out into other professions, or sons chose other callings as they realized that they could no longer earn a decent living from small-scale farming.

Rural districts are constituted by farms and nonfarm areas. The nonfarm rural areas had a poverty rate of 13.6 percent in 1990. Individuals living in these areas comprised 27 percent of the American population in poverty, an overrepresentation considering that they account for only 22.4 percent of the total population. Children's poverty is more persistent in nonmetropolitan areas,[19] poverty in general is deeper, and the poor are less likely to seek social assistance (Jensen and Eggebeen, 1994).[20] Basically, rural poverty is a proxy for lack of local opportunities (Garrett, Ng'andu, and Ferron, 1994), as rural unemployment rates are higher (U.S. Department of Agriculture, 1990).

Moreover, as Devine and Wright (1993) point out, rural or nonmetropolitan area poverty is confounded by racial and geographic variables. For instance, while the south contains 34 percent of the overall population, 44 percent of the nonfarm rural districts are located in the south. Moreover, 96.8 percent of all blacks who are disadvantaged and who do not reside in large urban areas live in the south where they constitute 41 percent of the nonmetropolitan poor. Elsewhere, 92 percent of the poor who live in nonmetropolitan areas are white. Thus, except for the south, rural poverty is a white phenomenon.

CONCLUSION

The roots and nature of poverty in the United States and Canada differ from that of countries on other continents where low income is endemic. What is probably most striking about North American poverty is that it exists amidst affluence, democracy, and an **ideology** of egalitarianism. Poverty that is visible in terms of degraded urban areas, homelessness that spills into city streets, and shacks that dot the countryside are demoralizing factors for most citizens. Visible poverty represents the scars of a society's otherwise silent disease. At least from a moral and social point of view, it depresses the quality of life of an entire area, whether rural or urban.

In simple economic terms, each individual can be an asset or a liability to his or her country. In this vein, the disadvantaged are a liability from several perspectives. First, they disproportionately have recourse to various social assistance programs that are subsidized by taxpayers' money. Second, the unemployed do not pay taxes and do not contribute to the national and local budgets. Third, the disadvantaged often live in government subsidized housing projects that they have no incentive to maintain in good condition; these costly projects deteriorate and become an added financial burden for the administrative level that manages them. Fourth, people who are poor people do not enjoy the means to purchase a great variety of goods and services; hence, they do not contribute to the creation of jobs and to economic growth. Fifth, poverty has dire consequences, some of which are ill health, delinquency, and teenage childbearing—and all of these entail tremendous economic costs.

The price of poverty[21] nationally is generally calculated in terms of reduced economic competitiveness stemming from lower educational achievement, higher welfare and Medicaid costs, and the loss of tax receipts to the government. But the price of poverty is above all else a human one. At the very least, each poor citizen experiences material deprivation, shattered aspirations, and diminished access to quality schooling, housing, and even medical care. Depending on where they live and what kinds of persons they are, poor individuals can also be affected by ill health, functional illiteracy, deficient self-esteem, and social isolation, as well as being victims of crime. In this text, after examining the causes of poverty in the following two chapters, we endeavor to show both its economic and especially its human price.

Chapter 2

Systemic Causes of Poverty

There are multiple causes of poverty and none can explain independently all the individual situations of economic disadvantage; causes tend to cluster and to reinforce each other. They can be divided into two types: systemic and personal. **Systemic** refers to social and economic variables, such as overall changes in the structure of the economy. Personal refers to attributes of the poor. As a general rule, personal causes are preceded by systemic causes; systemic phenomena generate both poverty and the personal sources of poverty (Haveman and Wolfe, 1994). Were the economic and social causes of poverty eliminated, the personal causes, while not vanishing entirely, would be radically reduced.

The systemic causes examined in this chapter are tied to the globalization of the economy, the evolving structure of the North American economy, unemployment and underemployment, the heavy national debt, inadequate social assistance payments, and more recently but as a lesser cause, low-skilled immigration. The key systemic variables of racial segregation and discrimination are discussed in Chapter 8.

GLOBALIZATION OF THE ECONOMY

The 1970s witnessed the slow emergence of the economic movements which culminated in the transformation of world policies in the early 1990s, beginning with the **GATT** signed by 111 countries in 1993. Various free trade agreements ensued between Canada and the United States, and at an even more international level, between several Western European countries, to form a unified common market,[1] with a sole currency as one of its goals.[2] There has initially been some resistance to the terms of the free trade agreements on the part of some nations: by European countries such as Denmark, Portugal, and Spain; and in North America, by Canada. These countries face, at least in the short run, a far greater potential for the dislocation of their economies than do their more powerful neighbors such as France or Germany and, on this side of the Atlantic, the United States. In Canada, many manufacturing jobs were and are being lost to the United States and, with **NAFTA,** to Mexico, because Canadian salaries and social benefits are superior to those in the other two countries and thus reduce corporations' profitability (Menzies, 1996).

Since the 1970s, multinational conglomerates have become more numerous, and companies with industrial and management subsidiaries in different countries have multiplied. Examples are Toyota plants in the United States and Canada, and McDonald's outlets in Russia and China. Moreover, the electronics revolution has hastened the process by making it easier for companies to communicate with their international subsidiaries, and to relocate production while retaining high-skilled financial services in a few privileged cities (Dreier, 1993). Financial markets and related specialized services are the most globalized, a development which has had implications for income distribution: financial centers employ comparatively few low-skilled individuals and therefore do not contribute as much as other industries to the economic well-being of the less educated population. Furthermore, as a few key cities ("global cities"[3]) on each continent emerge as command posts for financial markets and for the flow of services as well as investments, other cities decline economically (Sassen, 1994). In Canada, Toronto (and to some extent Vancouver) have supplanted Montreal, where unemployment and poverty are higher than in the other two cities. Toronto has become a center specializing in **producer services,** particularly banking and finances, as well as health services (Todd, 1993).[4]

One of the consequences of globalization is that national economies are now more at the mercy of world-wide fluctuations, and governments are less in control of the internal organization of the labor market and of the financial sector in their countries (Cerny, 1996). As Nelson states (1995:14), "Under post-industrial capitalism, markets are freer and more influential." This became particularly obvious during the crises created by the first increases of **OPEC** oil prices in 1973 and in 1979, which brought both recession and inflation, with inflation in turn eroding the value of wages. Efforts to stimulate employment have become more dependent upon international competitiveness and economic development, and consequently may not target national areas or populations most in need of jobs (R. A. Rhodes, 1994; M. Rhodes, 1996).

Governments have failed to evolve policies that are adapted to the new realities or even to curb certain financial practices that threaten the social fabric. Amidst international controversy, Canada has, however, recently moved to protect certain aspects of its culture, such as the content of publications and television programs, as has France. It also has guarded its health care system against encroachment by other nations. In most Western countries, government policies and inaction have generally failed to protect the jobs of the most vulnerable blue-collar workers with little education and, in the case of the United States, the jobs of inner-city residents (Goldsmith and Blakeley, 1992). The globalization and consequent restructuring of the national economy have dragged many families into indigence (Duncan, Smeeding, and Rodgers, 1993).

EVOLVING STRUCTURE OF THE ECONOMY

With the changing global economy, most industrialized and postindustrialized societies face essentially similar structural problems (Noble, 1995). Perhaps the most salient and obvious change resides in the dramatic growth of the service sector and the retrenchment of the manufacturing sector. Other changes include increases in part-time employment, low-paying jobs, two-wage-earner families, higher educational requirements, and job relocation, as well as the ascendancy of corporate executives and shareholders' financial profits. All are discussed in the following subsections.

Relative Loss of Manufacturing Jobs

Large economies are constituted by three primary sectors: exploitation of natural resources (agriculture, mining, forestry), production of goods (such as cars, homes, and clothing), as well as the service sector (retail, finance, health, entertainment and leisure, restaurants, hotels, education, and research). As industrialization progressed last century, the first sector, particularly agriculture, became more efficient and productive. Fewer individuals were needed to feed the nation, and the farming population diminished substantially. Then, for several decades from World War I until the 1970s, industries predominated in terms of the number of occupations they offered and the proportion of the work force they employed. Steel, auto, and garment manufacturers contributed to the wealth of cities. These industries also had the advantage of staving off poverty: the skills they required easily matched those of young workers fresh out of high school. Manufacturers offered well-paying, entry-level jobs, employment security, and benefit packages to workers with relatively little education. In American cities, they employed large numbers of African-American youths who became heads of families and solid members of the working and middle classes in their communities.

But, after the 1970s, because of a combination of factors[5]—the energy crises, technologization, the overvalued American dollar, and lower exports (Strobel, 1993)—growth ceased in this sector, and there were periods of retrenchment. Furthermore, manufacturers moved out of large cities which were chiefly inhabited by minorities. For instance, between 1970 and 1985, Chicago lost 250,000 manufacturing jobs (Skogan, 1990). Despite these losses in certain geographic areas, the manufacturing sector itself remains healthy; its output has increased in dollar terms and still represents nearly 22 percent of the GNP (Nelson, 1995:87). The number of industrial jobs has not declined since the mid-1970s, but their *proportion* among all jobs has declined, their location has changed, the type of goods manufactured has diversified, and, with the introduction of computers, the production process has become far more specialized.

This evolution has had a marked impact on the availability of jobs, particularly in inner cities and among African Americans. First, in order to sustain a growing labor force, the number of manufacturing positions should have expanded much more than it did. Second, the number of jobs offered to youths with only a high-school education decreased when some industries relocated and then began to be more selective. As low-skilled occupations disappeared or were moved to the suburbs, to the south, or to other countries with inexpensive labor forces, opportunities for high-school graduates shrank and youth unemployment rose (Persky, Sclar, and Wiewel, 1991).

Since 1970, the proportion of males working in manufacturing has declined from 30 percent to 19 percent. While employment in the trade and service sectors has grown from 39 percent to 48 percent, this increase was not sufficient to offset the losses in manufacturing. Although all low-skilled workers have suffered,[6] young African-American males in the inner cities have been particularly affected. In 1974, 46 percent of jobs held by young black males were in the manufacturing sector, compared with only 26 percent in 1984 (Bound and Johnson, 1992). This means that an increasing proportion of employed young African Americans are working in sectors that do not provide adequate salaries. Hence, these shifts in economic sectors account for 25 to 33 percent of the decline in the wages of low-skilled and young workers,[7] and account for 33 to 50 percent of the decline in employment among young African Americans who have not completed high school (Panel on High-Risk Youth, 1993).

Expansion of the Service Sector

At the same time, the service sector expanded to meet a rising demand for producer services in banking, computers, and law, and for consumer services to meet growing expectations in terms of lifestyle, education, and health, as well as the demands of an aging population. These two subsectors have constituted 84 percent of all employment growth between 1979 and 1987 (Harrison and Bluestone, 1988). While such numbers are impressive, they nevertheless bring economic problems in their wake because the service sector has a double profile as an employer.

On one hand, some service occupations, especially those in producer services (lawyers, computer technicians, financial advisers) as well as a few in consumer services (educators, physicians) require advanced educational credentials and reward their holders with commensurate salaries. In the United States, the number of high-paying producer service jobs grew from 6 million in 1970 to over 16 million in 1991; in Canada, the number grew from 0.5 to 1.6 million (Sassen, 1994). On the other hand, an even greater number of service occupations, including most of those in consumer services, offer low salaries and often no more than part-time employment. One can think of retail, beauty shops, laundry, repair, catering, and food chains—the latter has been referred to as the McDonaldization of employment. In the United States, the number of such jobs grew from 8 million in 1970 to nearly 14 million in 1991; in Canada, it grew from 0.6 to 1.9 million.

All the combined figures in the growth of the service sector and the retrenchment of the industrial sector indicate that individuals with little education have no choice but to be satisfied with low-wage occupations, if they are to be employed at all, and many of them subsequently join the ranks of the working poor. Therefore, it is not surprising that recent technological changes have increased inequalities based on skills and educational credentials (Panel on High-Risk Youth, 1993). At least in part due to the growth of the service sector, the share of middle-level jobs is decreasing, while that of both high-paying occupations (producer services) and low-paying occupations (consumer services) is increasing (Economic Council of Canada, 1990).

Increase in Part-Time Employment

In the face of a more competitive and high-tech economy, many jobs have been downsized into part-time ones (Rifkin, 1995). In addition, part-time employment is particularly suited to the structural needs of employers in the consumer service sector, especially retail.[8] Therefore, the proportion of wage earners who work part-time because they cannot find full-time employment has grown from 33.7 percent to 53.5 percent (Tilly, 1991). In Canada, between 1981 and 1989, 44 percent of all new occupations created were part-time or temporary (Economic Council of Canada, 1992:30). By 1993, 18 percent of all Canadian workers were part-time employees, up from 13 percent just three years earlier (Canadian Council on Social Development, 1993).[9]

Part-time employment is directly correlated to poverty, especially in instances where it is the sole source of familial income (Levitan, 1988). Furthermore, women are overrepresented among part-time employees, because such positions constitute a solution to potential conflict with their familial responsibilities, and because they congregate at the lower echelons of the consumer service sector. In fact, 44 percent more women than men occupy part-time jobs involuntarily (Handler, 1995:43). Single mothers who hold these occupations because of a lack of other opportunities are inevitably poor. Among household heads employed less than half the year, one out of four is poor,[10] while among those with full-time employment, only 1 in 30 is poor (Schiller, 1995:86). When a household has more than one wage earner, the likelihood of poverty is further diminished (U.S. Congress, 1992).

Part-time employment of teenagers has increased dramatically in Canada since 1980, from 51 percent to 68 percent for males and from 58 percent to 75 percent for females. In the United States, 43 percent of all 16-to-19-year-olds in school are also working (U.S. Bureau of the Census, 1993d). A growing number of adolescents are combining school and work, mainly to defray the costs of their media-propelled consumer needs. Others who are out of school may not be able to find full-time employment and have to settle for part-time jobs. Young people experience more unemployment than any other age bracket. In 1991, unemployment for the 15-to-19-year-old age group was beyond that of people ages twenty-five and over by 6.7 points (Kerr, Larrivee, and Greenhalgh, 1994:44).

Increase in Low-Paying Jobs

There has been a 50 percent increase in low-paying jobs in the 1980s (Nelson, 1995). In Toronto alone, the number of positions at the minimum wage level jumped by 40 percent from 1991 to 1996.[11] Workers whose earnings are minimal are naturally far more at risk of becoming poor; in fact, 36 percent are poor (Danziger and Gottschalk, 1988). Inadequate salaries affect not only part-time employees; in 1992, 18 percent of *full-time* workers who earned low salaries were poor (Handler, 1995). The majority of low-wage earners escape poverty only because of extenuating circumstances. These include small family size (44 percent); at least one other worker in the household (27 percent); the availability of other sources of income, such as investments (13 percent of the cases); or home ownership. The situation of minimum-wage households is precarious: the arrival of an additional child or the sudden unemployment of the second worker easily upsets the balance and may necessitate recourse to welfare. Nevertheless, it is striking that *only 12 percent of full-time workers who are poor use welfare.*

Low-paying jobs generally do not require advanced skills. Hence, it is unlikely that workers in these occupations will soon free themselves of the threat of poverty: their occupations do not increase their skills, nor do they usually have the educational requirements to pull ahead—unless, of course, they are teenagers living with their families and attending school. The situation regarding low-wage earners appears to be worsening. Real wages declined over the 1980s for the employed poor and near poor, even though the economy was expanding (Blank, 1993). In 1991, Canadian families earned an average of 2.6 percent less than in 1990, and the income of single-parent families dropped by 4 percent within just one year (Canada Year Book, 1993).

Increase in Two-Wage-Earner Families

It has been estimated that 50 to 70 percent more families with two wage earners would fall below the poverty level without the earnings of the second worker (Gardner and Herz, 1992). These estimates indicate that women's employment, practically nonexistent in married families four decades ago, is now essential for economic survival. Feminine employment is the ingredient that keeps many households out of indigence. In fact, real family income has remained largely stable since 1973 despite an increase in the number of wage earners per household[12] and in the average hours worked by each wage earner (Blank, 1993). However, there are costs as well as benefits to having both adults at work in households with children. These include day care, transportation, and clothing. If these costs are subtracted from total family revenue, the financial advantage brought by the second wage declines, particularly in low-income households.

In Canada, wives' contributions to overall family incomes have increased from 15 percent in 1970 to 29 percent in 1990 (Rashid, 1994). Wives' employment is usually higher when husbands are employed, perhaps a result of **assortative mating** on the basis of education or income. Assortative mating suggests that men and women with little education, or who originate from low-income families, tend to marry amongst themselves. Such families have a higher risk of both male and female unemployment. In 1990, in contrast, 80 percent of families with the highest incomes had both husbands and wives employed, up from 36 percent in 1970. Women with superior incomes thus help propel their families' total earnings into the top two deciles. In contrast, in 1990, only 21 percent of families in the lowest decile were dual-earner families, in part because many of households in this income category are headed by a mother alone (Rashid, 1994).

Higher Educational Requirements

With the technological revolution in computers firmly entrenched in the workplace, whether in secretarial work, banking, sales, or hotel reservations, employees need to possess technical skills or be able to learn these skills on the job. It is estimated that two-thirds of all new positions created during the next decade will require at least thirteen years of formal education, and 45 percent will require more than sixteen years. Even manufacturing has been affected by these trends. For instance, in 1960, less than 4 percent of manufacturing employees were professionals and 6 percent were managers; in 1990, these numbers had risen to 12 and 14 percent, respectively (Nelson, 1995:45).

Education is directly related to income (Murphy and Welch, 1993).[13] In 1990, in Canada, *full-time* workers with nine or more years of schooling but no diploma averaged $27,289 compared with $32,850 and $49,861, respectively, for persons with a trade certificate or some university education and those with a university degree (Gartley, 1994). Therefore, today, the failure of some youth to even complete high school is both a personal and societal tragedy (Ensminger and Slusarcick, 1992).

Currently, persons who are computer literate are the first to secure a position, especially if they also possess mathematical or literacy skills. Needless to say, youth who have attended low-quality schools in impoverished neighborhoods or rural areas, where the only computer available may be in the office, are not prepared to compete favorably in this labor market. Therefore, new educational requirements at the job entry level contribute to the perpetuation of poverty in some segments of the population. But basically, the poverty created by a lack of educational credentials stems largely from the fact that families bear the entire burden of preparing their children for, and providing them with, an education (Saporiti and Sgritta, 1990). This is an anomaly because, ultimately, society reaps the benefits of parental investment in children's education (Zelizer, 1985):[14] children become tomorrow's labor force and tax base (Qvortrup, 1995).

Job Relocation

Job relocation has contributed to the poverty of inner-city neighborhoods in the United States. As the neighborhoods deteriorate further, additional employers flee the area and move to suburban districts. Even employers based in safe middle-class cities often relocate to the suburbs where property taxes are lower. In other instances, companies move to the Sun Belt where wages are inferior and unions are weakly represented. While this situation allows companies to remain competitive in terms of high profitability, it also exerts a downward pressure on wages in general. Other companies move part or all of their operations to countries with very low-cost of living. A great proportion of these countries' workers are women, a division of labor which maintains a preponderance of low wages. Nevertheless, these women still earn far more than their less fortunate counterparts (Lim, 1990). Health benefits are not expected by this population, thus again increasing corporations' profit margins. While such relocations help the host countries, they deplete the labor markets in North America, at least temporarily—that is, until the economies of the host countries improve to the point where they can import North American products and services (Krugman, 1995).

There are also economically motivated political reasons why jobs are relocated. One is to appease the leaders of countries that constitute a vast potential market. China is a case in point. According to the American Federation of Labor, in 1995 alone, more than 500,000 American industrial workers had their jobs exported to China (Simons, 1996). To avoid the high tariffs that the Chinese government places on American-made goods entering its borders, some corporations are planning to manufacture their products in China (for example, cars by General Motors). In order to expand the market, even electronic companies such as Motorola and Intel have shifted jobs to China. If they did not, China would turn to other nations willing to manufacture on its soil, such as France or Germany. All these moves represent losses for employment growth in North America.

Moreover, technology developed in North America often is exported along with these relocations and is shared with the host country. This situation constitutes a serious risk for the future competitiveness of the North American economy; it may lose its technological edge because the host countries simply borrow, adopt, and disseminate the technology at lower costs. There is also the danger that this advanced technology may be used for military purposes by nations that entertain expansionist and imperialistic dreams.

Emphasis on Financial Profit

For several years, large corporations and even small enterprises have taken advantage of technical advances to reduce the size of their work force, slashing hundreds of thousands of jobs at all levels. These layoffs have received a new label: downsizing. Companies undergo pressure to reduce their production costs in order to be more competitive both nationally and internationally and retain substantial profit margins. When asking, "profit for whom?," it is evident that it is largely for the stock market and shareholders. Companies' loyalties no longer rest with their employees but with their shareholders. In other words, the capitalist ethos has drifted into a paper economy of superprofits. Financial transactions are given preeminence, and the best graduates of business schools flock into finance, marketing, and management strategies rather than into the design and development of products (Nelson, 1995).

However, shareholders and brokers are not the only beneficiaries of corporate profits. While the middle class seems to be shrinking in terms of its wage base and while the poor become poorer, chief executive officers (CEOs) of the same large companies that are downsizing reap higher incomes (salaries, dividends, and other fringe benefits) than they did five years ago. For instance, in 1995, the ratio of earnings of a typical CEO to that of a typical worker was as follows: American CEOs earned a whopping 120 times the average salary; Canadian CEOs 36 times, British 33 times, German 21 times, and Japanese 16 times.[15] Hence, companies benefit their shareholders and their CEOs, and contribute to the widening gap between the rich and the poor. In doing so, they create unemployment, reduce job benefits, and deepen poverty (Korten, 1995).

Moreover, the huge sums of money that are borrowed by companies for speculative purposes and to finance takeovers and mergers could be put to work for the benefit of the entire population by developing environment-friendly manufacturing and services, thus creating jobs rather than producing a costly paper trail. Unfortunately, speculative activity creates superprofits that are not possible to achieve in the manufacturing and personal services sectors (Sassen, 1994). Thus, it is unlikely that corporations will curtail this activity voluntarily; because of deregulation, there is little that national governments can do at the moment unless a political will to change emerges.

UNEMPLOYMENT

There is no doubt that when unemployment rises, poverty becomes more acute, especially visible poverty. The number of homeless people increases. So does the number of individuals who rely on various forms of government assistance and charity-supported institutions, such as shelters and food banks. Companies can create unemployment in two ways. First, they can lay off workers—a direct source of unemployment. Second, they can stop hiring new workers—an indirect yet salient source of unemployment given that the supply of new jobs is as important as the retention of already existing ones. Companies also create underemployment with part-time and temporary positions.

In the past seven years, unemployment reached the two-digit level even in countries that had been bastions of economic growth, such as Germany. The United States has recovered more rapidly than other nations from the recession of the early 1990s. However, Canadian unemployment rates are 40 percent higher than American rates, although they have slipped slightly from a two-digit peak. In Canada, one cause—albeit a politically controversial one—for this stubborn unemployment situation stems from NAFTA. Although it may have salutary economic benefits for Canadians down the road, it currently exists mainly to the advantage of American corporations.

Indeed, with NAFTA, because American wages and prices are lower, several American subsidiaries that were located in Canada have moved out now that they can sell their goods directly into Canada with few or no export tariffs.[16] This also allows them to avoid the taxation costs of Canadian social benefits. At least for the time being, the social benefits (particularly the health care safety net) that Canadians enjoy make companies less competitive and less profitable for their shareholders if they remain in Canada. Upon moving, they create unemployment in Canada but open jobs for Americans. It is a difficult balancing act that has yet to be resolved in favor of both countries equally.

Now that some of the factors related to unemployment have been introduced, some statistics describing the situation itself are examined. The unemployment rate in June 1997 was below 5 percent in the United States, but well above 9 percent in Canada. In 1993, the unemployment rate for white males of all ages was 7.1 percent, but was 17.6 percent for white males age sixteen to nineteen. For black males, the unemployment rate was 13.8 percent, but it was as high as 40 percent for young African Americans between the ages of sixteen and nineteen.[17] Unemployment among youth is exacerbated by lack of education. In 1996, in Canada, 17 percent of male and 30 percent of female dropouts were unemployed.[18] In Toronto, between 1981 and 1991, because of the increase both in youth unemployment and minimum-wage jobs, the number of children older than twenty-four who live with their parents has skyrocketed by 144 percent. An added problem for youth is that employers often require experience and favor those who have already held a job, even if part-time, or those who have done volunteer work. Once again, students from disadvantaged districts, both rural and urban, may have few employment and volunteer opportunities in their neighborhoods, and are unlikely to have contacts who could help them secure jobs (Wacquant, 1995) The difficulty and cost of transportation often prevent them from venturing to areas that offer part-time employment. The problem is compounded when the youth are black, for instance, and the job opportunities are located in a predominantly white neighborhood.

Using U.S. Bureau of Labor Statistics, Schiller (1995:63) calculated that the rate of poverty doubles and even triples as soon as the head of the household is unemployed. Only 5 percent of two-parent families are poor when the father is employed, but 12 percent are when he is unemployed. When women head the family, 26 percent are poor when the mother is employed compared with 57 percent when she is unemployed. In addition, the longer unemployment lasts, the more likely people are to become indigent because, after a certain period, they have exhausted whatever savings they had accumulated and whatever help they could receive from their families.

NATIONAL DEBT

We rarely think of government debt at the national and regional levels as a source of poverty because the problem is hidden under other rubrics. Debt arises when yearly deficits accumulate because a government spends more than it generates in revenues from taxes, fines, and investments. The government is then forced to borrow, and the interest it disburses on the debt constitutes a drain on the national budget. Payments on the debt are a main cause of yearly budgetary deficits. Yet governments prefer to reduce welfare payments and cut back on various job creation programs rather than subsidize the debt in less costly ways, such as having their reserve funds or central banks assume a larger share of the financial burden.

Currently, all Western governments are striving for balanced budgets to prevent further increases in their national debts. As a result, large numbers of civil employees have lost their positions, the military establishments have reduced their personnel, and social programs—particularly those affecting health, education, and welfare—have been slashed. These numerous cutbacks create unemployment, as well as a reduction of services that affect the most vulnerable members of society. In turn, this unemployment raises the deficit and the cycle is perpetuated. In Canada, for instance, according to a 1991 forecast, the federal deficit would have been $23.9 billion instead of $29.8 billion if the unemployment rate had been 8.5 percent rather than 10.3 percent (Canadian Council on Social Development, 1993:78).

LOW SOCIAL ASSISTANCE PAYMENTS

Decreases in welfare assistance contribute to a deepening of poverty and homelessness among the already disadvantaged (Devine and Wright, 1993:31). Social safety nets are most likely to be weakened during times when the impoverished need assistance the most. Aid for Families with Dependent Children (AFDC) state-administered benefits are not generally indexed for inflation; their purchasing power declined accordingly by 43 percent from 1970 to 1992 (Strawn, 1992). Taking the state with the median level of payments as a baseline, this decline translates into a loss of more than $3,400 a year. In addition, the eligibility criteria for social assistance have been tightened, which may be one of the reasons why, in 1990, only 60 percent of needy children's families were receiving AFDC benefits. Children are indigent because the cost of their care and financial support falls entirely on families (Sgritta, 1994); in turn, eligibility criteria for welfare are based on parents' characteristics rather than children's needs. Furthermore, low income rental units dipped from 6.8 million in 1970 to 5.5 million in 1990, while the number of disadvantaged families had grown by 3 million to a total of 9.6 million (Garbarino, 1995:141). This discrepancy between supply and need contributes to insecurity and instability, as well as homelessness, among indigent families. In February 1997, there were 11.9 million individuals on AFDC, which is 2.5 million fewer than the March 1994 welfare peak (DeParlee, 1997). It is too early to tell if this reduction is due to cutbacks or to better employment opportunities, and if it means that more poverty is being left unattended.

It can be argued that welfare payments are not a cause of poverty because they are given to people who are *already* poor for other reasons. One can answer that when assistance in general is insufficient or occurs only after marginally secure people have depleted all their resources, it fails to prevent poverty. For instance, AFDC payments are so inadequate that they raise only about 10 percent of recipient families over the poverty line (Danziger, Sandefur, and Weinberg, 1994:10). More generous income supplements to the working poor are important as a preventive measure and, consequently, are less expensive, particularly in the long run. They are also less detrimental psychologically than outright welfare handouts. Moreover, people who are just above the poverty line generally hold insecure jobs at minimal salaries. An income supplement would allow them to accumulate some savings while employed, and would be beneficial for the economy as well because their purchasing power would increase.

LOW-SKILLED IMMIGRATION

Nearly all immigrants who arrive in Canada and the United States come in search of employment or "the American dream" of financial security and political freedom. A greater proportion than ever before originate from economically distressed countries or countries that are struggling on the way to "development." Consequently, immigrants as a group generally improve their situation by moving to North America, although there are few studies comparing their pre- and post-immigration economic status. The surge of illegal immigrants, particularly of those who can easily return to their native countries in Latin America if desired, seems to indicate that they improve their living conditions. If not, they at least improve those of their children who often benefit from better schooling, health care, and job prospects than were available back home.

Immigrants in the United States currently experience higher rates of poverty and social assistance than was the case in the past and compared with the rest of the population (Borjas and Trejo, 1991). This stems from their having less education than American-born or Canadian-born citizens (Borjas, 1993).[19] Fewer than 25 percent of Mexican immigrants and 46 percent of Central American immigrants hold the equivalent of a high school diploma or more (Goldenberg, 1996:5). Undocumented Mexican immigrants' educational skills and incomes are inferior to those of their documented counterparts. Immigrants' elevated rates of poverty may also stem from the fact that a great proportion settle in inner-city neighborhoods that are socially and economically disadvantaged. Their children's assimilation, therefore, takes place within an already deprived milieu where education is not valued by youth and opposition to the mainstream culture is normative. This is appropriately referred to as *downward assimilation* (Portes, 1995b). Were they instead able or encouraged to settle into secure working- or middle-class neighborhoods where social resources are adequate, their poverty rate, and particularly that of their children, might decline.

Immigrant workers have increased the potential labor force of school dropouts by 25 percent, that of high school graduates by 6 percent, and that of college graduates by 10 percent.[20] Immigrants who accept substandard wages displace other minority workers, as in the case of members of formerly black unions of well-paid janitors in southern California (Mines and Avina, 1992). Currently, in Canada, immigrants in general are less likely to be on social assistance than nonimmigrants. However, recent **cohorts** experience higher recipiency rates than previous ones.[21]

Unskilled immigrants, whether from one region to another or from another country, can no longer expect to secure the types of readily available and well-remunerated jobs that existed during earlier waves of immigration (Lieberson, 1980). It has been suggested that governments may have to be more selective in terms of immigration policy (Briggs, 1996). However, at least in Canada, the mere mention of selectivity gives rise to charges of racism and elitism. Moreover, porous borders and interminable coastlines make it difficult to curtail illegal immigration.

CONCLUSION

The key causes of poverty are global and affect everyone in each of our societies; however, affluent as well as reasonably well-remunerated individuals are advantaged by these social factors. Indeed, the current structure and culture of the economy is sustained only because it strongly benefits approximately 25 percent of the population. Were it to threaten the welfare of professionals, executives, and well-paid employees, one would see an entirely *different discourse* emerge quite rapidly. But as long as only the poor and the economically marginal are devastated, the overall situation remains unchallenged. The disadvantaged do not have a voice, do not have power, and they vote less often than other citizens. In addition, they are not major shareholders of corporations, and their buying power is too minimal to affect governmental and corporate policies.

Many current causes of poverty, such as the globalization of the economy, are perceived favorably or as inevitable by some economists, politicians, and corporation heads (Korten, 1995). The goal of international competitiveness becomes a major underlying factor in the discourse emphasizing personal causes of poverty, such as school dropout. Within this ideological context, school dropout is socially defined as detrimental because it threatens to reduce future competitiveness on the global market. But there are other reasons why it is detrimental—human reasons—which are not given pre-eminence. We can think here of the fact that a lack of education narrows life options for individuals in terms of health, employment, and family life; it also closes avenues of enjoyment by reducing options in the domain of leisure activities. These human conse-quences are in themselves powerful enough reasons to develop a system that encourages youth to remain in school longer and corpo-rations to be more responsible to the needs of the citizens of their country.

It will be difficult at best to even minimally reduce poverty when preeminence is given to protecting international competitiveness via corporation downsizing, and to balancing federal budgets in order to reduce the national debt. These two types of cutbacks, particularly in Canada, raise the level of unemployment and underemployment, and reduce the effectiveness of the social safety nets; thus an increase in and a deepening of poverty ensues. As Handler (1995:39) points out, the problem of poverty is really the problem of work—or the lack thereof as well as lack of well-paid employment. When extensive poverty exists, governments emphasize remedies aimed at personal causes even though these causes are themselves largely created by systemic conditions.[22]

Chapter 3

Personal Causes of Poverty

The personal causes of poverty are generally the ones favored for discussion both by the public, the media, and policymakers. They have human interest value (Hilgartner and Bosk, 1988). Anything that has to do with people's *lives* fascinates the public. Everyone has an opinion on these issues, particularly when they are aired on talk shows. These personal causes imply that individuals who bear certain demographic characteristics, such as single motherhood, are responsible for their poverty and for all the consequences flowing from it, including a child's delinquency, for instance.[1] An emphasis on the personal causes of poverty leads to the reasoning that, were these persons to change their attitudes and behaviors, poverty would be eradicated. One can thus appreciate why, in decades of budgetary constraints, welfare programs for mothers with dependent children are popular targets of suspicion and cuts. While welfare fraud hotlines or "snitch lines" exist in some areas, there is no counterpart for corporate and professional fraud—yet, these types of fraud are far more costly to the economy than the few disadvantaged mothers who may cheat the system![2]

Too little attention is paid to the more global causes described in Chapter 2. It is easier to discuss what to do about teenagers who beget children than it is to try to curtail corporations' profits in order to save jobs that could eventually trickle down to teenagers, and offer them an alternative to early childbearing. Corporation megaprofits are a far more important cause of economic disparities than teenage motherhood. But broader social matters require some training to grasp or, at the very least, the careful weighing of a multiplicity of variables that seem far out of most persons' immediate interest. But because one cause is more difficult to understand, less visible, less popular, and less interesting than another does not mean that it is less pertinent. In fact, as suggested above, it can be far more important.

In the Introduction of this book, it was mentioned that some of the personal causes of poverty also double as consequences, while systemic causes are located at a broader level and influence or exacerbate personal causes. In this chapter, the following personal causes of poverty are examined: single parenting, both as a result of divorce and out-of-wedlock births, including to teenagers; then, poverty in the family of origin, lack of education, school dropout, and delinquency are discussed, as well as mental illness and other health problems. Several of these topics will be revisited in subsequent chapters as consequences of poverty.

SINGLE PARENTING

There are two forms of single parenting. The first occurs as a result of separation, divorce, or widowhood—what has been labeled the broken home. Second, and becoming increasingly salient, is single parenting as a result of childbearing outside of marriage. This category of parents is herein referred to as the never-married.

Forty-four percent of American marriages end in divorce as do 30 percent of Canadian marriages; these rates are higher (closer to 50 percent) if they are calculated using the yearly proportion of new divorces divided by new marriages. Yet another measure—per thousand population—indicates that Americans, Canadians, and British have the highest divorce rates in the world at 4.7, 2.9, and 2.9, respectively.

In the United States, over half of the current generation of children will live in a single-parent family before age sixteen (Rodgers, 1996). It is expected that this proportion will reach 60 percent for the more recent cohort born since 1985. In 1991, 25 percent of American children, 21 percent of British children, and 17 percent of Canadian children under eighteen lived with a single parent.[3] Sixty percent of children residing with a single mother had separated or divorced parents and 35 percent had a never-married mother.[4] These statistics contrast sharply with those of the 1970s when 73 percent of children living with a single mother had separated or divorced parents, and only 7 percent had a never-married mother.[5]

Currently, nonmarital births constitute 67 percent of all births among African-American women and 17 percent among white women (U.S. Bureau of the Census, 1993a). Marriage rates have decreased more dramatically for African-American women than for other women,[6] in part because of a decline in the proportion of young black men holding well-remunerated occupations that would allow them to support a family.[7] Testa et al. (1993) found that when fathers who reside in inner-city Chicago are employed, they are twice as likely as unemployed fathers to marry the mother of their first child. South (1996) also reports that the availability of employed males accelerates both white and black women's transition to marriage. In summary, between 1970 and 1993, the number of families headed by a mother more than doubled, from 3 million to 8.7 million (Rodgers, 1996). While only one family in ten was headed by a mother in 1960, the ratio had risen to one in four in 1993.[8]

Single Parenting and Poverty

These statistics on single-parent families would not be so alarming were it not for the context of poverty that accompanies them (see Cooksey, 1997). In Canada, in 1996, 21 percent of all children lived in poverty, but 65.8 percent of children in single-mother families were poor (Vanier Institute of the Family, 1994).[9] Similarly, in 1993, 23 percent of all American children were poor. Breakdowns by race and ethnicity add another dimension to this dismal picture. Of all non-Latino white children, 10.5 percent were poor, but 35 percent were poor in single-mother families. For children of Puerto Rican descent, 41 percent lived in poverty compared with 68 percent of those in single-mother families.[10] Among Mexican-American children, 31.5 percent of the total were disadvantaged versus 55 percent in single-mother families. Among African-American children, 38 percent were poor compared with 57 percent in single-mother families (Lichter and Landale, 1995:349). In 1989, the median income for a black family with two parents was $30,650, but it was only $11,630 for a black family headed by a single mother.[11]

In 1989, in the United States, only 7 percent of two-parent families' incomes were below the poverty level, and 17 percent were marginal incomes, that is, the incomes were slightly above the cutoff point. Among single-parent families, 18 percent of father-only families were poor, while another 21 percent were marginal.[12] In contrast, 43 percent of mother-headed families were poor, and another 26 percent were marginal—and we know that mother-headed families constitute the majority of single-parent families (Meyer and Garasky, 1993).[13] The figures were somewhat higher in Canada where 58 percent of single-parent families were poor in 1991.[14] Furthermore, the level of single-parent families' poverty may be deepening in both countries. For instance, in 1976, a single parent with one child needed to work forty-one hours per week at minimum wage to reach an income at or above the poverty line, while similar parents currently need to work seventy-three hours weekly (Canadian Institute of Child Health, 1994:119). Moreover, single-parent families tend to remain poor longer than other categories of the disadvantaged.[15]

International comparisons are enlightening, although it is difficult to obtain up-to-date statistics for some countries. The latest available complete set of data was for 1987, and looked at poverty for households containing children and headed by a person age twenty-five to fifty-five. Consequently, for nearly all countries, the focus on family heads between age twenty-five and fifty-five results in an underestimation of poverty. Indeed, households headed by a person younger than twenty-five are more often poor but are not included in these data. The international statistics reveal that 24 percent of two-parent households were poor or marginal in the United States, compared with 17 percent in the United Kingdom, 16 percent in Canada, 10 percent in France, and 5 percent in Sweden. For single-parent households, the North American rates were generally far higher than those of European countries: 53 percent were poor in the United States and 45 percent in Canada, compared with 25 percent in what was West Germany, 18 percent in the United Kingdom, 16 percent in France, and 6 percent in Sweden (Canadian Institute of Child Health, 1994:21).

The United States and Canada are the two Western countries where single-parent families have extremely elevated poverty rates, and where there is a vast income difference between single- and two-parent families. A near exception is Germany: although the poverty rate of German single-parent families is less than half that of their North American counterparts, there is a wide gap in income between single- and two-parent families. In contrast, in 1987, both types of families in the Netherlands had an equal poverty rate, at 7 percent, while the rates were 5 percent and 6 percent, respectively, in Sweden (Oderkirk, 1992). These figures indicate that single parenting is a cause of poverty in only some societies, such as Canada and the United States. It is, however, relevant to recall that European countries are not burdened by the high **incidence** of teenage single parenting experienced in North America.

Gottschalk and Danziger (1993) have demonstrated that, had the 1960s proportion of female-headed families remained constant, poverty would now be a third less among blacks and a fifth less among whites. For his part, Smith (1989) believes that the increase in female-headed families explains all of the *increase* in child poverty since 1968.[16] Although this conclusion may be correct, it was reached before the economic recession of the early 1990s and before the consequences of downsizing and the spurt in part-time jobs came into effect. Nevertheless, it is certainly a fact that the density of single parenting in the United States and Canada severely exacerbates income inequality (Nielsen and Alderson, 1997).

Divorced Single Parenting

A longitudinal study of tax files by Finnie (1993) demonstrates that, in the first year after divorce, Canadian women's household incomes plummet by about 50 percent while men's decline by 25 percent (see also Smock, 1994). When income-to-need ratios are utilized—that is, when the figures are adjusted for family size—women's incomes drop by 40 percent while men's increase slightly. Women's poverty rises from 16 percent predivorce to 43 percent postdivorce. Even three years after divorce, women's incomes remain far below what they had been during marriage and far below their ex-husbands' current incomes. Similar results hold for the United States (Duncan and Hoffman, 1985). Hao (1996) provides additional information on the economic gap that exists between men and women after divorce: he documents that divorced fathers accumulate a median wealth of $22,930 compared with only $600 for divorced mothers.

These statistics implicate divorce as a direct cause of poverty; they do not, however, preclude the fact that many families experiencing a divorce were already disadvantaged. This may be particularly so for minority families (Bane, 1986). Approximately 70 percent of divorced women remarry,[17] thus a resulting concern is that before children reach the age of eighteen, they have a nearly 50 percent chance that at least one of their parents will divorce again (Furstenberg and Cherlin, 1991:14). We do not know how repeated divorce affects the family's financial status. The impact on a family's economic situation of the increasing phenomenon of stepfamily formation by cohabitation rather than by formal marriage also needs to be studied (Bumpass, Raley, and Sweet, 1995). Currently, indications are that although male cohabitants earn less than married men, they nevertheless contribute to a reduction of child poverty by 29 percent in cohabiting families (Manning and Lichter, 1996). But the instability of such unions leads to questions concerning the long-term economic and psychological outcomes for children in these families (Raley, 1996).

Never-Married Parenting

The increase in the proportion of children born to never-married mothers carries important ramifications in terms of well-being because *never-married mothers are much poorer than divorced and widowed mothers* (London, 1996), *and they remain on welfare longer,* both in Canada (Dandurand, 1994) and the United States (Ellwood, 1989). Hao (1996:281) documents that about 68 percent of never-married mothers possess no wealth or are in debt. Moreover, their chances of marrying are lower, and when they marry or cohabit they are more likely to divorce, furthermore contributing to their long-term poverty (Bennett, Bloom, and Miller, 1995). Black and Puerto Rican women give birth within informal cohabitations more often than whites, and these unions are more unstable than marital ones (Landale and Fennelly, 1992; Landale and Forste, 1991). This situation further increases these minority groups' poverty.

As indicated earlier, it has been suggested that between 50 to 70 percent of the increase in welfare cases between 1989 and 1992 was related to the increase in births to unmarried mothers (Gabe, 1992). Many are adolescent, which usually compounds the disadvantage.

Although American teenage parenting has slightly decreased in the past two years, the United States still has by far the highest level of teenage births *and* abortions of the Western world. In 1985, when such rates were even lower than current ones, there were 52.4 births per thousand 15-to-19-year-old females, with a rate of 42.6 for abortions. This compares with 29.5 and 19.2, respectively, for the United Kingdom, 23.2 and 14.2 for Canada, 11.1 and 6.8 for Sweden, and 6.8 and 4.5 for the Netherlands (Wadhera and Strachan, 1992). *Although teenage single mothers account for only 30 percent of all single mothers,* their situation is of great concern because *they tend to be poorer and remain on welfare longer than their older counterparts* (Bane and Ellwood, 1986). In 1991, 93 percent of families headed by a 15-to-19-year-old woman were poor (Lindsay, Devereaux, and Bergob, 1994). Disproportionate numbers of single teenage mothers originate from families that were already disadvantaged and, in addition, drop out of school. When they marry, they experience a high divorce rate.[18]

Forty-seven percent of poor children have a mother whose first birth occurred when she was under age twenty compared with only 17 percent of nonpoor children under age six (National Center for Children in Poverty, 1990). In 1988, 60 percent of the women on welfare had been nineteen or younger at the birth of their first child (see Testa, 1992). In fact, 50 percent of all single teenage mothers go on welfare within a year, and 77 percent do so within five years of their first child's birth (Congress of the United States, 1990:52). Never-married mothers may also be more socially isolated than other mothers, even among African Americans (Franklin, Smith, and McMiller, 1995). Isolation may be especially acute when unattached mothers live in areas of concentrated poverty.

Moreover, a longitudinal study titled "Adolescent Family Life" (Testa, 1992) determined that African-American and Puerto Rican adolescent mothers remained on welfare or AFDC longer than both non-Hispanic white and Mexican-American teenage mothers. Testa (1992:90) reports that, "Whereas over one-half (54 percent) of non-Hispanic white respondents and 39 percent of Mexican respondents moved off AFDC rolls at least once during the three-year study period, only 24 percent of Puerto Rican and 20 percent of black respondents did so." These results stem in great part from shared aspects of Puerto Rican and black poverty: these minority groups often live in neighborhoods of high poverty concentration, substantial levels of welfare dependency, and limited employment opportunities. Their poverty is more all-encompassing than that of most whites. Whites and Mexican Americans tend to exit welfare more frequently via marriage while blacks who exit do so by obtaining a job—and perhaps by cohabitation, but there is little research on this last topic. Respondents whose mothers were also on welfare reported leaving AFDC rolls at a 49 percent lower rate than other respondents, and those who reported that many of their neighbors were also on welfare left at a 33 percent lower rate (Testa, 1992).[19]

Very young families are much in the news these days, as well as much in the minds of politicians as they attempt to rein in the budgetary deficits at the national and local levels (Congressional Budget Office, 1990). Government expenditures for families that began with a birth to an adolescent mother reached $16.65 billion in 1985 alone (Hayes, 1987). Furstenberg, Brooks-Gunn, and Morgan (1987) report that adolescent mothers who remain with their parents for the first few years after giving birth are definitely at an advantage. Beyond that, they become dependent (see SmithBattle, 1996). In the mid-1980s, at the national level, 12 percent of all grandmothers coresided with grandchildren (Baydar and Brooks-Gunn, 1991). Thirty percent and 9 percent, respectively, of black and white grandmothers were in such arrangements. In the late 1980s in Baltimore, 60 percent of adolescent mothers were coresiding with their mothers.[20] Nationally, 31 percent of black single mothers with small children receive no help from their parents compared with 23 percent of similar white mothers (Eggebeen and Hogan, 1990).

Effects on Children

Although children's poverty is discussed at greater length in Chapter 7, it is relevant here to put the consequences of single parenting and poverty in context, with a brief summary of research results concerning the children exposed to divorce and single parenting. These children on average suffer more from behavioral and psychiatric problems, low self-esteem, and anxiety than children from two-parent families.[21] Adolescents are more frequently delinquent,[22] and they generally do less well academically.[23] As adults, they are more likely to divorce[24] and become single parents themselves,[25] to reach lower occupational levels,[26] to experience a somewhat diminished well-being,[27] and to have a shorter life expectancy compared with adults from two-parent families.[28] For both African Americans and whites, men whose parents divorced during their childhood are more likely to experience intergenerational **downward mobility** than those whose parents stayed together (Biblarz and Raftery, 1993).

Most of these results have been replicated in several Western societies. Even in countries with little poverty, such as Finland, single parenting is generally detrimental for children (Aro and Palosaari, 1991).[29] Many of these disadvantages remain in stepfamilies (Dawson,1991).[30] In North America, it is estimated that much of the negative effect of single parenting on children stems from poverty (Morris et al., 1996), which, in most cases, is also related to the mothers' lower educational levels (Garasky, 1995). Thus, poverty could be alleviated if the parents had more education and could, presumably, obtain occupations that were reasonably well remunerated. By controlling alternatively for income and family structure, Wu (1996) has established that *both* low income and family structure (single parent or divorced) are related to a higher **prevalence** of out-of-wedlock pregnancies among the offspring. Daughters of never-married mothers are particularly at risk of becoming single mothers (Burton, 1990).[31] Moreover, a downward economic turn in family income, particularly when already at low levels, is also causally implicated in the formation of never-married-mother families. Therefore, poverty is both a cause and an effect of single parenting. In contrast, divorce is a cause of poverty, but it is not a unique effect of poverty because divorce is found at all economic levels, although poor families are more disadvantaged by it.

Furstenberg, Hughes, and Brooks-Gunn (1992) found that the longer a mother remains on welfare, the lower her child's academic achievement and the higher the rate of subsequent teenage parenthood; thus, an extended period of welfare constitutes a risk factor for the intergenerational transmission of poverty. Another long-term consequence of single parenting, in this case divorce, stems from the tendency of young adults to leave home earlier than young people from families where parents are still together. Remaining home longer helps youths complete their education and become more competitive in the job market. It also allows them—although not all offspring who reside at home do this—to save some money and accumulate assets. Boyd and Norris (1995) report that 68 percent of unmarried adults age eighteen to twenty-nine were living at home in 1990 when their parents were together, but only 51 percent were when their parents were separated or divorced. Of the latter, 59 percent remained home when neither parent was remarried and 56 percent when only the father was. In contrast, 47 percent lived at home when the mother was remarried. Of those age eighteen to nineteen, 88 percent still resided at home when both parents were together, but only 75 percent did when parents were apart. At the 20-to-24-year-old age level, the rates were 61 percent and 40 percent, respectively. These figures raise concerns because a Quebec study indicates that at least 60 percent of single 16-to-26-year-olds who live alone are poor (Lazure, 1990).

POVERTY IN THE FAMILY OF ORIGIN

In this section, we examine child poverty mainly in terms of the risk for adult poverty incurred by children from already disadvantaged families. Children from impoverished families suffer from a multiplicity of deficits that may be caused partly or entirely by their poverty. They often live in less affluent neighborhoods, attend schools—at least in some cities—where dropout is the norm rather than the exception, and are frequently involved in juvenile delinquency. In other words, both the familial and the neighborhood/ school environments reinforce each other negatively and depress youngsters' own human and social capital, resulting in low educational aspirations, poor study and work habits, deficient social skills, and a tendency to segregate themselves with same-status peers.

These youth are often unprepared for the labor market's requirements. Many offer such a poor self-presentation when they arrive at a potential job site that they are passed over in favor of other applicants having more adequate social skills. Some may try a few times and then "quit" until they are older and more mature, or until they start a family and are forced by welfare agencies to look for work more assiduously. Many of these youths have "nothing to lose" by becoming parents in their teens. With the birth of a child, young parents add to their own parents' financial burdens or go on welfare, thus beginning a third generation to be raised in poverty. Although most will exit welfare to a job, that job is unlikely to pay well and many will join the swelling ranks of the working poor.

Another reason that youngsters who were raised in disadvantaged families remain poor themselves, or perhaps leave poverty but are not able to accumulate assets, is that indigent people less frequently own their homes than individuals in other income brackets. This means that rent money is forever lost in a bottomless pit with no return while comparable payments made by homeowners go toward reimbursing their mortgages; eventually, a home becomes an investment, an edge against poverty and inflation, a resource for one's old age, and property that can be passed on to the next generation.[32] Ownership also allows parents to take a home equity loan later on to defray the costs of their children's college education, something which is more frequently encountered in the United States than in Canada.

Although at least half of the children from disadvantaged families eventually break through the web of poverty, the fact that another half remains trapped is of great consequence. Individuals most likely to remain in poverty are those whose families have been on welfare for most of their youth; whose parents at the same time suffered from addictions or disabilities or had been in the penal system; whose mother began childbearing as an adolescent and never married; or whose parents were already poor before the parents' divorce. It is therefore not surprising if Solon et al. (1988) have found that a woman's probability of receiving welfare was 66 percent if her sister had also been socially assisted.

SCHOOL DROPOUT AND LACK OF EDUCATION

All relevant studies indicate a powerful association between education and employment as well as income and status.[33] High salaries congregate at the top levels of achieved education, although there are some exceptions, mainly among skilled technicians who earn more than MA or PhD recipients. In 1992, employed dropouts' median income was $14,200, compared with $21,700 for high school graduates, and $40,000 for college graduates (Schiller, 1995:156). Looking at the role of education from another angle, 26 percent of adults without a high school diploma were poor, compared with 10.4 percent of those who had graduated, 7 percent of those with some college, and only 3 percent of those with a college degree (Schiller, 1995). Moreover, the gap between the real earnings of college graduates and those of persons without a college degree has widened since 1973 (Murphy and Welch, 1993).

In 1991, at least 18 percent of twenty-year-old Canadians had left school without graduating—22 percent among males and 14 percent among females (Statistics Canada, 1991a). There are geographic differences, with proportionately more dropouts in the eastern provinces (Gilbert and Orok, 1993). Recent data indicate, however, that many dropouts soon return to complete high school, or earn equivalency credits (Clark, 1997). Parental attitudes make a difference in this landscape. Only 14 percent of children whose parents valued education dropped out compared with 49 percent of children whose parents did not think that high school completion was important. A greater proportion of dropouts than graduates had failed a grade in elementary school, and their grades in high school tended to be lower. More dropouts (12 percent) had been convicted for criminal offenses than graduates (3 percent). In fact, discipline problems, dislike for school, and low aspirations are more characteristic of dropouts than of other students.

In particularly disadvantaged areas, the chances of completing high school can be in good part predicted from a child's low marks in grade one and a boy's aggressiveness at the same age (Ensminger and Slusarcick, 1992). Therefore, early prevention programs would be far less costly in the long term than is the current dropout rate. The valuing of academic success has to be recaptured and encouraged via the peer group early in life. Prosocial behavior has to be rewarded, and disadvantaged children's adaptation to and appreciation of school have to be facilitated.

School dropout may occur very early and not only in the junior or senior years. For instance, two studies report that 50 percent of students who leave do so before grade ten, thus just before reaching age sixteen or even fifteen (Carnegie Council on Adolescent Development, 1989). In a second study of 1,242 black first-graders living in a high-risk area, more than half did not go on to graduate (Ensminger and Slusarcick, 1992). Of these, 40 percent of the females and 35 percent of the males had left before the end of grade ten. Therefore, in poor neighborhoods, not only do nearly half of the student populations fail to graduate, but anywhere from 25 to 40 percent of adolescents do not go beyond grade nine or ten. In a society such as ours, where educational requirements for jobs are increasing rather than decreasing, these statistics are particularly alarming. They herald more long-term unemployment, more indigence, a deeper entrenchment of the poorer class, and higher governmental burden.

In fact, in the late 1980s, it was estimated that one year's cohort of dropouts in Los Angeles schools cost $3.2 billion in lost earnings and $400 million in social services (Catterall, 1987). Similarly, Marsden et al. (1991:6) estimated that approximately 187,000 students leave school due to poverty and that this failure to graduate will cost Canadians an estimated $620 million in unemployment insurance and an additional $710 million in social assistance payments; these authors also conclude that, were these students to remain in school, "the federal and provincial incomes taxes would rise by $7.2 billion and consumption taxes by $1.15 billion."

ADDITIONAL FACTORS: DELINQUENCY AND ILL HEALTH

Teenage delinquency, *when it persists*, leads to poverty, even though it generally originates from poverty, as discussed later in Chapter 10. *Repeated* delinquency is related to inferior educational attainment, difficulties in social integration, and diminished employment prospects. Longitudinal studies indicate that adults who were habitual delinquents have inferior employment records, less adequate housing, and less satisfactory marital situations than adults who were one-time teenage offenders (Moffitt et al., 1996). Adult criminality closes access to a multitude of jobs that require a clean police record. Time spent in jail makes it difficult to obtain a job after release because the ex-convict lacks experience and a steady employment history. There is actually little information concerning the economic status of convicts' spouses and children. These families are certainly at risk for poverty, if only because one potential breadwinner is unemployed. Moreover, children of criminals are often less well adjusted socially, and this situation may contribute to delinquency, criminality, and poverty in the next generation.

Serious emotional problems such as severe depression and schizophrenia (see Glossary for definition, and Chapter 9 for more in-depth discussion) often prevent individuals from holding jobs.[34] Although psychiatric patients generally live with parents or spouses, their consequent dependence may depress the economic resources of the family unit, particularly when they have a spouse and children. Mental illnesses are discussed at greater length in Chapter 9. Suffice it to say here that social causation factors, such as stressors related to poverty, are far more important than **social selection** factors in explaining the large numbers of mentally ill persons among the ranks of the poor (Dohrenwend et al., 1992).[35] Mental illnesses, particularly of the less severe and nonchronic type, are more likely to be caused by poverty than to lead to poverty.

As we will see, there is a close connection between poverty and physical illness: disadvantaged people have a shorter life expectancy, more illnesses, and even more accidents than the nonpoor. Furthermore, once ill, people cannot work, and if their earnings were meager before, they will soon fall into the category of the poor. For others, prolonged illness leads to poverty for the first time in their lives (Arber, Gilbert, and Dale, 1995). In the United States, illness carries yet another danger from which poverty can result: medical expenses can lead to a severe loss of resources. Few disadvantaged people benefit from private medical insurance: 22 percent of the poor compared with 79 percent of the nonpoor (U.S. Bureau of the Census, 1993d). Thus, the disadvantaged are at double risk: first, of becoming ill, and, second, once ill, of not being able to afford medical care. The near poor, for their part, face much the same predicament and can easily slip into poverty once ill.

CONCLUSION

There are multiple causes for poverty. Some operate like vast umbrellas at the societal level, and others operate at the personal level while being influenced or exacerbated by the larger socioeconomic forces. In turn, poverty has profound social, cultural, and personal consequences, many of which are analyzed in subsequent chapters. First, poverty encourages the decay of neighborhoods (Chapter 4), saps the quality of education (Chapter 5), and victimizes families (Chapter 6). Second, women, children, and the elderly are particularly affected by poverty (Chapter 7). Third, in concert with discrimination and segregation, poverty reduces the quality of life of visible minorities (Chapter 8). And last, poverty also contributes to ill health (Chapter 9) and delinquency (Chapter 10).

While this volume focuses largely on the consequences of poverty, we frequently return to its causes in the many discussions which follow. Indeed, one key element of this text resides in the combination of systemic and individual perspectives or, more precisely, socioeconomic, cultural, and psychological levels of analysis. The many detrimental effects of poverty on individuals and families are examined, while the other larger social units in which their lives evolve, particularly neighborhoods and schools, are also discussed.

Chapter 4

Urban Neighborhoods in Poverty

With this chapter, we turn to neighborhoods, repositioning our focus on what is intended to be the main thrust of this volume: the consequences of poverty. In 1959, 56 percent of the poor lived in rural areas, 17 percent in the suburbs, and 27 percent in cities. But by 1985, only 29 percent of the poor resided in rural areas and small towns (Goldsmith and Blakeley, 1992:46); the majority of the North American impoverished population is now urban, so that when speaking of neighborhoods in poverty, we generally are referring to urban ones.

Cities have inherited an increasing number of disadvantaged people, particularly in their core neighborhoods. The centers of American metropolitan areas have become poorer and more racially segregated (Kasarda, 1993). In 1989, 18 percent of the population in the center of cities and 37 percent in central impoverished areas were poor—and these figures do not include those who are just above the poverty level, or near poor. It is therefore not surprising that the bulk of the research on poor neighborhoods focuses on urban areas. But this also means that we do not have sufficient research information on nonurban disadvantaged neighborhoods and on their comparative effects on families and children, both poor and nonpoor.[1] Moreover, there are no empirical ways of determining what a *social* neighborhood truly is for any family or individual.[2] This limitation forces us to follow the tradition of referring to the physical area or grids of streets in the midst of which a person lives.[3] Census tracts and zip codes are often used for this purpose.

In most towns or cities, there have always been areas with a predominance of either rich people or of poor people, or, yet again, of middle-class persons or laborers. Economic opportunities and matters of choice in terms of lifestyle have contributed to the stratification of cities. Furthermore, cities have been divided along ethnic and racial lines, either by choice or because of discrimination. Segregation has generally led to economic disadvantage for the group that is discriminated against. In cities of the past, economic segregation was spatially relative, given that the poor and the rich could simply walk a few blocks and find themselves in each other's neighborhoods. But mass transit evolved, automobiles became commonplace, and the size of urban areas increased so that the geographic distance between various social classes, but particularly between the very poor and the others, grew. Additional forces such as racial segregation and the outmigration of the upper and middle classes compounded this distancing. In the United States, racial and class segregation overlap to a great extent.

THE CANADIAN EXCEPTION

At the outset, it should be stressed that much of this chapter's contents do not apply to the Canadian situation—which is not to say that Canadian cities do not exhibit segregation. As in the United States, all large Canadian cities contain some very deprived areas economically speaking (Ram, Norris, and Skof, 1989), including some that harbor higher deviance rates. Even so, the latter are not comparable with the American situation. Moreover, in Canada, ethnic segregation usually prevails over racial segregation; it is more voluntary, occurs generally *within white groups*, and never approaches total segregation, except in Quebec among Francophones who form the majority of the population. In terms of race, First Nations have the highest index of segregation. They are followed in this respect by blacks in Halifax whose forebears arrived in Nova Scotia and other Maritime provinces as free persons and others as slaves for their Loyalist masters.

Toronto and Montreal, the two largest urban zones, are the most ethnically and racially segregated (Driedger, 1991). This segregation, however, does not necessarily correlate with economic boundaries, and is voluntary. The greater Toronto area, for instance, is home to three distinct "Chinatowns," each with a different mix of household income, and only one of which is predominantly Asian in terms of residential occupancy. With the recent waves of upper-income Chinese immigration, particularly from Hong Kong, the Chinese population has grown substantially in Canada—specifically in Vancouver and Toronto—and resides throughout many diverse neighborhoods that are predominantly white.

People of black origins numbered only 224,620 in Canada in 1991, or 0.8 percent of the population (Statistics Canada, 1991b). Most live in Toronto and Montreal where, as a group, they are more visible. African Canadians are, however, scattered throughout both cities, even in previously all-white suburbs. But there are boroughs in Toronto and even Montreal with larger black populations than others, as well as substantial contingents of other visible minorities. These boroughs are very racially mixed.[4] At the same time, black segregation is becoming more prevalent, although it takes place within geographic pockets rather than on a large scale. For instance, one observes enclaves of African Canadians in largely white and Chinese upscale neighborhoods where a few older rental apartment buildings have changed tenancy within the past five years.[5] While black segregation is voluntary, it is dictated by the availability of inexpensive housing among the less affluent, who form the bulk of this group. Blacks in general are noticeably underrepresented as home and condominium owners because of lower economic means.

The Canadian black population is quite diverse in its origins and is largely composed of fairly recent arrivals from Caribbean and African countries, in the latter case from Nigeria, Somalia, and Ethiopia, among many others. Immigrants from Somalia and Ethiopia came as refugees, and many had to become dependent on social assistance and subsidized housing, factors that contribute to economic segregation.

THE DEVELOPMENT
OF HIGH-POVERTY NEIGHBORHOODS

A poverty area is so defined when at least one of every five households is officially classified as poor; when at least two of five households are so classified, this becomes a high-poverty area. In the last two decades, the number of Americans living in poor neighborhoods has more than tripled,[6] so that some neighborhoods in inner cities harbor a very substantial concentration of poverty

(Kasarda, 1993). About 87 percent of residents of poor urban areas are members of minority groups (Jargowsky and Bane, 1990a). Even though the American population as a whole has more non-Hispanic white than black and Hispanic people, census tracts with a high concentration of poverty tend to be predominantly black or Hispanic—in the latter instance, particularly Puerto Rican or Mexican American (Massey and Denton, 1993). In 1989, 71 percent of blacks who were poor lived in areas of poverty, compared with 40 percent of whites who were poor—the latter including a large proportion of Hispanics (Goldsmith and Blakeley, 1992:48). Whether or not they are poor, 57 percent of black children live in poor neighborhoods compared with only 7.5 percent of white children (Brooks-Gunn, Klebanov, and Duncan, 1996).

From the 1920s through the 1960s, large migrations of southern African Americans took place toward the industrialized cities of the northeast, as detailed in Chapter 8. Black workers were hired in well-paying blue-collar industries. The middle class solidified and African-American neighborhoods, although racially segregated, were not rigidly stratified by social class. Following fair housing legislations, many middle-class blacks fled the inner cities after 1968, seeking more favorable living conditions. The black entrepreneurs who, before the 1930s, had had a white clientele, more and more catered to other blacks in the "protected markets" of the segregated neighborhoods (Butler, 1991). This situation "failed to give African Americans an economic interface with whites" (Boyd, 1996:141), and contributed to their economic insularity as well as eventual downfall when other middle-class blacks left the areas and the concentration of poverty increased.

But by far the most powerful factor in the creation of inner city poverty and the retrenchment of the middle-class among blacks[7] resided in the fact that the industries that had traditionally employed African Americans scaled down in the last two decades and other employers moved out of urban areas (Wacquant, 1995). As a result, the supply of well-remunerated jobs available to inner-city residents slowed down to a trickle (Bluestone and Harrison, 1982). The secondary businesses that tend to accompany manufacturing firms also became more scarce. The result was increasing unemployment among the black working class, particularly among young black males just coming out of high school. Job prospects were destroyed. For their part, Puerto Ricans immigrated in the 1950s and 1960s to work in industries such as the needle trade in New York (Valdivieso and Nicolau, 1994). But the garment industry largely left New York City and new minority immigrants—from the Dominican Republic, for instance—increased competition for unskilled occupations so that Puerto Rican unemployment skyrocketted.

As joblessness rose in inner-city neighborhoods, so did poverty (Wilson, 1996). Moreover, the advent of an increasing proportion of low-paying and part-time jobs also contributed heavily to poverty. With spiralling rates of unemployment and underemployment, work lost its social integration function.[8] As legitimate opportunities for employment were lost, many young men turned to illegal activities. Therefore, the neighborhoods with a large concentration of impoverished people inherited a strong element of criminality which became more violent with the availability of firearms and the expansion of gangs into the drug trade, particularly cocaine and, more recently, crack cocaine. While these phenomena were occurring, the prevalence of single motherhood was increasing in these same neighborhoods, in part related to the unemployment of young African-American males. Thus, the districts developed a triple concentration of disadvantages, each feeding upon the other: poverty, criminality, and single-parent households (Sampson, 1992).[9]

More and more inner-city census tracts in major American metropolises became poor and black or, more recently, Hispanic. This means that, as adjacent census tracts fell like dominoes to this concentration of poverty and segregation,[10] it became more difficult for their inhabitants to be in touch with institutions and individuals who could help them find legal employment (Sampson, 1993). In fact, most inner-city residents can no longer walk out of their poor neighborhood because even a transit ride takes them into another equally disadvantaged and racially segregated area.

It is important to keep in mind, in this discussion, that poverty coupled with social disorganization is a recent phenomenon. As Wilson (1987) points out, *even poor areas of inner cities exhibited all the features of social organization before the 1960s.* There was some joblessness, as well as some criminality, and a minority of black families were headed by women. However, the streets were

still relatively safe, there was little welfare dependency, and most
African Americans were legally employed.

DEPLETION OF NEIGHBORHOOD RESOURCES

As neighborhoods accumulate a larger concentration of residents
who are poor and a higher level of criminality, many retail and
service establishments fail financially and close down. Others relocate to areas that are safer,[11] and where residents are more affluent.
Not only does this cycle further deprive neighborhoods of much-
needed employment opportunities, but it also bars access to services
and even to some basic necessities such as well-stocked grocery and
drug stores with affordable prices. The economic resources of the
area are further diminished when about 70 percent of the residents'
consumer dollars are spent elsewhere. This in turn contributes to the
lack of successful retail and business outlets in the district. Moreover, a proportion of the residents' income is used for illegal and
destructive goods such as drugs and weapons—all underground
market economies that depress the area's tax base.

This diminished taxation base in turn disadvantages schools in
terms of resources. Qualified teachers prefer to be assigned to areas
that are safer, that service a more motivated student body, and that
offer more competitive salaries. With unemployment and teenage
pregnancy, school dropout increases as youngsters see no reason to
pursue an education that will probably not lead to a job. Moreover,
their role models are parents, older siblings, and neighbors who
themselves have left school. The vicious circle closes in on itself as
lack of employment opportunities undermines morale. In turn,
demoralization further restricts opportunities to pursue an education
that could help greater numbers of residents escape poverty, if not
necessarily escape from the area.

"Planned shrinkage"[12] of social services has contributed to
urban decay in several cities. It has become common for community
services that provide health care, safe leisure activities, or life skills
education to either close or scale down. Inner-city residents' access
to medical care is limited, even though a proportion are on welfare
and have recourse to Medicaid. But the health care they receive is
frequently of inferior quality than that benefiting the nonpoor who

are privately insured. Above all, the social resources at the disposal of ghetto and barrio residents became dramatically insufficient compared with those available in districts with a lower ratio of poverty and criminality (Wacquant, 1995). The term social resources refers to: exposure to positive role models for youth in the form of steadily employed citizens with whom they can interact, and who hold a variety of occupations; exposure to employment opportunities; positive or at least neutral contact with police personnel; and direct or indirect community supervision of young individuals as well as youth groups.

Sampson (1993) hypothesizes that social disorganization follows when a community is no longer able to maintain social control and to supervise teenage peer groups (Sampson and Groves, 1989). Certain values may emerge that allow for a greater tolerance of criminality and deviance—or a resignation to it. The concentration of female-headed households not only means that children are less well monitored when their sole parent is employed, but also that large numbers of unattached young males roam the district with few responsibilities and too much free time on their hands (Land, McCall, and Cohen, 1990). A heavy concentration of out-of-school and unemployed young males generally precludes effective social control of their activities and of those of male children who grow up imitating them. These young males, neither responsive to their mothers' demands nor to their children's needs, are a far more important element of community disorganization than the presence of female-headed families.

As the poor become more entrenched in some areas, and as there is frequent mobility of individuals in and out of the neighborhood—thus instability—higher levels of criminality frequently ensue.[13] This means that a great proportion of poor neighborhoods, albeit not all, are also relatively unsafe. The most obvious deficit of poor areas, then, is that of criminality and its accompanying effects: victimization and fear (Garbarino, 1995). In fact, the poor are far more often victimized than the rich, especially when they live in dangerous neighborhoods (Rose and McClain, 1990). This is most evident in what is referred to as "black on black" violence, which occurs for the simple reason that African Americans are far more likely than others to live in dangerous areas. When there is a large concentration of female-headed families in a neighborhood, the rate of victimization is two to three times that of areas with a predominance of two-parent households (Sampson, 1993). The absence of adult males in the household often leads to the perception of women and children as easier targets for theft and sexual assault; adolescents also become easier recruits for delinquency.

Skogan (1990:2) describes the physical and social dimensions of what he terms "disorder" in a neighborhood. There is a great deal of trash in vacant lots; there are vandalized buildings, graffiti, boarded-up windows, and stripped cars in the streets. According to Skogan, disorder "is signalled by bands of teenagers congregating on street corners, by the presence of prostitutes and panhandlers, by public drinking, the verbal harassment of women, and open gambling and drug use" (1990:2). When neighborhoods are plagued by disorder, social control in public places is no longer exercised by the alienated members of the community. As a result, these areas become attractive to criminals and delinquents and less effectively policed by authorities. They become "deviance service centers" (Clairmont, 1974). Children who live in such neighborhoods are labelled "at risk."

POOR NEIGHBORHOODS AND NEGATIVE SOCIALIZATION OF CHILDREN

In impoverished and disorganized neighborhoods, particularly those where large housing developments are located, it becomes difficult for adults to establish linkages among themselves that could allow for mutual assistance to collectively monitor each other's children—what Coleman (1990:319) refers to as intergenerational closure. Generally, parents in such areas are deprived of adequate power of supervision over their children.[14] In contrast, neighborhoods that foster a degree of relationship among children's parents constitute a social capital that is utilized to create positive human outcomes in children (Coleman, 1988).[15] In poor neighborhoods, lack of such social capital further reinforces personal risks for parents and children.[16] Furstenberg et al. (1993) have shown how social capital in an area can allow impoverished and socially marginal families to keep their children from "falling through the cracks."

This ties in with results from Steinberg et al. (1995) who have documented how adolescents who benefit from **authoritative parents** enjoy even better outcomes when their friends' parents are also authoritative. As the authors conclude, "parenting therefore appears to be more than the individualistic process that contemporary society makes it out to be." It is a group phenomenon. Unfortunately, research conducted at the parent/child dyadic level rarely questions whether obtained results might be confounded with such community level processes. In subsequent chapters, we will return to the consequences for children and families of these diminished social resources, which, themselves, are both a result of poverty and a contributor to it. The concept of social resources suggests the presence, as defined by Coleman and Hoffer (1987:7), of a "functional community which augments the resources available to parents in their interactions with school, in their supervision of their children's behavior, and in their supervision of their children's associations, both with others their own age and with adults."

Research bears out the expected negative results of living in disadvantaged inner-city districts (Wilson, 1991a, 1991b). Jencks and Mayer (1990) provide a taxonomy of the theories explaining the effect of neighborhood in general on child development and on outcomes such as school achievement. There are some differences in the findings depending on the samples and the year the studies were carried out, but, overall, research generally points to negative effects on adolescent outcomes of living in neighborhoods with a large concentration of unemployment and unskilled jobs.[17] But it is not yet known whether African-American males or females[18] or other ethnic/racial groups are particularly affected, as well as whether it is the concentration of poor or the relative lack of middle-class neighbors which is the important variable (Duncan, 1994).

Some indicative results are emerging, however. For instance, Kupersmidt et al. (1995) compared children with familial vulnerabilities living in relatively low-socioeconomic areas to similar children living in more affluent neighborhoods. They found that the latter neighborhoods served as a protective shield against the development of aggression in high-risk children. They were less likely to associate with deviant peers, and, therefore, inadequate parental supervision was not as detrimental as it would have been in a low-income area. In an experiment whereby black inner-city residents relocated, children who had moved to suburban apartments were more likely to go on to college and, once adults, to earn higher salaries than children who had moved to apartments in the city (Rosenbaum, 1991). Overall, it seems that a certain percentage (a critical mass) of low-income neighbors increases the risk for behavioral problems in children as young as five. In contrast, the presence of affluent neighbors raises a child's chances of completing high school (Brooks-Gunn et al., 1993).[19]

Ensminger, Lamkin, and Jacobson (1996) also found that living in a middle-class neighborhood influenced the likelihood of graduating from high school among black males. But theirs and most of the other relevant studies detected little impact on females. The authors reason that females may be "more restricted to home and its immediate context because of the perceived dangerousness of the area" (p. 2411), thus precluding neighborhood effect.[20] However, Hogan and Kitagawa (1985) reported that the more poor and segregated a district was, the higher the rates of early sex and pregnancy among African-American adolescents.

The neighborhood effect, particularly for males, remains even after controlling for individual variables such as ethnicity, maternal education, and single-parent families. Brooks-Gunn et al. (1995:14) suggest that "collective socialization may be operating, in that the absence of affluent neighbors confers risks to both young children and adolescents. Whether this effect is due to the presence of role models, the absence of planful or efficacious families, or other mechanisms, is not known." Families enjoying a decent income generally sustain better links to mainstream society's opportunities, and maintain more socially appropriate values and ways of behaving than families whose members are chronically unemployed. Therefore, a critical mass of stably employed and well-remunerated neighbors generally offers an environment conducive to a collective socialization that is operating within the mainstream context. In contrast, we surmise that *in segregated and poor neighborhoods, there is also a collective socialization taking place; it is, however, often in opposition to the values and behaviors of mainstream or middle-class society* (Ogbu, 1994). In addition, in some extremely poor urban areas, up to 66 percent of men and 44 percent of women under age forty-five have been involved in the drug trade to improve their incomes (Fagan, 1993); this intrafamilial activity may directly exert a negative influence on children's outcomes.[21]

Poor neighborhoods, within this theoretical perspective, socialize many children *away* from schooling, jobs, and two-parent family formation, due to a complex array of negative factors including lack of opportunities as well as segregation and insularity. Another difference between collective socialization in nonpoor and poor areas is that, in impoverished neighborhoods, collective socialization more often than not counters parental socialization and defeats it (Gorman-Smith, Tolan, and Hunt, 1997). In contrast, there is greater, albeit not perfect, congruence between parental and neighborhood socialization in middle-class districts so that one supports the other. There are fewer **cross-pressures** exerted on children, and this allows them to assimilate appropriate values and behaviors more easily.[22] There are, however, wide differences in these respects among middle-class and affluent neighborhoods. In other words, in some well-to-do enclaves, no collective socialization by adults takes place; parents are largely absent and permissive; adolescents spend their time away in cars and at various "hot spots." Hence, one should not err in the direction of attaching an aura of superiority to a district simply on the bases of lack of *street* criminality and income superiority.

With elevated rates of delinquency and substance abuse, children, rich or poor, are more likely to succumb to temptation because of the deviant alternatives presented to them by peers. In fact, one of the best predictors of delinquency is contact with delinquent peers (Quinton et al., 1993). For its part, social distance from delinquent peers protects youngsters—along with higher intelligence and lower novelty seeking impulses (Moffitt, 1994). These three factors combined accurately predict absence of behavioral and delinquency problems in children who might otherwise be vulnerable because of detrimental neighborhood influences (Fergusson and Lynskey, 1996).

POOR NEIGHBORHOODS
AS RISK FACTORS FOR CHILDREN

We have hypothesized that, in impoverished areas that are also disorganized, there is no effective community of neighbors and relatives who look after the well-being of all the children and act as agents of social control for youth. In fact, quite the opposite occurs for children and adolescents in ghettos. They are, on average, *less well educated, socialized, supervised, and protected* according to mainstream norms than other children. This quadruple deficit results from several overlapping factors that are examined below where the meanings of these four risks are explained. Before proceeding, it should now be obvious that poor children in disadvantaged neighborhoods cannot be compared with poor children who live in areas that are either mixed or more affluent. The latter children are at a far lower risk of negative *life course* outcomes than those who are the focus of this chapter. Moreover, we underscore the fact that more research is needed on neighborhood effects, how they operate, and on what aspects of life they are particularly effective. It is especially important to disentangle family effects from school effects, peer influences, and other adult effects (Jencks and Mayer, 1990), not to omit media influences. The latter have yet to be considered in the new research on neighborhoods.

As stated above, four risks confront children in areas of poverty. First, children, *whether poor or nonpoor*, who live in overwhelmingly impoverished neighborhoods, are collectively disadvantaged at the educational level—this is the focus of the next chapter.

Second, such children, especially when their parents are also poor, are often not adequately socialized in terms of the development of the social skills needed in the workplace, of personal life skills, and general work habits. Many are surrounded by negative examples in these respects, whether at school, in their neighborhood, at home, or all three. As well, few adults are at their disposal who can *proactively* teach them appropriate skills and habits. What their parents succeed in teaching them is often undermined by other forces around them, and these include what they see on television and videos. In other words, they live in an ineffective community with respect to proper socialization into mainstream America— where the employment opportunities are.

Third, poor children in disadvantaged districts are generally not as adequately supervised as children in other neighborhoods for many of the same reasons discussed above. Peers often belong to gangs that rule the area, and therefore largely escape the supervision of responsible adults. Moreover, these neighborhoods are also disproportionately populated by single-parent families. Studies indicate that, on average, children from such families are less well monitored (Fischer, 1993). Single mothers are frequently beset by problems that worry them, and take away attention and time that could be devoted to their children. When these mothers are employed, their children may return to an empty home after school, or to the homes of equally unsupervised peers, or they may "hang out" on street corners or abandoned buildings where risks abound. Supervision is one of the elements that is generally found to be lacking in cases of early childbearing, drug use, and juvenile delinquency. However, it is emphasized here that *supervision by parents in individual families may no longer be the key element*; rather, it is a collective level of supervision that is necessary.[23]

Fourth, children and adolescents who live in areas of poverty are often not adequately protected. Lack of collective supervision leaves them free to roam buildings and streets that are dangerous. It also allows them to be prey to temptations that may be too difficult to resist at that age, particularly because they are exposed to peers who may not resist the lure of deviant activities. These children are not adequately protected from bullying, sexual abuse, substance abuse, delinquency, and early childbearing. Even when parents monitor them adequately, the neighborhood violence they witness still affects them, creating stressors against which there is no protection (Aneshensel and Sucoff, 1996; Schwab-Stone et al., 1995).

For instance, in Chicago in 1993, 67 percent of homicides occurred in public places (Garbarino, 1995:76). Because of better emergency care, many serious assaults that would have ended in death a decade earlier now result in permanent disabilities, and therefore do not appear as homicide statistics. They are, however, generally committed in public places. This visible form of violence becomes a salient part of the community's experience and consciousness, often creating a war or siege mentality among children and parents alike (Garbarino, Kostelny, and Dubrow, 1991). In disrupted inner-city areas, perhaps one-third of all school-age children have witnessed a homicide, and perhaps as many as two-thirds were present during an assault (Bell and Jenkins, 1991). In Los Angeles, 45 percent of seventh-grade Mexican-American boys and 34 percent of girls know of someone close to them who has died violently;

65 percent can name friends who are in gangs; and 39 percent of boys and 63 percent of girls have a close relative in jail (Rumberger and Larson, 1994:147).

To complete this bleak picture, a study of inner-city high schools found that 22 percent of the nondelinquent students and 83 percent of those with a police record possessed a handgun. Eighteen percent of students still in school were drug dealers, and the majority of these owned a firearm: 75 percent actually carried a gun with them to school (Sheley and Wright, 1995). Many youngsters who bring arms to school do so out of fear, to protect themselves, although once it is known that they carry a weapon, they may become targets. Or, yet, they may use the weapon with deadly effect instead of settling scores with their fists or swear words as in the past. Young black males are particularly likely to be both aggressors and victims of lethal violence, hence their elevated rates of incarceration and death by homicide.[24]

HOMELESSNESS

Homelessness[25] is not entirely unique to high-poverty neighborhoods because homeless people often sleep in public parks and retail areas in affluent districts. But shelters for the homeless are generally located in or near areas of concentrated poverty. As such, homelessness becomes a problem of disadvantaged neighborhoods, particularly so since abandoned buildings are often used by "squatters," and street life serves as a focal point for "vagrants." Only about 12 percent of the homeless are estimated to reside outside of metropolitan areas (Children's Defense Fund, 1991).

Homeless people as a group are more varied than in the recent past because entire families are currently involved. The homeless are the poorest among the poor, even though this may be a transitory condition in the case of two-parent families. A majority of the homeless either have been poor all their lives, or poised at the margin of poverty. Many have never been on welfare, perhaps because of inability to secure benefits (Toro et al., 1995). At any point in time, there may be as many as 700,000 homeless; perhaps as many as 1 to 6 million Americans each year experience a period of homelessness. One out of five homeless persons remains so for several years (Aday, 1993). The lifetime prevalence has been estimated at anywhere between 12 and 26 million (Link et al., 1994).

In addition to poverty, various disabilities and addictions (Rossi, 1990) contribute to retaining people into homelessness once it has begun (Toro et al., 1995). Over 50 percent of the homeless have never married, while most others are either separated or divorced (Rossi and Wright, 1993). Most homeless men and women have no relatives or even friends who can take them in during hard times, possibly because their families are equally poor, but most frequently because they have lost touch with them. The magnitude of the personal problems many suffer from may have worn out their welcome with their families. It is also possible that many of their families are equally **dysfunctional.** At the very least, the problems of the homeless certainly prevent their reintegration into society at large. Domestic violence is often a cause of homelessness for women and their children, and may serve to isolate them from at least a part of their family. Psychiatric problems[26] as well as various addictions[27] are endemic and certainly contribute to social isolation. Moreover, the trend to deinstitutionalize the mentally ill, without the safety net of community care that had been promised by politicians, has widely exacerbated the problem.

THE NONPOOR IN DISADVANTAGED NEIGHBORHOODS

There is yet another side to poor urban neighborhoods that is not sufficiently documented. It consists of those middle-class and adequately-remunerated working-class individuals and their generally well-functioning families who reside in these districts. Recall the definition of what constitutes a high-poverty neighborhood: an area where two or more out of every five households are deemed poor. There may be two types of such neighborhoods. First, there are those where the rest of the households are also periodically poor or always only slightly above the poverty level. Such neighborhoods are the truly poor ones and are the most bereft of social resources. Second, there are neighborhoods where perhaps one or two out of every five households earn an income that is at least twice that of the poverty level, and where at least 10 percent earn $50,000 and above. For instance, in Harlem about 12 percent of individuals earn more than $50,000 and at least one-third earn between $22,000 and $50,000.

Recognition of the second type of high poverty leads to two related considerations. First, some inner-city neighborhoods are finally attracting the attention of national chains of retailers that have saturated the suburban markets and need to diversify geographically by establishing profitable outlets in underserviced areas. For example, several such stores opened in Harlem recently, and supermarkets are being built—thus giving access to goods and food at competitive prices within the neighborhoods and opening up dozens of retail positions for the local population. Similar initiatives are underway in other states. It would be important to study how such developments change the culture of the neighborhood.

The second consideration is that research has failed to highlight those individuals who reside in such areas and continue to be successful. Studies are needed that compare samples of very poor families with samples of stably employed working-class and middle-class families, all residing in neighborhoods with a high concentration of poverty. (Currently, designs simply hold family income constant in the study of neighborhood effects.) Comparative designs would allow us to document the frustration and difficulties that the latter category of families experience, particularly in the education of their children. Above all, such samples would shed light on the coping mechanisms and the strengths inherent in families living amidst poverty and disorganization, yet not poor themselves. One would also want to know the role that these families play toward their community: do they contribute to its social organization or even reorganization, or do they simply withdraw inwardly and isolate themselves amidst threatening disorganization?

CONCLUSION

Poor neighborhoods are created by an economic system that deprives residents of reasonably well-paid and legitimate employment opportunities. These areas, in turn, are a drain on a society's resources and morale. Their residents disburse a low level of taxation, while at the same time utilizing welfare, medical, police, judiciary, and penal resources. These neighborhoods contribute little to society, and society has to support their residents in a demeaning and disempowering way because it has denied them the opportunities for self-support. Thus, society contributes relatively little in human terms to the residents of impoverished neighborhoods. Moreover, the demoralizing concentration of social problems leaves the impression that such areas are lost. Because of their isolation, they can easily be dismissed by the rest of society as if they were part of a foreign country.

While disadvantaged neighborhoods have been created by the systemic forces of discrimination, segregation, and economic abandonment, once the consequences of these forces have solidified, the neighborhoods become a system that feeds upon itself and often expands into adjacent areas. In fact, the number of poor districts in each American city has increased since 1970. While they are a blight on a country's map, they are above all a disaster for the residents, particularly the trapped elderly, the children, and their hapless parents. Obviously, "throwing money" at institutions such as area schools would help, but would offer an insufficient solution if a revamping of the educational system is not accompanied by a social rebuilding of the neighborhoods themselves. Job creation, the instauration of health and community activities, the cleanup of crack and prostitution houses, and the interruption of the flow of drugs and arms are all necessary to rebuild these neighborhoods. A tall order, true, but the longer these changes are postponed, and the more entrenched poverty, crime, and illiteracy become—perhaps spreading to adjacent districts and schools—the greater will be the human and economic cost to society and to individuals for each year of delay.

Chapter 5

Schools and Education
in Poor Districts

This chapter on schools serves as a bridge between the previous one on neighborhoods and the following on families. There is a close interplay between the three sites—neighborhoods, schools, and families—in terms of the effect of poverty on child socialization, development, daily life experience, and well-being. This chapter discusses the state of schools in deprived neighborhoods;[1] the quality of the school personnel; students' experiences as well as outcomes; and the relationship between schooling and parental resources. The situation of minority students who are economically disadvantaged and segregated in poor districts is examined. Ogbu's (1991) useful distinction between voluntary and involuntary minorities to explain school achievement is also discussed.

SCHOOLS IN IMPOVERISHED NEIGHBORHOODS

The location of a school determines its resources (Rivkin, 1994). Schools in poorer districts are disadvantaged because of the local funding system based on property taxes. In 1991, the forty-seven largest urban school districts received $875 less per pupil annually than suburban districts; in a class of twenty-five pupils, this results in a $22,000 shortfall. As the Panel on High-Risk Youth (1993:7) notes, "When the relatively greater need of urban children for special services is taken into account (for health needs, language instruction for non-English-proficient students, etc.), the resource differences are even more critical." Many rural areas suffer from the same problems.

In *Savage Inequalities*, Kozol (1991) describes district after district where, in the same urban area, schools serving primarily students who are both poor and members of minority groups receive much less than schools in affluent districts. For example, in 1988, Chicago spent $5,000 per inner-city high-school student, compared with $8,500 to $9,000 per suburban student (p. 54). In Illinois, $2,100 was spent per child in the poorest district versus over $10,000 in the richest (p. 57). The range in the state of New York in 1987 was from $5,500 per pupil in New York City to above $11,000 in many suburbs of Long Island (p. 83). In Texas, a very wide gap existed between poor and some particularly well-endowed schools—from $2,000 to $19,000 (p. 223).

But these numbers are not sufficient to describe the often dreadful conditions of these underfunded institutions. Lack of finances translates into classrooms without teachers; classrooms through which up to seventeen substitutes parade in a semester; and teachers who are so unqualified that they neglect their pupils academically, abuse them psychologically, and destroy their self-esteem. Lack of finances also translates into word processing being taught without a computer; 200 students sharing thirty textbooks, or using textbooks that are outdated by over twenty years, or having no textbooks at all; courses that have to be held in lavatories; several classrooms sharing a noisy gym for want of space; 1,000 students crammed into a school designed for 500; science labs without water or even electricity; heaps of garbage behind the school yard; sewage backing up in the toilet and kitchen facilities; holes in the roof; ceiling tiles falling down. Unfortunately, this list could go on.

Kozol points out that the preparation provided by these disadvantaged schools is so inadequate that "the odds of learning math and reading on the street are probably as good or even better. The odds of finding a few moments of delight, or maybe even happiness, outside of these dreary schools are better still" (p. 59). The destruction of young minds in these institutions and neighborhoods is so systematic that, in some schools such as in Camden, New Jersey, of 1,400 students, only 200 graduate—and of those, only sixty achieved a high enough SAT score to qualify for college (Kozol, 1991:149). This is a rate of 4 percent compared with nearly 99 percent in the better institutions. In Chicago, according to Kozol, only 3.4 percent of high school students who graduated could read up to the national average (p. 58), and at the city's community colleges, which receive most of their students from Chicago's public schools, only 1,000 of 35,000 college students obtained degrees (p. 59).

Children who attend these institutions are treated as if they were expendable, as if they were lost before they entered the schools, while, in reality, it is the dreadful poverty of these places that puts students at further risk. As Polakow (1993) points out, these are "at-risk" schools that destroy the human potential of their students. Bowles and Gintis (1976) already observed over twenty years ago that schools in high-poverty areas did not encourage their students to develop the self-presentation skills that are favored by employers, and thus from the start disadvantage their students in the labor market. This long and continuing history of educational deprivation is one of the elements we refer to in Chapter 8 when we discuss the current consequences of *past* discrimination.

These observations altogether may well mean that some of these schools contribute to a decline in their pupils' IQ levels (Jensen, 1977). In contrast, in normal situations, years of schooling tend to increase IQ levels (Ceci, 1991), and absence from a good school for a prolonged period results in lower scores. For instance, black children who had moved to Philadelphia from abysmal pre-desegregation schools in Georgia benefited from an increase in their IQs of one-half of a point for each year of schooling in Philadelphia (Lee, 1951).

But inner-city schools face yet another problem. Middle-class and stable working-class families in poor neighborhoods often enroll their children in private or religious institutions in adjacent areas. This means that the less academically-oriented students or those with less affluent parents are left behind in ghetto schools, forming a critical mass that impedes their progress and demoralizes their teachers. In addition, even in schools that are more racially integrated, individual classrooms can be segregated. This occurs when a disproportionate number of minority students are placed in low-achievement classes via the tracking system. African-American students are frequently victims of this system because the test results on which tracking is implemented overwhelmingly disqualify them: as a group, they score lower on IQ and achievement tests.

This result is not surprising because, as has been discussed, black students often reside in very disadvantaged neighborhoods and originate from families where the parental education level is on average lower, and family resources are generally minimal. Thus, because of their environment, these children have been deprived of opportunities to develop the cognitive skills necessary for achievement in primary school and for optimization of their intellectual abilities (Farkas, 1996). One should carefully note that, while I accept the fact that on average black pupils score lower on IQ tests than whites, albeit only by a few points, the explanation herein suggested is *purely environmental*. It has nothing to do with racial and genetic inferiority as may be implied by Herrnstein and Murray (1994).

QUALITY OF SCHOOL PERSONNEL AND DISADVANTAGED FAMILIES

Low resources affect not only class size, but they also affect the quality of teachers. For instance, Ferguson (1991) has shown that both large class size and teachers' lower test scores depressed students' performance. One can also hypothesize that these same characteristics of school personnel impact negatively on students' well-being as well as on the family-school fit. Teachers' salaries are, not surprisingly, related to student achievement (Card and Krueger, 1992). Qualified teachers may be more sensitive to the existence of a variety of family types and functioning as well as to **socioeconomic status (SES)**. Better quality schools can increase the alliance between school board, teachers, and community (Hill, Wise, and Shapiro, 1989). Such alliances are particularly useful to improve the child-school **goodness of fit** for children from deprived backgrounds, particularly when the family is experiencing a transition into poverty.

Competent and understanding school personnel impact positively on family dynamics when a supportive and cooperative relationship is established with parents. In contrast, unskilled school personnel unavoidably affect children and their parents negatively (Knapp and Turnbull, 1991). This situation more frequently occurs in schools where a large proportion of minority students is enrolled (Bridges, 1992). We know that teachers make more frequent requests for involvement from disadvantaged parents,[2] in part because their children need more help, because of learning or behavioral problems (Sui-Chu and Willms, 1996). In fact, when children's grades are low, parents have more contact with the school (Muller and Kerbow, 1993). These requests and contacts place a strain on parents, and this experience may be particularly detrimental when the personnel are not well trained.

Carta (1991:441) contends that "the classroom holds the greatest potential for producing academic risk for children from deprived environments" above and beyond family characteristics. She emphasizes that teachers' attitudes and techniques make a large difference. Schools are more effective when a value consensus toward learning exists among teachers, parents, and students, and when there is coordination among staff members (Goldenberg, 1996).[3] According to Coleman and Hoffer (1987:62), "This ordinarily requires both that parents be strongly oriented to their children's learning in school and that children themselves adopt these parental values, rather than those they pick up from the mass media or elsewhere. Thus, it would seem to depend on a high concentration in the school of students from families that both have middle-class values and are able to transmit these values to their children." Religious schools often provide a functional community that leads a rescue of children from poverty and dropout. However, schools produce a human deficit when the teaching style and educational content fail to capitalize on the students' personal and cultural resources,[4] and instead emphasize their deficiencies or inferiority.[5] Suitable culturally sensitive programs can be initiated in all schools, as they are currently done on an experimental basis here and there (Diaz, Moll, and Mehan, 1986).[6]

Education manuals emphasize the "partnership" that exists between teachers and parents. This is especially important for minority children, particularly when they are also poor (Berger, 1991). Yet the term partnership implies equality, and this is generally not what teachers seek. They do not want parents to question their professional qualifications and classroom behaviors—especially when these are not up to par. Neither do they appreciate parental interference in the curriculum. White, Taylor, and Moss (1992) criticize the concept of parental involvement evoked by educators as being of little benefit when parents are simply used as backup staff. They suggest that more attention should be devoted to programs that provide assistance to parents and family members. Moreover, as Kerbow and Bernhardt (1993) point out, the traditional concept of parental involvement implies that it depends solely on parents' motivation, while, in practice, there are several elements that either encourage or discourage parents from being involved, as will be discussed later in this chapter.[7]

DISADVANTAGED STUDENTS AND SCHOOLS

After all this has been said, it is not surprising that low-income students do not enjoy as positive a school experience as do their higher-income peers (Swadener, 1995). They do not need to come from dysfunctional families to be at risk; just being in disadvantaged schools endangers them (Montgomery and Rossi, 1994). The inferior school environment presented to low-income students is conducive to an eventual decision to drop out (Fine, 1991). Studies describe how disadvantaged students are more often ignored by teachers,[8] are more frequently punished,[9] and are disproportionately channeled into low-ability groups and special education classes.[10] This income differential is then compounded by race differentials (Jackson, 1997; Reed, 1988). We know that disadvantaged students' school performance is on average lower,[11] and several possible explanations for this deficit have been offered.

First, there are indications that this negative school experience begins upon initial contact, in kindergarten or first grade, when there is a lack of fit between child human resources and school demands. In turn, lack of success and personal unhappiness leads to disengagement and cumulative disadvantage over the years to culminate in dropout (Alexander, Entwisle, and Dauber, 1994).[12] Second is the matter of behavior. Brantlinger (1993) has compared the responses of well-to-do versus poor high schoolers and found that the latter reported more acting-out problems and felt more ostracized and rejected (also see Elias, 1989). A study of 500 disadvantaged Hispanic students at risk of dropping out discovered that they had generated 25,000 disciplinary contacts in two years (Rumberger and Larson, 1994:144). Another longitudinal study of children in London, England, found that even after controlling for family background, children in disadvantaged schools compared with those in better schools exhibited more problems such as delinquency (Rutter, Maughan, and Ouston, 1979). Moreover, the negative or positive effect of schools carried over and above any neighborhood effect that existed. This study noted that successful schools emphasized academics, structure, preparation, homework, and a prosocial atmosphere. But also, these schools had a larger percentage of their students with at least average intellectual abilities; delinquency rates were higher in schools with a large percentage of students lacking in intellectual skills. Kellam (1994) reports that, in one study, low-ability classrooms experienced rates of aggressiveness of 60 percent or more compared with 5 percent in higher-ability classrooms.

FAMILY ROUTINE AND ORGANIZATION

On another front, research indicates that children are more successful at school and better adjusted to its requirements when family life is similar to the middle-class climate of school organization (Hansen, 1986). Children in families that have a schedule, where they eat breakfast, where rules are followed, and where educational activities are encouraged, become more easily integrated into the school system (Rumberger et al., 1990). Impoverished households with no employed adult are less likely to provide such a structure. In households where everyone gets up whenever he or she wants, does not dress until later or not at all, eats meals whenever hungry, watches unlimited hours of television, and where reading material is absent, daily life is a world apart from school routine and even goals. Hence, children from these families may experience more difficulty fitting in at school, as well as more trouble learning, because the two lifestyles may actually clash (Comer, 1988).

If the children have an easy temperament, are cooperative, and are at least of average intelligence, they may overcome this lack of congruence between family and school. Scarr (1985) posits that children who come from disadvantaged families, but are intelligent and "spunky," are more likely to be noticed and encouraged by teachers than are their less personable counterparts from a similar background. The children may in turn bring some organization into their family life, generally unwittingly, or they may insist on arriving at school on time and hence consciously set about changing household patterns. At that point, the child may open a window of opportunity for the family, especially when parents have little education and are chronically unemployed. Parents who are functionally illiterate, as are many high school dropouts,[13] may begin reading more easily when, with the encouragement of teachers, they share their children's interest in their first grade books, for instance.

But when disadvantaged children are less intelligent or have temperamental difficulties, they may be unable to integrate themselves into this alien world, especially if their parents cannot help them with their lessons. Such parents may have felt equally alienated at school when they were themselves small. These children immediately elicit teachers' negative attention, and here is the start of what can be a long and ongoing struggle between parents and teachers, or at least tension between the two, and the beginning of the journey toward school failure for the children.

PARENTAL RESOURCES
AND INVOLVEMENT IN SCHOOLING

Parental involvement in schooling is positively related to children's achievement,[14] and is consequently a key concern in research (Epstein, 1987). It is also a concern of teachers, who expect parents to support them and to prepare children for school. Lareau (1989) has documented how parents are unequal vis-à-vis schools, teachers, and curriculum. Building on Coleman's (1988) theory of resources, Lareau illustrates the gap that exists between educated and affluent upper-middle-class parents and a much less educated, more disadvantaged group of working-class parents, many of whom were unemployed at the time of her study. This research demonstrates how the differences among parents' social class positions (or SES) result in an unequal set of resources that can impact differentially on children's school performances,[15] and especially on parents' ability to be involved in their children's education.[16]

According to James Coleman (1988), there are three types of resources (which he calls capital) that a family provides to its children: financial capital; human capital which includes parents' intelligence and education;[17] and social capital, which refers to the quality of the parent-child relationship, as well as to the quality and quantity of the relations that parents and children maintain within the community. Each of these resources is important in different ways. Muller (1995) reports that, when maternal employment (which provides financial resources) deprives the child of adequate supervision (social capital), the child performs less well in mathematics (human capital). However, when maternal employment is accompanied by adequate supervision and involvement, the child receives the full advantage of resources available to his or her mother. Consequently, the child's academic achievement benefits, and so do other types of child outcomes or child human capital (Muller, 1993).

In Lareau's (1989) sample, upper-middle-class parents, who are well-educated executives or professionals, are competent to help their children when they encounter learning difficulties. Such parents also feel self-confident with teachers, and do not hesitate to request changes that could benefit their children, or to question teachers' decisions.[18] In their own social networks, they have access to professionals, such as other teachers, psychologists, and tutors, whom they can consult on school matters. These parents are also more aware of school requirements,[19] and are better equipped to meet teachers' requests because they have more material resources at their disposal (Zill and Nord, 1994). These resources allow them to provide their children with educational facilities, such as computers, tutors, and art or music lessons, and perhaps summer camps, as well as to pay for babysitting if a conference with teachers is required (Stevenson and Stigler, 1992). Lareau also mentions that these same parents often bring work home from the office, which allows their children to have at least some idea of their parents' employment activities. In contrast, less advantaged parents may not even be able to provide the example of what holding a steady job entails. They are used to the separation of work and home, and they apply this separation to school and home as well. Most see teachers as professionals who are more competent than they are, and they do not question their decisions. This is especially so among immigrant minorities who place much emphasis on respect for authority figures.

Low-income parents generally value education, at least at an abstract level, as highly as do their wealthier counterparts. In fact, Muller and Kerbow (1993) report that minority parents verbalize higher expectations for post-secondary education than white parents. But, as Fernandez Kelly (1994:215) points out, "the translation of values into action is shaped by the tangible milieu that encircles them." Not surprisingly, many disadvantaged parents entertain lower expectations for their children in terms of actual school achievement than do higher income parents,[20] because, while aspirations follow cultural norms, expectations are grounded in reality (Connell, 1994). Mothers living alone tend to expect less (Entwisle and Alexander, 1996). There is, therefore, a gap between poor parents' ideals and practices. The problem resides both in the realities of parents' daily existence and in the fact that they generally lack the skills or resources to support their children when they encounter school difficulties (Gibson and Ogbu, 1989).

As illustrated by Lareau (1989:109), less educated parents who want to help their children are often rebuked because the youngsters lack confidence in their parents' competence. Furthermore, parents may feel intimidated by teachers, and it is a well-known fact that parents of lower-class origins voluntarily attend conferences with teachers far less frequently. Often, lack of day care or babysitting prevents them from meeting with teachers. Also, working-class parents do not benefit from a flexible work schedule allowing them to participate in school activities, such as volunteering, which would position them within the system and give them an "inside track."

Several researchers have emphasized the differences that exist between children of diverse social classes in terms of summer activities. Middle-class children benefit from summer activities that are compatible with school routine, and that are permeated with a higher level of cultural capital (DiMaggio, 1982). In contrast, disadvantaged children often spend their vacations in pursuits that increase their distance from what is required for school performance (Heyns, 1988). Not surprisingly, research indicates that these children lose a few points on the IQ scale as well as on tests of mathematical ability during vacations; a knowledge vacuum is created, and they have more difficulty than advantaged children in readapting themselves to school routine once classes resume (Entwisle and Alexander, 1992). It is important to refer to a fairly substantial literature in sociology, initiated by Kohn (1969), indicating that parental values concerning their children's socialization vary depending on their class situation, and more specifically on their occupations.[21] These parental values influence the quality of the home environment and of parent-child interactions (Menaghan, 1994), which in turn are related to school achievement.[22] For instance, Menaghan and Parcel (1995) demonstrate that single mothers who are employed in high-wage jobs provide their children with a home environment compatible to that available in similar two-parent families. In contrast, single mothers who earn little or are unemployed experience a reduction of the quality of life they can provide their children.

To some extent, parents who are the more advantaged in terms of resources are in a better position to provide an environment that is congruent with the school system. Only a tiny fraction of children from affluent families do not graduate from high school (McClelland, 1996). In contrast, parental economic disadvantage is consistently related to inferior academic achievement, school failure, and dropout (Ceci, 1996; Ramey and Ramey, 1990). Radwanski (1987) documented how students with low abilities were more likely to stay in school if their families were of high socioeconomic status, compared with low-ability students from low-status families. But, more to the point, low-ability adolescents from high-SES families were more likely to stay in school than high-ability adolescents from low-SES families. In this context, Slavin (1994:114) points out that "the life of a middle-class family in the United States or Canada is probably more like that of a middle-class family in Italy, Ireland, or Israel than it is like that of a poor family living a mile away." Low-SES status is, in Hanson's (1994) words, a predictor of "lost talent."

LOW-INCOME MINORITY STUDENTS

In a nutshell, there is a middle-class home-school goodness of fit that does not exist to the same extent for less advantaged families. This is more obvious when impoverished families are also members of a visible minority. Such parents and their children may be doubly disadvantaged: not only are they poorer than the average family, but cultural and structural differences in their lives may also make it difficult for them to understand teachers' requirements and to help their children. When schools do not have personnel from their ethnic or racial group, parents may feel that the institution is a foreboding, alien world. They may be afraid to talk to teachers and may not understand their vocabulary. Unless they form an organized group, such parents are usually unable to influence the system so that it can assist their children. They may value school highly because they see it as the door to future opportunities for their youth (Yeo, 1997). But there often is a gap between their values and their ability to implement them in compliance with a system that is so different from their life at home (Kagan et al., 1985).

Even when income is held constant, black children score generally lower than whites on aptitude tests. This disadvantage that afflicts on average even affluent blacks may result from the stress of overt and subtle forms of racism that minority children experience. Moreover, cultural segregation, social insularity, low-quality schooling, and detrimental neighborhoods all contribute to the lower scores of African-American children (Gougis, 1986). As will be discussed in Chapter 8, these disadvantages translate into income differentials when the children reach adulthood.

Currently, Hispanics have the highest dropout rate, although this varies by country of origin, with Mexican Americans constituting 63 percent of Hispanic dropouts (Valdivieso and Nicolau, 1994). Comparatively few Hispanic parents have completed high school—and parental education is the best predictor of a child's school performance. The Hispanic population is the fastest growing ethnic group in the United States, and by 2020 it is estimated that the number of Hispanic youths will have increased by 65 percent (Rumberger, 1990). It is also projected that by 2050, 25 percent of the American population will be Hispanic (U.S. Bureau of the Census, 1996). This changing demographic profile predicts higher overall rates of school dropout over the next ten years (Rumberger and Larson, 1994).

Apart from lower parental SES (Warren, 1996), one of the main factors of failure to achieve by some visible minority students resides in school segregation. A study by Orfield (1993) indicates that although school segregation has somewhat diminished for black students (depending on the criteria used), Hispanics have become more segregated. This is in great part due to their spectacular numerical increase in various cities where they have settled in Latino or minority neighborhoods. Orfield (1993) looked at schools that were 90 percent or more populated by minority students. In 1968-1969, 64 percent of African Americans attended such schools, compared with 34 percent in 1991-1992, thus a substantial decrease. During the same period, the percentage of Hispanics who attended segregated schools rose from 23 percent to 34 percent. However, it should be noted that nearly two-thirds of both black and Hispanic students currently attend schools that are at least 50 percent minority populated, and 60 percent of white students attend schools where 90 percent of the students are white (Kerbow and Bernhardt, 1993). Therefore, while one type of segregation—entirely black schools—has diminished, it has largely been replaced by entirely white schools and by predominantly minority schools that enroll a combination of blacks and Latinos, with a smattering of newly arrived Asian immigrants. Inner-city schools are no less segregated than they were in the 1960s.[23]

There is currently a great deal of discussion and research toward the goal of designing a curriculum that is culturally sensitive to the needs of disadvantaged minority children. There are different interpretations, however, regarding the potential usefulness and fairness of what is meant by cultural sensitivity. Some argue that if it means understanding and respecting children's and families' cultures, and utilizing the cultural resources pupils bring to school, then the merits of such an approach seem obvious. A curriculum based on respect for minorities' traditions and cultural strengths that is then geared to facilitate children's adaptation and transition to the mainstream structure of employment, and of legal and civic affairs, is essential.

However, were cultural sensitivity to mean designing curricula with exclusively African-American or Mexican-American contents, to the detriment of learning mainstream knowledge, then, it is argued, such a situation could be unfair to minority students who need mainstream knowledge and skills, particularly at the junior and high school levels.[24] The world of work is mainstream middle-class; anchoring students in a tradition that radically differs from these requirements may close doors in terms of employment and life opportunities. Moreover, many minority group members, particularly those who are affluent, subscribe to mainstream values and lifestyles, and object to a curriculum that disadvantages their children in the workforce (Goldenberg, 1996).

INVOLUNTARY AND VOLUNTARY MINORITIES

In order to explain why minority groups such as African Americans, First Nations, and Mexican Americans do less well in school while others do better, Ogbu (1991, 1994) proposes that there are two types of minorities.[25] First are involuntary minorities, who were brought in as slaves or were conquered in their own territories and colonized. Second are voluntary minorities, who chose to immigrate to North America for a variety of reasons, but particularly to improve their economic conditions and their children's future. In the first group are African Americans (slavery) as well as Natives and Mexican Americans (conquest). Mexican Americans who have immigrated from Mexico belong to the second group, as do minorities who immigrated voluntarily from other countries, such as Vietnamese and Cubans.[26]

Involuntary minorities often have a long past of opposition to the majority group that is an integral part of their collective consciousness. Because of centuries of discrimination, segregation, and oppression, they have developed ways to resist the dominant culture in order to maintain their identity and self-esteem (Wacquant and Wilson, 1989) This is what Ogbu (1991:15) calls a secondary cultural system, that is "one in which the cultural differences arose *after* the group has become an involuntary minority. In other words, involuntary minorities tend to develop certain beliefs and practices, including particular ways of communicating or speaking as coping mechanisms under subordination." In contrast, immigrants have not experienced generations of lack of reward for effort, as African Americans have, for instance (Ogbu, 1988). Moreover, they tend to believe that their opportunities are better in the host country than back home (Suarez-Orozco, 1991). Blacks who were born in the United States cannot compare their living conditions with relatives "back home." Instead, their comparison groups are whites and other more fortunate blacks (Shihadeh and Steffensmeier, 1994).

Such differences in turn lead to diverging perspectives on education. Voluntary immigrants, such as various groups from Europe and Asia, consider schooling as their children's passport to success and learning English as a prerequisite for jobs. They accept being integrated for the purpose of functioning successfully in society while being able to retain their customs and language at home if they so wish. They then become bicultural (Kim and Choi, 1994), and develop a *positive* dual frame of reference. They encourage their children to respect teachers and to learn English properly (Gibson and Ogbu, 1989). In contrast, school is one institution that involuntary minorities may not trust, and standard English may be viewed as a mark of lost identity or assimilation. Involuntary minorities often invent other forms of language ("improper" English or even Spanish), as well as new vocabulary, and develop activities that are not part of the Euro-American way of life and, as such, give them a sense of resistance to mainstream culture. They are more likely to want to change the curriculum of the schools than to encourage their children to adapt to it. This pattern is referred to as reactive ethnicity (Portes and Rumbaut, 1990).

However, even among involuntary minority groups, opposition to the majority culture is not equally adhered to. Their upper- and middle-class and well-remunerated blue-collar members have already been successful according to mainstream norms and are more willingly assimilated. Many working-class and even low-income minority families similarly believe in schooling as the key to success, but they may not be able to promote these beliefs in their children because of detrimental neighborhood and peer effects (Steinberg et al., 1995). Even voluntary immigrants, such as Mexican Americans, who settle in segregated neighborhoods may see their children become assimilated into an involuntary-minority subculture, what Portes (1995b) calls downward assimilation. In such districts, school dropouts tend to have a disproportionate number of siblings and peers who have also dropped out (McPartland, 1994). Peers often accuse same-race students who achieve academically of "acting white" (Portes, 1995b). This is what is referred to as cultural inversion. The stigma of "acting white" is a very powerful method of peer group control. In a Washington, DC school, Fordham and Ogbu (1986) identified seventeen different behaviors and attitudes that African-American adolescents reported avoiding because they were "white," such as "speaking proper" English and being on time. These rejected behaviors become handicaps in terms of school achievement and employability (Mehan, 1992).

Basically, both the school and the peer group can be analyzed as institutions contributing to the maintenance of the stratification system. Schools and peer groups in deprived neighborhoods that are populated by involuntary minorities serve to retain everyone in "their place"—different from whites and poor. By the same token, schools and peer groups in middle-class districts contribute to the replication of the superior position that everyone already occupies. Schools and peer groups are, in this vein, conservative institutions—except for schools that strive to educate and graduate their indigent students and thereby overturn the system. Such schools and their student bodies raise children's mainstream social and cultural capital over that of their parents; the cycle of poverty is broken rather than perpetuated, and the children are integrated into society at large, at least economically. While schools have been analyzed as institutions in the reproduction of the stratification system—a phenomenon that is quite explicit in this chapter—consideration of peer groups as fulfilling a similar function constitutes a new perspective on the role of peers: peers act as levelers (Portes, 1995b).

CONCLUSION

In studies on children of the poor, the emphasis is placed on children's readiness for school and on the dysfunctional aspects of the families that have "caused" this lack of readiness. There are two obvious problems with this orientation. First, while it is true that families (or, more specifically, parents) are partly responsible for this lack of readiness, this should never be stated without the proviso that the ultimate cause resides in poverty and its correlates of insularity and segregation.

Second, one would like to see a greater emphasis on *schools'* readiness to integrate and teach children who are truly disadvantaged on several levels (Swadener, 1995).[27] As discussed in this chapter and in Chapter 4, inner-city schools are not ready for these children. In fact, in many instances, they are not ready for *any* children. This means that they would ruin more advantaged children if they had them enrolled, because these institutions are, at best, warehouses of youthful humanity.

Chapter 6

Disadvantaged Families

This chapter documents how poverty is an important contributor to family problems—although the element of risk varies depending on the outcome studied. For instance, poverty is a far greater contributor to adolescent childbearing than it is to adult divorce because a majority of teenage mothers come from disadvantaged families while divorce occurs in all social classes. Nevertheless, the consequences of poverty within the context of, for instance, a single-mother family are not identical in all these families. Individuals are unique, relationships between parents and children vary, social and personal resources differ, and the quality of neighborhoods is not uniform, so that the experience of each impoverished child and mother or father is specific to that dyad (Richters and Weintraub, 1990).

In this chapter, we begin with family size which is examined both as a cause and a consequence of poverty. This is followed by several sections focusing on teenage single parenting. These sections not only complement those on single parenting presented in Chapter 3, but they address issues specific to this age level. We then discuss the adverse consequences of poverty on family processes, that is, in terms of domestic violence, child abuse, and child neglect, as well as abuse of parents by children. Parenting skills and the dilemmas faced by mothers in poverty are underscored in the last sections.

Before proceeding, it should be pointed out that the rapidly evolving social, technological, and economic landscape of our societies contextualize the results herein presented and discussed. This means that research carried out in the early 1980s may no longer be applicable to the various linkages between poverty and family dimensions that are now observed. It also means that current research and conclusions may be outdated ten years down the road.

FAMILY SIZE

Family size can be both a cause and an effect of poverty. Declining family size over the decades has helped contain the overall poverty rate (Gottschalk and Danziger, 1993). For instance, today in Canada, in sharp contrast with the recent past, 20.7 percent of children have no siblings, and 44.8 percent have only one (Kerr, Larrivée, and Greenhalgh, 1994). Had family size not diminished, poverty would be more prevalent. Compared with other ethnicities, Hispanic Americans' birthrate is higher (Garcia-Coll and Garcia, 1995), which may contribute to their poverty as a group. As Schiller (1995:122) explains, "In both two-parent and one-parent families there is a dramatic increase in the incidence of poverty as family size increases. Among two-parent families, the poverty rate starts at 5.1 percent if there is only one child and jumps to 33.6 percent if there are five or more children." Of single-parent families with five children or more, 94 percent are poor. Schiller (1995) estimates that a further reduction of 6 to 12 percent in poverty could be achieved with yet another decline in fertility. But such a decline would be more relevant to the poor and the economically marginal than the affluent—an observation that may carry unpalatable policy implications if it leads to the argument that the poor should restrict family size while the affluent need not.

A large sib group contributes to the dilution of family resources, particularly at the economic level (Downey, 1995). When a family's income is adequate but low, additional children constitute a risk of impoverishment. A large sib group also increases the possibility that the children's educational and thus occupational achievement will be less than optimal (Ceci, 1996).[1] This is particularly likely to happen when children are closely spaced (Powell and Steelman, 1993). Therefore, a large number of children can be a two-pronged cause of poverty: in the family of origin and, later on, at the level of the second generation.

But, in addition to being a cause of poverty, larger families often result from poverty. Studies carried out in the 1980s reported unplanned births among 17 percent of the nonpoor families, 26 percent of the economically marginal, and 42 percent of the poor families.[2] Contraception and abortion are currently more widespread than a decade ago, and therefore these percentages of unplanned births may be lower today. But the gradient by socioeconomic status has not disappeared: lack of control over one's life in general due to poverty extends into the domain of family planning.

ADOLESCENT SINGLE PARENTING

The Situation

The proportion of infants born to *single* adolescent women, particularly to younger teens, compared with that of married adolescents, has risen steadily (Moore, 1992). The same observations holds for older single women compared with married ones.[3] This situation is problematic because babies of very young mothers are likely to begin life with less social and material capital than babies born to older, more educated, and married parents who hold at least one job between the two (Klerman and Parker, 1991). The lifetime marriage rate of women who have a child out of wedlock is lower, again reducing their chances of securing a second income, and thus reinforcing the web of poverty around them. Furthermore, teenagers who have children are at risk of giving birth to a larger number of offspring than average because they have activated a longer procreation span.

As the socioeconomic ladder is ascended, the incidence of teenage childbirth decreases quite spectacularly,[4] both for whites and blacks (Morris et al., 1996). However, at all social class levels, the rate remains higher for blacks than for whites, particularly for *unmarried* teenage births. This race differential may be the consequence of historical and cultural factors, but it certainly results from the last decades' economic downturns in the inner cities. Hence, the relative unavailability of young men who can support a family may be a factor in this differential (Wilson, 1987). Young African-American men are more often unemployed, or they earn lower salaries than their white counterparts. This double economic disadvantage does not make them suitable marriage partners according to Western gender roles. In extremely poor neighborhoods, 25 percent of young black males are either incarcerated, hold a legal record, or have been murdered. This situation creates a gap between the number of young black mothers and the availability of fathers who can support their children on a daily basis within a conjugal unit.

Male and female adolescents who hold low educational and vocational expectations may feel that they have little to lose by engaging in unprotected sex that might lead to pregnancy (Furstenberg, 1991, 1992). In contrast, youths who are pursuing their education, and who maintain reasonable expectations of finding a decent job after college or postsecondary training, are generally motivated to avoid early pregnancy. As Devine and Wright (1993:139) put it, "For the average middle-class girl, in short, having a baby is a quick path to downward mobility." For many impoverished adolescent women, having a baby out of wedlock may be the only form of social status they can look forward to (Fernandez Kelly, 1995): marriage is not an option, school does not respond to their needs, and job opportunities are unavailable. In such a context, motherhood, although usually not planned, is easily achieved, and carries short-term rewards (Anderson, 1990).

But perhaps too much ink has been spilled over motives and aspirations as well as "adaptations" to poverty, because these may not enter in the equation at all when adolescents begin having sexual intercourse as young as ages ten to fifteen. At such an age in our society, teenagers of all races are generally too immature to behave responsibly in terms of contraception, and, among the poor, to engage in sex as an alternative to their hopeless situation. At that young age when sex occurs, it is often an erratic game, simply a pleasurable activity, a dare, a copying of what older peers or siblings do, an oppositional or rebellious act, a gesture to please a boy, or even an accident resulting from awkward fumblings. Often, young girls who have had intercourse do not even know that this is what has occurred. Many of these youths are actually quite ignorant of specific sex acts and their consequences, even though they are surrounded by the results of the "facts of life."

Age-appropriate leisure activities are lacking in poor areas as are proper educational opportunities. Monitoring of young adolescents would obviously alleviate the situation, but is frequently impossible to achieve in disadvantaged neighborhoods that are overcrowded and disorganized. Impoverished parents may actually be less likely

to take "extreme steps" (Furstenberg, 1991:136) than their more affluent counterparts to prevent teenage pregnancy because they are aware
of the limited economic opportunities awaiting both sons and daughters, particularly among African Americans. In some very deprived
inner-city neighborhoods, parents simply tolerate or have to tolerate
early sexual activities (Sampson, 1992). Within this perspective, it is
less the "motive" of early teens that lead to pregnancy than the hopelessness that pervades their neighborhoods. Nevertheless, as seen in
Chapter 3, teen pregnancy simply compounds and increases poverty.
While it may be an "adaptation" to poverty,[5] it is certainly not, to
paraphrase Furstenberg (1992:240), a pattern that is in the interests of
those who engage in it or of the group that tolerates it.

Consequences for Offspring

Adolescent parents are overwhelmingly poor and unschooled.
They have yet to acquire the maturity and stability of personality
that are likely to benefit children. Therefore, a baby born to parents
between the ages of twelve to eighteen may suffer from multiple
disadvantages, each disadvantage compounding the other. This baby
is often labeled an "at-risk" infant: an infant at risk of being
deprived of an optimal development because of its parents' characteristics (Lamb and Teti, 1991; van IJzerdoorn et al., 1992). Other
infants are at risk because of personal characteristics, such as low
birth weight, hyperactivity, or deficient motor skills. A combination
of problematic parental characteristics, vulnerable infants, and a
deprived environment represents a cumulation of risk factors that is
particularly detrimental to child development. Such a combination
of disadvantages maximizes the likelihood of developing negative
traits and frequently prevents the actualization of competencies. It
can also be argued that teenage parenting, with its component of
poverty, may now result in more negative consequences for mothers
and children than was the case a decade ago, because the demands
of the current and future technological and economic contexts are
more exacting.

Adolescent mothers vary greatly among themselves,[6] and many
are quite competent (Roosa and Vaughan, 1984). Moreover, a good
proportion of their children grow up normally, and so do the mothers themselves (Furstenberg, Brooks-Gunn, and Morgan, 1987).

But, on average, a young mother is less likely to be as knowledgeable about child care or as mature psychologically as an older
woman (Karaker and Evans, 1996).[7] In fact, research indicates that
teenage mothers entertain more unrealistic expectations (Haskett,
Johnson, and Miller, 1994), are less perceptive of their young children's needs than older mothers,[8] and may be less qualified to help
their child acquire cognitive skills that could be useful at school.[9]
On average, children of young mothers develop more behavioral
problems and tend to be more impulsive (Brooks-Gunn and Furstenberg, 1986). In comparison, the children of older single mothers
who are educated and earn a reasonable income perform academically as well as comparable children from two-parent families (Ceci,
1996). Furthermore, adolescents whose single mother returns to
school and goes on to college experience far better educational
outcomes (Furstenberg and Weiss, 1997).

Adolescents do not seek prenatal care as frequently as older women,
and often their diets are not conducive to healthy fetal development.[10]
Consequently, a greater proportion of their infants are born under-
weight or with health deficits and neurological defects.[11] The combination of a frail baby and a still immature mother may result in
problematic child outcomes, and increases the risk of child maltreatment (Massat, 1995). Because teen mothers begin childbearing so
early, they are more likely than older women to experience multiple
life transitions, such as successive cohabitations and separations,
which make lives, including those of small children, less stable
(Capaldi and Patterson, 1991). Such frequent life changes require a
higher degree of adjustment than is needed in a stable family with
older parents (Eggebeen, Crockett, and Hawkins, 1990). This is unfortunate for children who are vulnerable due to personal characteristics,
because a stable home environment is even more important for their
optimal development than it is for children in general (Escalona, 1982).
Hence, a mother's multiple life transitions may present a danger to less
resilient children. In general, children whose mothers experience multiple transitions tend to drop out of school and live independently
earlier (Aquilino, 1996); they are thus more at risk of becoming
impoverished adults. Compared with married parents, twice as many
single parents report that they worry about making ends meet and are

concerned about their children dropping out of school and getting pregnant (National Commission on Children, 1991).

Yet another disadvantage of teenage parenting is that, in many cases, the adolescent tries to delegate her maternal duties to her own mother or even grandmother. However, it is worth noting that this expectation materializes in only a minority of cases,[12] even though a majority of adolescent mothers initially continue to reside with their families (Wasserman, Brunelli, and Rauh, 1990). Indeed, young grandmothers are frequently burdened by family responsibilities of their own and may be less than willing, or less able, to care for their daughters' offspring than expected (Burton and Bengtson, 1985). For their part, black teenage mothers are less likely to live with two parents than their white counterparts, and this means that their own mothers have fewer personal and economic resources to put at their disposal (Folk, 1996).

Young women whose own mothers started their families as adolescents are more likely to become teenage parents themselves, in part because the mothers' age and marital status at childbearing had placed the daughters at or below the poverty level, thus reducing their educational and occupational options (Morris et al., 1996). Furthermore, these mothers often had not graduated from high school. We know that both sons and daughters whose mothers completed high school remain in the educational system longer and are less at risk of early parenting than those whose mothers dropped out. In addition, a mother's own early childbearing is an example that cannot be overlooked, although children may not consciously plan to follow in their mother's footsteps. Early childbearing provides a background that makes it difficult for a mother to censure or supervise her adolescents' relationships and sexual activities: "Don't do what I did" is advice that is not necessarily credible or practical.

Types of Single Adolescent Mothers

Single adolescent motherhood is far from a homogeneous category resulting in similar outcomes for mothers and children everywhere. In this section, *we consider the age of mothers as a source of heterogeneity.* Adolescence itself is generally divided into early, middle, and late phases.[13] In this text, motherhood that occurs between ages eleven to fifteen is considered excessively premature for all parties concerned. One would hypothesize that such early reproduction is more substantially correlated with poverty, deviances, and poor family processes than either middle (ages sixteen and seventeen) or, especially, late adolescence (ages eighteen and nineteen).

Elster, Ketterlinus, and Lamb (1990) found that adolescent mothers had accumulated more instances of suspensions, truancy, drug use, and fighting in school than other adolescents. This suggests that single parenting is part of a problematic syndrome for at least a group of adolescents who, even though they are rather antisocial and impulsive, end up with the responsibility of a helpless baby whom they may neglect and even abuse (Huesmann et al., 1984). One needs to know if this syndrome of deviance is related to the age at which pregnancy occurs. In the same vein that early age at onset of delinquency tends to be part of a larger package of problems for boys,[14] one can wonder if excessively premature motherhood is not indicative of a similar syndrome among girls. It is indeed possible that 11-to-15-year-old girls who become mothers are more antisocial or problematic, are less easily socialized, or are less well supervised and parented themselves, and/or come from more dysfunctional families than girls for whom motherhood occurs at a later age. Another possibility is that the peer group of mothers under the age of sixteen is more deviant, or that the males they associate with are more problematic, irresponsible, and exploitative.

Whatever the answer to these questions, it can be concluded that *for one category of teenage mothers, single parenting appears to be linked to deviance and social pathology. Their offspring's outcomes should then be much more problematic than those of nondeviant adolescent mothers.* One would also expect that this type of motherhood is more related to poverty, both as a cause and as an effect, and thus related to its intergenerational transmission. The corollary is that parenting by older and well-balanced adolescents is probably less detrimental for all involved and, in some cases, may actually be based on a rational decision, especially when the young women pursue their education. This line of reasoning is particularly applicable to older single women who are financially secure and choose to become mothers, either because they prefer to remain independent or because of a lack of suitable marital partners.

Single Fathers: The Real Problem?

The focus of research on poverty related to single parenting is unfortunately placed strictly on the young mother. Relatively little is known about the father, largely because he often plays a peripheral role in his infant's life. Few studies include him, not only because relatively few studies include fathers in general,[15] but also because nonresident fathers can be difficult to locate. A father's involvement with his child may be positive both for mother and infant, or conversely, a father may be a salient source of problems in a young mother's life (Nitz, Ketterlinus, and Brandt, 1995). In some cases, the father's involvement may carry negative consequences for the child if he is an inappropriate role model (Thomas, Farrell, and Barnes, 1996). When the mother is a teen, the father is not necessarily an adolescent himself (Sullivan, 1989a). The older the nonresident father is, the fewer his contacts with his child, in some cases because he already has other children. A young father's involvement is greater when the child is an infant,[16] in part because of the social significance of the transition to fatherhood, particularly among disadvantaged adolescent youth (Liem and Liem, 1990). The baby may be no more than a symbolic object for masculine status and may soon be forgotten.

There are several research and policy implications as well as questions that need to be addressed concerning the fathers of adolescent mothers' babies. My personal perspective leads me to advance that young or not-so-young male progenitors are more of a social problem than are the girls to whom we always refer when discussing "adolescent parenting." Some literature clearly indicates that an undetermined proportion of young mothers have more or less been manipulated or conned into sexual activity by the males in question (Anderson, 1993). *Yet, when we discuss single adolescent parenting and stigmatize it, the focus is always directed onto the young women because they are the ones who are left with the babies and, henceforth, constitute the statistics and the "social problem."* The fathers are invisible, untouched, and unblamed—and they rarely pay child support.

Welfare is being cut, and, in order to receive it, adolescent females will soon be forced to complete high school (an excellent idea in terms of anticipated outcomes for mother and child) or to work (not necessarily a good idea in terms of outcomes). The fathers, however, may remain unemployed and out of school if they so wish. Identifying the fathers and, when they can afford it, forcing them to pay child support is a reasonable idea. Unfortunately, it is not a policy that will reduce the mothers' poverty to any great extent because the fathers are too frequently uneducated and unemployed (Lerman, 1993). But if a culture of male responsibility in terms of sexuality and procreation could be injected into the peer group, the rates of early parenting would drop and so would poverty. One should not expect that the responsibility for reducing the incidence of out-of-wedlock teenage pregnancy be an exclusively feminine one.

FAMILY CONFLICT AND VIOLENCE

Marital Conflict and Spousal Abuse

Male unemployment and insufficient family earnings can become sources of friction, general tension, and irritability between husbands and wives (Elder et al., 1992). Men feel diminished, experience psychological duress due to their unacceptable status and defeating job searches, and may react more abrasively or withdraw emotionally from their wives (Conger et al., 1990). These behaviors may undermine the spousal relationship and contribute to marital instability (South and Spitze, 1986). For their part, wives may become resentful of their lack of financial resources, and when employed, may complain that they are shouldering the entire family's economic burden. Poverty frequently leads to depression (Vinokur, Price, and Caplan, 1996), and there is some evidence that symptoms of depression may include outbursts of anger and violence directed by males against their wives (Julian and McKenry, 1993). Thus poverty may lead to marital dissolution indirectly, via depression, marital conflict, tension, and even abuse (Kessler, Turner, and House, 1988).

Poor couples who live in disadvantaged neighborhoods are more at risk of spousal abuse (and as will be discussed below, child abuse) than similar couples who live in economically secure environments. They may benefit from a network of family members who are not disadvantaged and who can help them to some extent, at least morally. In addition, the absence of visible violence in relatively affluent areas may act as a deterrent against domestic abuse. In fact, poor neighborhoods exhibit higher rates of violence of all sorts, and this includes spousal abuse.

Unfortunately, cases of spousal abuse that come to the attention of the police are not categorized by income levels in national statistics. It is only in the research carried out by social scientists that correlations with low income appear.[17] It is also important to note that few studies focus on ethnic differences. In view of income differentials and segregation, which result in African Americans living in neighborhoods where more violence exists in general, it is not surprising that one study indicates substantial levels of cohabitant and spousal abuse among blacks (Uzzell and Peebles-Wilkins, 1989). Not unexpectedly, Centerwall (1995) has documented that once controls are brought in for SES, differences between blacks and whites in domestic homicides disappear.

Child Abuse

The daily stressors of poverty exacerbate difficult temperaments and may activate predispositions to violence, while simultaneously inhibiting controls against violence. In conditions of poverty, coping mechanisms are unduly taxed by daily irritants that cumulate to form a frangible situation. Depending on the temperament of the individuals affected, and the characteristics of the child who is targeted (Elder, Caspi, and Nguyen, 1994), explosive as well as apathetic behaviors may result. Moreover, looking at it from the angle of affluence, money can compensate to some extent for inadequate personal resources: it can buy services and support that in turn can prevent child abuse and neglect. There are many studies linking parents, daily stressors and psychological distress to distant and punitive parenting.[18] McLoyd (1995) shows that among single mothers, the adverse effects of poverty increase maternal depression and, in turn, punishment of adolescents.

Child abuse and neglect are more common among the impoverished, especially in neighborhoods with a high concentration of poverty and violence (Pelton, 1991; Volpe, 1989). It is possible that child abuse is more easily detected among the poor—particularly those who are clients of social agencies—than among other income groups who may also harbor this problem. Despite this cautionary caveat, a true relationship still exists between poverty and child abuse (McLoyd, 1995). In fact, Garbarino and Sherman (1980) found that living in a high-risk neighborhood correlates with child abuse, even after controlling for family characteristics. The lack of an effective community means that each set of parents or each single parent is socially isolated,[19] lacks support, and is deprived of elements of social control that might prevent them from lashing out at their children. It is also possible that overcrowded housing conditions facilitate child sexual abuse by older siblings and by sisters' or mothers' boyfriends.

In addition, child abuse may be precipitated by the marital conflict and domestic violence that poverty engenders: husbands who batter their wives often assault their children as well (McCloskey, Figueredo, and Koss, 1995). Mothers who are under duress as a result of marital conflict may treat their children in a harsh and rejecting manner, and even abuse them. Children who are or have been abused do less well in school on average (Eckenrode, Laird, and Doris, 1993). They are also more frequently delinquent and aggressive (Sternberg et al., 1993).[20] This means that child abuse may reinforce poverty by contributing to its transmission to the next generation via school dropout and delinquency.[21]

Child Neglect

Child neglect is more common than abuse and one can easily understand that it can be indirectly or directly caused by poverty (DiLeonardi, 1993).[22] To begin with, people who are economically disadvantaged, particularly if they belong to a segregated minority group, often have little choice in the matter of where to live. When forced to remain or settle in a disadvantaged neighborhood, their children are immediately at risk for physical and psychological harm, not to omit bad example. The dangers are so numerous that parents have to be extremely vigilant, which is not a normal state, either for parents or children (Garbarino, Kostelny, and Dubrow, 1991). Moreover, when parents are under stress or hold jobs that keep them away from home a great deal of the time, children go unsupervised. This becomes child neglect, not because of parental ill will, but because of detrimental circumstances. If such neglect is temporary, it may produce little negative effect in a "good" neighborhood because the neighborhood offers fewer dangerous activities for children to engage in. In a disadvantaged and dangerous area, however, neglect can have disastrous consequences; as discussed earlier, it can lead to excessively premature motherhood, among others.

Next, parents who suffer from lower cognitive abilities and deficient coping skills are likely to be particularly disorganized by poverty and less able to care adequately for their children, compared with disadvantaged parents who possess adequate or even superior personal skills. When insufficient personal skills are combined with poverty, it becomes easy to be a neglecting parent in our type of society. Indeed, keeping children out of harm's way is part of the definition of being a dutiful parent, while inadequate supervision constitutes neglect. Yet in neighborhoods with little collective adult supervision of youngsters and high levels of criminality, it is extremely difficult for parents to supervise their offspring. The children may resent being monitored, may compare themselves unfavorably with peers whose parents are permissive ("cool") and/or uncaring, and may be swayed into premature independence by a deviant peer group. Pelton (1991:3) correctly points out that *poverty sets up a double standard* of *parenting* "in that we implicitly ask impoverished parents to be *more* diligent in their supervisory responsibility than middle-class parents, because greater protection is required to guard children from the dangerous conditions of poverty than from the relatively safer conditions of middle-class homes and neighborhoods."

Abuse of Parents by Children

There are two additional types of abuse that might be influenced by poverty in some families: ill-treatment of parents by their adolescent children, and elder abuse. The latter involves the abuse of senior parents by their adult offspring who often depend on their aged parents for support (Pillemer, 1985). The literature is wanting concerning both topics. This gap in our knowledge is particularly vexing because it would be important to determine whether these two types of abuse follow the general pattern whereby poverty creates or exacerbates problems of abuse and violence.

The question of parent abuse by children may be timely because children and adolescents are, on average, less disciplined, more delinquent, more aggressive, and exhibit more behavioral problems—particularly among the poor—than before (Ambert, 1997a). One could well predict that parents could easily become victims of aggressive and out-of-control children, particularly in decades when respect for parents is less valued than in the past, even by parents themselves (Alwin, 1986), and when peer groups, often of the deviant type, have become more influential. Personally, I am perplexed by this relative absence of research in view of the fact that I have witnessed widespread verbal abuse of parents by children and particularly by adolescents. I have also witnessed frequent occurrences of physical assaults on mothers, even by children as young as four or five. Several of these observations took place in public areas, such as subway platforms, for everyone to see, a sign that children do not fear public opprobrium in this respect. Moreover, my fieldwork has revealed mothers who were regularly assaulted by their adolescents, and two mothers bore terrible marks of recent beatings. The mothers involved were single and poor.

PARENTING SKILLS AND POVERTY

Studies indicate that authoritative parenting is the most beneficent parenting style for the development of positive child and adolescent outcomes—a topic to which we return in the next chapter.[23] When a great proportion of youth in a school or a neighborhood have authoritative parents, each child benefits. Such a school or neighborhood provides social capital to each individual youngster and his or her parents. Each parent inherits a lower burden in terms of supervision when all the children belong to homes that can be trusted to monitor their own offspring and to keep an eye on peers' behaviors.

Two caveats deserve to be underscored. First, as indicated in the following chapter, a more disciplinarian approach carries benefits in dangerous neighborhoods with high delinquency rates. Second, physical discipline does not preclude parent-offspring affection and warmth (Simons, Johnson, and Conger, 1994). Thus, one can suggest that African-American neighborhoods characterized by high adult involvement with all the children in the area, even if it is disciplinarian in nature, will produce positive results for all children and all families.

Poverty and unemployment sap adults' energy, self-esteem, and ability to be supportive and firm. Such adults may easily become erratic, physically harsh, or overly permissive parents. Unemployed parents often lose credibility in the eyes of their adolescents and, consequently, authority over them (Flanagan, 1990). We have seen that the stress of poverty often creates marital conflict which, in turn, contributes to a disruption of parenting skills. A conflictual marital relationship also correlates with lack of expressed warmth toward children.[24] Fathers who are unemployed or who are economically strained tend to become less warm than mothers toward their children, as well as toward their wives. As Elder et al. (1992:26) explain it, "With tempers on edge, the badgering of parents for money to buy things or to go places may lead some fathers to vent frustrations on their children." A vicious circle ensues where fathers' and children's irritability and hostility feed upon each other, resulting in difficult behaviors and perhaps depressed feelings in offspring. But when mothers remain consistently nurturing, paternal hostility produces little vulnerability in terms of child outcome (Elder et al., 1992; McLoyd, 1989). Single parents who are poor are particularly at risk of developing detrimental parenting practices. Their children then suffer from a triple disadvantage: poverty, having only one parent, and inconsistent or inappropriate parenting.

As will be discussed at greater length in Chapter 11, the genetic factor in this equation should not be overlooked. There is a small proportion of adults who are chronically poor because of their own personal frailties, whether mental illness, deficient cognitive abilities, alcoholism, or antisocial personalities. These adults are unlikely to be ideal parents when poverty exacerbates their deficits. Furthermore, their children may have inherited some of their parents' frailties and may be difficult to raise, making it even more problematic for their parents to care for them adequately, particularly in a neighborhood that is marred by a concentration of delinquency. Such parents and children would be less vulnerable were they living in a more stable and resourceful neighborhood.

Adequate financial means may be more important to individuals who are already genetically at risk than to individuals who are endowed with more personal resources. Well-balanced persons who become unemployed and poor can draw from personal strengths to reorganize their lives and escape from the web of poverty. They are also far more likely to maintain appropriate levels of parenting. In turn, because of heredity and adequate home environment prior to poverty, their children may be equally resilient.

PARENTAL DILEMMAS

Most books focusing on the consequences of poverty not only present the negative results of poverty, but also unwittingly paint a somewhat negative picture of the affected individuals as well as of their families. While a minority of poor families disproportionately provide this society's criminals and chronic delinquents, the fact remains that the majority of poor families struggle on as law-abiding citizens and try to raise their children conscientiously. Poverty places a heavy burden on these deserving parents and their children. Some of the problems they face are similar to those of the rest of their more dysfunctional counterparts. For instance, both they and other poor may live in a neighborhood that is unsafe. However, while a minority of their counterparts contribute to the lack of safety in the area, the rest of the poor struggle to keep their children safe, to prevent them from joining gangs or getting prematurely pregnant, to maintain them in school, and to encourage them to find jobs.

It is unfortunate that deviant minority elements too frequently endow an area with a threatening atmosphere. The danger for the other families is that the neighborhood subculture and structure become dominated by these deviant persons, some of whom come from outside the district to deal in drugs and prostitution. The negative structure and subculture may come to pervade the daily life of all the families, and they have to be extremely vigilant in order to protect their own safety and particularly to safeguard their children's upbringing (Garbarino, 1995). In detrimental neighborhoods, both poor and nonpoor families whose children complete high school without either a juvenile record or early childbearing have had to invest of themselves in these children far more than would have been necessary in a better neighborhood.

Mothers who have succeeded despite all odds are more attentive to their children's whereabouts and activities and, as Furstenberg et al. (1993) have observed, possess superior communication skills. They are better able to obtain their children's cooperation and transmit their values and goals. These authors note, "Often, these same parents had a greater capacity to cope with high levels of stress, were more imaginative and persistent in finding solutions to day-to-day problems, and were generally more positive and easygoing when facing troubles" (p. 236). They have to spend a great deal of time with their children, taking them out of the neighborhood for leisure activities, perhaps even for school. Some mothers walk their adolescents to and from high school to make certain that they *do* go to school or that they get there safely (Lorion and Saltzman, 1993). Furstenberg and co-authors (1993:243) label them "supermotivated" mothers.

Parents who are thusly motivated *and* raise successful children (for indeed, there are equally motivated parents whose children fail) are endowed with certain strengths of character that some of their children may also have inherited. Therefore, the personal resources that such parents utilize to raise their children may be mirrored in responsive counterpart qualities in their offspring, who are by nature motivated to be cooperative and to stay out of trouble (Ambert, 1997a). Unfortunately, other equally resourceful and motivated parents live in an area that is too dysfunctionally powerful, and negates all the possible effects of good parenting and positive child predispositions; their children likely would have done well had they lived elsewhere. Finally, in still other cases, resourceful and motivated parents' children did not inherit similar resourcefulness, are not resilient, and are therefore vulnerable because of the area they live in or the school they attend.

CONCLUSION

From a moral perspective, one can suggest that conscientious parents who are poor, and particularly those who live in an area with a high concentration of social problems, are more meritorious than other parents because their burden is so much heavier. The comparison with conscientious parents who have disabled, chronically ill, or particularly difficult children is appropriate. All of these parents labor under heavy environmental and even genetic constraints from which the majority of parents in our society are shielded. Being a good parent under such circumstances is a far more difficult and stressful experience. It may also be a particularly painful one when either the negative environment, the child's vulnerabilities, or the combination of the two lead to negative outcomes, such as delinquency, despite parental efforts.

It is therefore appropriate to conclude with the observation that clinical interventions with poor mothers to lessen their depressive moods and rectify their childrearing practices are well intended and often effective in the short run. However, in the long term, they can be effective only if the mothers' poverty is alleviated,[25] and if they can benefit from supportive networks at their community level. Depression and stressful parenting are largely caused by poverty-related duress, social isolation, and hopelessness. Simple depression tends to be caused by burden and stress rather than by genetic liabilities. Thus, treating the symptoms without alleviating the larger causes in the environment may provide jobs to specialists and absolve policy makers of guilt, but it does not redress fundamental problems. The afflicted individuals remain afflicted (Huston, 1995). Attempting to change individuals without changing the conditions that have made them dysfunctional in the first place is illogical. Similarly, trying to send mothers back to work without job availability, decent salaries, and day care is a recipe for failure. It is a recipe for creating future negative child outcomes that will perpetuate poverty and delinquency in the next generation.[26]

Chapter 7

Women, Children, and the Elderly

Women are more affected by poverty than men, not only because their occupations are often less secure, carry lower wages, or are only part-time, but also because they are the caretaker parent in a majority of single-parent families, and do not generally receive much support from their child's father. Moreover, when older, women are more likely to live alone than men, which places them at greater risk of impoverishment. The elevated rates of poverty among women have given rise to concepts such as the femininization of poverty and the pauperization of women.[1] Like women, children constitute a large segment of the disadvantaged, either because they belong to indigent two-parent families with an unemployed or low-wage breadwinner, or because their single parent is poor. Older persons constitute a third category that suffers disproportionately from poverty, even though their economic situation has improved vastly in recent decades. Current cohorts of elderly have lower incomes than middle-aged persons and, in the case of women, are not likely to have benefitted from a long employment history with commensurate pension benefits. Because women live longer on average than men, elderly poverty is largely synonymous with feminine poverty.

In this chapter, we first look at women's poverty with a particular emphasis on consequences for mothers. Children's poverty is then examined, and finally the economic situation of the elderly is discussed, with a focus on elderly women, particularly those belonging to minority groups. Some of the issues initially addressed in Chapter 6 are herein complemented.

WOMEN

Women cluster in a very small number of the several hundred occupations listed by the Bureau of Labor Statistics,[2] particularly in the clerical and sales sectors (Harris, 1996). These positions are less well remunerated than those occupied by males and many have recently become part-time, resulting in reduced incomes. Consequently, a gendered wage gap exists. In 1990, in Canada, employed men and women earned an average of $30,253 and $18,046, respectively; women's earnings represented only 59.7 percent of men's. For full-time employees, women's average income was 67.4 percent of that of men (Gartley, 1994), in part because men who are employed full-time put in an average of 40.4 hours a week compared with 35.2 for women. Moreover, employers frequently underpay women compared to men for similar work (Holzer, 1996). Women generally enjoy less seniority and fewer promotions than men because of discriminations[3] and child-related interruptions in their careers. The gender gap for part-time employees is even wider because women work fewer hours than men, and they congregate in personal service and retail jobs that are not adequately remunerated.

Consequently, women in the age group eighteen to thirty-four have experienced a shift toward lower wages: in 1979, 29 percent earned low salaries. The proportion had increased to a staggering 48 percent by 1990 (Fitzgerald, Lester, and Zuckerman, 1995). Aside from these variables pertaining to the gendered structure of the labor market, a second source of poverty among women resides in divorce and single parenting, as detailed in earlier chapters. Hence, women are tied to poverty by roles, including motherhood, that are inadequately rewarded by society.

Contrary to what one might expect on the basis of economic need alone, single mothers tend to be less often gainfully employed than married mothers. Women are also more likely to be employed when they are married to nonpoor men rather than poor men (Morris et al., 1996). Moreover, the higher are husbands' incomes, the higher are wives' incomes (Cancian, Danziger, and Gottschalk, 1993). This correlation stems in part from spouses' relative educational **homogamy**. Among single mothers who worked in 1994, 76 percent of blacks but only 29 percent of whites held full-time occupations— perhaps because the latter receive more financial help from their families or their children's fathers (Morris et al., 1996). There are two additional variables that combine with gender to increase

women's poverty: advanced age and minority status. Both are discussed later on in this chapter.

MOTHERS IN POVERTY

Their Burden

Women in poverty carry a heavy burden and stigma: they are
often single parents as well as poor and, therefore, as discussed in
the previous chapter, many raise children in circumstances that are
difficult at best and impossible at worst. Moreover, society blames
mothers for all the ills affecting their offspring (Ambert, 1992).
These women are therefore especially vulnerable to feelings of
inadequacy as parents. Indeed, their children have elevated rates of
all kinds of problems, both as a result of the many risks accompanying poverty, and because of marital conflict and sudden poverty in
cases of divorce. Welfare reforms and cost-cutting measures victimize impoverished women far more than they do men; when these
women are on welfare, it is generally as mothers. Most would be
above the poverty level were they childless. In 1987, more than half
of women on welfare mentioned being in poor health and 41 percent
suffered from specific health problems (Wolfe and Hill, 1993). A
circular process exists whereby a woman who is in ill health or
whose child is disabled works fewer hours than others (Payne,
1991). This in turn reduces her income, which can be expected to
further magnify her health problems.

Impoverished mothers who live in neighborhoods, especially in
housing projects, which have a high concentration of poverty and
criminality, are particularly vulnerable to failure as mothers *because
the circumstances under which they raise their children are simply
unfair* (see Kotlowitz, 1991). The deck of cards is stacked against
them from the very outset (Halpern, 1990). Their ability to control
their children effectively is thwarted by the circumstances of poverty (Sampson and Laub, 1994). In view of this situation, it is not
the elevated rates of negative child outcomes that are surprising, but
the fact that they are not higher still, and that so many of these
mothers' children grow up to be decent citizens—a tribute both to

the resilience of some children and to their mothers' extraordinary diligence and devotion. These mothers are deprived of the resources that a middle-class woman takes for granted in raising her children: a comfortable financial situation, a safe environment, spacious housing, professional consultations, hired help such as babysitting, reasonable schools, age-appropriate leisure activities, and a peer group that is usually more easily supervised. Without these, how can parents raise their children adequately in our cities? Yet most mothers with low incomes do not benefit from these advantages, particularly in inner-city areas and housing projects.

When such women are members of a minority group that is segregated in decrepit neighborhoods, their burden is magnified because they have far fewer opportunities for employment and for relocating to a better district. In addition, their maternal role may be more difficult than that of the majority of mothers because they often lack credibility in their children's eyes due to their poverty (Fernandez Kelly, 1995)[4] and, in some cases, due to their never-married status.[5]

The Matter of "Proper" Childrearing Practices

One issue in the literature on child development that becomes particularly thorny when discussing impoverished mothers focuses on "proper" childrearing practices. These practices are the ones endorsed by professionals, especially psychologists and social workers. Studies find that authoritative childrearing benefits children and adolescents across all racial groups (Steinberg and Darling, 1994). There is also a substantial debate concerning the possibility that physical punishment leads to maladjustment in children, adolescents, and even adults later on in life. In fact, in some fields, it is no longer a debate but an article of faith. Some research documents a relationship between corporal punishment and low self-esteem (Sternberg et al., 1993), or delinquency, aggressiveness, and other problems (Straus, 1994). However, this rather substantial research corpus rarely considers the material circumstances in which the families live, the type of peers surrounding their children,[6] whether the parents are loving or rejecting in their approach (Florsheim, Tolan, and Gorman-Smith, 1996:1229), and whether children perceive the punishment as a sign of parental rejection or concern

(Baumrind, 1994; Simons, Johnson, and Conger, 1994). There are indications that physical punishment is harmful psychologically only when youth perceive it as a form of parental rejection (Rohner, Bourque, and Elordi, 1996) or when the overall parent-child relationship is negative (Larzelere et al., 1989).

These results and discussions are relevant here because poor mothers, and particularly black mothers, are on average more disciplinarian or **authoritarian** than authoritative. They are more punishment- and no-nonsense oriented (Mason et al., 1994). But, then, this harsher type of discipline may be counterbalanced by African Americans' strong family value orientation, because it does not generally lead to negative behavioral outcomes among black children. It may actually have beneficial results (Deater-Deckard et al., 1996). In dangerous neighborhoods, this style of parenting may be appropriate to secure children's compliance and safety (Lamborn, Dornbusch, and Steinberg, 1996), and may be perceived as a form of concern. When peers are problematic, more controlling measures are adaptive and act as a deterrent (Mason et al., 1996). Respect for adults in authority may keep vulnerable youth out of trouble. Therefore, one needs to evaluate "proper" parenting practices within the context in which they are applied (Cauce, Gonzales, and Paradise, 1997).

Impoverished minority mothers frequently value not independence and creativity in their children,[7] but obedience and respect for authority—*as is the case, for that matter, in most countries of the world*. The valuation of independence and creativity is a middle-class Western phenomenon (Chao, 1994).[8] In poor neighborhoods, independence and creativity may constitute risks because they may be harnessed for deviant and even criminal activities. As Cook and Fine (1995:132) note, poor mothers have few childrearing options and cannot afford to make errors; for "errors" lead to delinquency, drug addiction, early pregnancy, and even death. Therefore, success in childrearing goals are seen in terms of "sheltering their children from the pitfalls of self-destruction, such as drugs, crime and cyclical government dependency" (Arnold, 1995:145). Loftier goals are a luxury in such environments. After enumerating the risks and limitations that low-income mothers, particularly those of color, have to overcome, Cook and Fine (1995:137) pointedly ask: *If you were in their place,* "then what kinds of child-rearing practices would you invent?"

The basic tasks of feeding, housing, and shielding their children from danger are at the forefront of these mothers' thoughts, energies, and parenting. In contrast, food, housing, and safety are not as salient and do not represent a daily struggle for more fortunate mothers. These do not become preoccupations and are more or less taken for granted. Can we blame mothers who are poor and live in unsafe environments if they neither have the time nor the inclination to converse with their small children and least of all read to them? If they fail to give them a daily routine that matches what they will encounter at school? If they use controlling parenting practices? If they severely punish disobedience, because they fear that disobedience could lead to delinquency, injury, or even death? What else are these women supposed to do in the contexts in which they live?

Mothers as Victims

Several states have attached penalties such as the reduction of welfare checks when children are truant. These policies greatly complicate mothers' roles and add to their stigma (Jarrett, 1996). Both in Canada and in some states, there is a movement afoot to allow civil suits against parents whose children have caused property damage or physical injury. While the rate of such youth crimes *may* diminish slightly as a result, the reduction will not be commensurate with the psychological price that will be exacted from parents. In fact, when children and adolescents commit crimes, they rarely do so with their parents' approval (Moffitt, 1994). These crimes generally constitute disobedience to parental rules as well as legal infractions. They are activities that teenagers engage in when parents' backs are turned. Do parents, particularly mothers, now have to pay financially for their growing children's crimes when they are already heavily penalized socially and psychologically (Ambert, 1997b)? It is first necessary to restore effective moral authority to parents, which many social agencies, professionals, the media, and even laws have inadvertently taken away. Only then could one justifiably chastise parents for their children's transgressions (Ambert, 1997a).

Disadvantaged mothers are generally victims of larger social circumstances, such as insufficient wages and unemployment that create their poverty. Government policies and the bulk of the literature in child development actually blame them for their children's failures. If only these mothers supervised their children more . . . if only they taught them how to be more responsible . . . if only they read to them . . . if only they went to work . . . if only they were home when their children came back from school . . . then their children would turn out all right and social problems would be solved. This is a wish list that is both unrealistic and unfair. The items on the list are also contradictory: mothers on welfare cannot *both* work *and* supervise their children if there are no day care or after-school programs available to them at a reasonable cost. It is not a question of sanctifying, romanticizing, or excusing impoverished mothers here, but merely facing reality: most social problems are largely created by the biggest of all—poverty—*not by mothers.*

Granted, as they become single parents, women and their coprogenitors do create poverty. But this result occurs because their lives are embedded within the social and cultural context of North America. If they lived in Holland, for instance, their poverty rate would not be higher than that of married mothers. Moreover, in the welfare states of Western Europe, rates of single mothering resulting from out-of-wedlock adolescent childbearing are very low, in part because poverty is less endemic due to social policies. Adolescents attend school longer, thus postponing and reducing unemployment among youth. Because of the cultural climate, women have better access to contraception and to abortion, and are also more knowledgeable about these options. But the current more favorable situation of those European countries in terms of reduced poverty is also grounded in history. Compared with the situation in North America, these countries do not harbor large groups of involuntary or conquered minorities who have suffered from a long past of discrimination, and, consequently, whose members are disproportionately poor.

CHILDREN

The Extent of Child Poverty

In Western societies, but particularly in North America, children are socially constructed as the sole responsibility of their parents,[9] especially their mothers. It does not follow, however, that parents should be solely responsible for children's economic well-being (Qvortrup, 1994a:16); indeed society is ultimately the recipient of grown children's economic contributions—not parents as was the case in the past. Unfortunately, the role of the State in children's economic welfare remains deficient (Cheal, 1996; Sgritta, 1994). The end result is that children's poverty is tied to their family's income, which, in turn, depends on the overall economic context, such as unemployment, low salaries, and the evolution of the service sector (Lichter and Eggebeen, 1994). It is also related to insufficient welfare payments, lack of day care resources, and living in a single-parent household (Heyns, 1991).[10] In the latter case, only one wage is available at best. For children born to never-married mothers, their poverty is increased by the absence of support from their fathers: only 4 percent of unmarried fathers pay any child support (Devine and Wright, 1993:70). Were all those factors removed, child poverty would nearly disappear. It is possible, however, that without the decline in fertility and the increased educational attainment of women in recent years, the number of poor children would even be higher (Gottschalk and Danziger, 1993). The growing labor force participation of mothers may also have contributed to a decrease in child poverty, particularly in low-income two-parent families where two wages stave off indigence.

With the exception of Australia, the United States and Canada boast the highest level of child poverty in the industrialized world (Smeeding and Rainwater, 1995). Twenty-one percent of Canadian children were poor in 1996, up from 15 percent in 1981. The poverty rate of American children has also increased from 15 percent in 1970 to nearly 23 percent in 1993.[11] By race, these rates had increased from 10.5 percent to 17.8 percent for white children, 41.5 percent to 46 percent for black children,[12] and 27.8 percent to 41 percent for Latino children (U.S. Bureau of the Census, 1995). Latino children's spectacular increase in poverty is mainly observed among Puerto Ricans and Mexican Americans, rather than Cubans, for instance. Overall, 58 percent of all disadvantaged children belong to visible minorities. Children under the age of six are even more likely to be poor than older children because their parents are younger and earn less (Strawn, 1992). All in all, children constitute

40 percent of the economically disadvantaged. The remainder is largely constituted by their mothers and elderly women.

Duncan and Yeung (1995) indicate that 24 percent of all American children spend at least one year during which their family is on welfare; one-fourth of these children's families receive assistance for eleven years or more. For their part, 70 percent of black children are on social assistance for at least one year (Armey, 1994). But these statistics on incidence of welfare do not tell the entire story, because each year a large proportion of poor children are not on welfare, particularly in rural areas. Therefore perhaps as many as 50 percent of all children are at or below the poverty level at least once during their childhood and adolescence (Duncan and Rodgers, 1988). With the erosion of earnings among low-income families and the financial gains of upper-income households, the gap between rich children and economically marginal as well as poor children is growing (Duncan, 1991).

To complete this dismal picture, one needs to consider that a great proportion of disadvantaged families with children are situated *far* below the poverty level. In 1991, on average, the income of a Canadian *poor couple with children was 30 percent below the poverty line;* in other words, the couple earned $8,000 less than the poverty cutoff.[13] For their part, single parents' incomes were 40 percent below the poverty line (National Council of Welfare, 1993). We are therefore talking of *dire* poverty.

Consequences of Poverty for Children

Child poverty is a particularly pernicious form of deprivation because it denies human beings the chance to develop adequately and securely *from the very beginning of their lives.*[14] Moreover, as Kitchen et al. (1991:4) point out, children are in no way responsible for the creation of their own indigence. They depend strictly on an improvement in the material and cultural circumstances of their parents to enjoy more favorable life opportunities. The effects of poverty on children are contingent upon a combination of factors, some of which result from other vulnerabilities (Lester et al., 1995). These factors include the age of the child, the extent and length of the poverty spell, family structure and functioning, race/ethnicity, neighborhood quality, parental education and mental health, as well as child characteristics and resources. Any child characteristic such as low birth weight or deficient cognitive abilities can combine with poverty to produce additional negative effects for the child.

Poverty generally covaries with other factors that place children at a disadvantage in certain domains of their lives. These **covariables** are discrimination, single-parent families, detrimental neighborhoods, antisocial peers, lack of monitoring, and parental distress, to name only a few. The greater the number of risk factors accompanying poverty, the more negative the effect (Sameroff and Seifer, 1995). Young children who live in persistent economic hardship develop more problems than those whose poverty is temporary (McLeod and Shanahan, 1993, 1996). In turn, the latter have more problems than children who have not experienced disadvantage.[15]

Individuals who become indigent for the first time as adults are deeply affected by this misfortune. But they at least have had the chance to mature according to the requirements of their society, and they often have acquired skills that allow them to cope and eventually to leave poverty. However, children born into indigence or who are poor for many of their formative years are often denied the opportunity to actualize their abilities, to receive a good education, to live in a safe neighborhood, and even to be fed adequately, which in turn can produce health deficits that will persist, imperil their well-being in old age, and ultimately reduce their life expectancy. Last but not least, children who experience poverty at *any point* are three times more likely to be poor in adulthood than children who have never been disadvantaged (Hill and Duncan, 1987), and are also more likely to earn less—even under favorable labor market conditions (Corcoran, 1995). In other words, the consequences of child poverty and its covariables far outlast the initial period of poverty itself and may be lifelong.

Negative Child Outcomes

In this and in subsequent chapters, we examine the vast literature attesting to a causal relationship between poverty and additional negative child outcomes (Dubow and Ippolito, 1994).[16] To begin with, disadvantaged children are in poorer health and have more frequent accidents than other children.[17] Babies more often suffer from low birth weight (LBW), and consequently are vulnerable to a number of neurological and health problems. The mothers' general health status and inadequate nutrition are the main culprits in this regard. A Montreal research program provided an enhanced diet to 500 low-income mothers who were pregnant with their second child. The new babies experienced a 50 percent reduction in LBW compared with their mother's first child (Higgins et al., 1989). Mott (1991) reports that the lower a baby's birth weight, the longer it takes for the mother to enter the work force. This delay could be caused by both the mother's and infant's health. A low-birth-weight infant raises more concerns so that it may be more difficult for the mother to find an appropriate caretaker while she works. Therefore, the arrival of a low-birth-weight infant may exacerbate the economic situation of a family that is already indigent or may plunge into poverty an economically marginal two-parent family for which the mother's income is essential.

The mortality rate of children and adolescents is 56 percent higher among low-income Canadians than among Canadians with the most affluent incomes: 70 versus 58 per 100,000 population (Canadian Institute of Child Health, 1989:98) It is estimated that 12 million American children go hungry at some point each month (Jackson, 1993). Even poor children covered by Medicaid rarely receive proper medical attention because, in some states, Medicaid does not cover the entirety of needed expenses (Wolfe, 1995). Moreover, children on Medicaid are less likely to experience continuity of care (St. Peter, Newacheck, and Halfon, 1992). The level of psychiatric problems for children on welfare far outstrips that of other children: 31 percent versus 14 percent in Ontario (Offord, Boyle, and Racine, 1989). Over 40 percent of children who live in subsidized housing underachieve in school, and over a third are perceived to be in need of professional help for behavioral and emotional problems. Children who are poor are seven times more likely than other children to be identified by teachers for conduct disorders. Even if we halve this figure to account for a possible teachers' bias against disadvantaged children or their parents (or against minority children or children in single-parent families), the difference remains substantial and is confirmed across the world.

Disadvantaged children often stand out from others in a multitude of other ways that are psychologically painful. For instance, they may be ashamed of living in a housing project. They may not want to let their peers know where they live and may not wish to invite them home. Their clothes may not be fashionable. They are unlikely to have the pocket money received by other children. They may be unable to participate in popular extracurricular activities with their peers, and this disadvantage can lead them to be ostracized. Their parents may be less well dressed, may not have a car or they may have an old and rusty one, and may be unemployed. They may receive free meals at school. All or any of these socially visible experiences are humiliating and painful to bear, although they may be less so in a school where a great proportion of the children are equally disadvantaged.

HOMELESS CHILDREN

Homeless children suffer from poverty within poverty. It is difficult to estimate the number of the homeless, and, for most families, homelessness is an even more transient situation than other kinds of poverty (Link et al., 1994). Some families are homeless because they can no longer afford their lodging or have been evicted. Others have left their homes because of domestic violence or family breakdown (Shinn, Knickman, and Weitzman, 1991). Mental illness and substance abuse among adults[18] and running away among adolescents are also important contributing factors. In the past, homelessness was largely a male phenomenon that has since spread across genders and ages, and includes entire families, whether with single or two parents.

In order to disentangle the effects of homelessness from those of poverty, studies have compared homeless children with poor children who live in their own homes (e.g., Schteingart et al., 1995). Much of this research involves children placed in emergency shelters with their families or in hostels where the homeless are temporarily lodged. However, there is little information on children whose families are turned away by overflowing emergency shelters, a situation which may occur in as many as 25 percent of the cases in many American cities.[19] What happens to these families is not known. Rafferty and Rollins (1989)[20] report that families are often "bounced" from one shelter to another, further disrupting their functioning and especially the children's education, given that they may be moved to a shelter that is in a different district. In their study of homeless families in New York City hostels, Rafferty and Rollins (1989)[21] found that 60 percent had been in at least two different shelters, 29 percent in at least four, and 10 percent in seven or more.

What is it like to live in a shelter? Families often sleep in close proximity to other families; facilities such as bathrooms are shared; few amenities are available, such as refrigerators in which a family can preserve its own food. There is virtually no privacy. According to Rafferty and Shinn (1991:1175), "Homeless parents often encounter difficulties balancing their own physical, social and personal needs and those of their children. The loss of control over their environment and their lives places them at increased risk for learned helplessness and depression." In fact, a large proportion of homeless mothers suffer from mental disorders (Zima et al., 1996).

Comparisons between poor children in shelters and those in their own homes have revealed that the two consistent disadvantages of homeless children reside in health and education. There are few consistent differences in terms of emotional and behavioral development. However, it is important to note that these studies are not longitudinal and therefore may not detect preexisting conditions and long-term consequences. For instance, it may take months of homelessness to produce emotional and behavioral dislocation while, in contrast, school and health problems result more rapidly and are easier to document.

In terms of health, homeless mothers more frequently give birth to tiny babies. In a study conducted in New York City, 16 percent of homeless mothers, 11 percent of women in public housing, but only 7 percent of women in the general population had LBW infants (Chavkin et al., 1987). This in turn was related to a far higher incidence of infant mortality among homeless women—over twice that of women in general. Homeless children are ill more often than other poor children. Their incidence of respiratory infections is especially elevated as a result of crowded conditions and the sharing of inadequate sanitary facilities. We can also presume that noise, overcrowding, and parents' distress depress their immune systems so that they easily contract pneumonias and viruses. This health crisis is exacerbated by a lower level of access to medical care among homeless children than other poor children.

The second domain in which homeless children are at a particular disadvantage is schooling. To begin with, their rate of absenteeism is higher (Rafferty and Rollins, 1989). They are also more likely to repeat grades (Rafferty and Shinn, 1991). We know that poor children do not, on average, achieve as well in school. Homeless children are even more affected in this respect, which may lead to far higher dropout rates down the road, especially among those who have repeated one or more grades and whose schoolmates are out of their age bracket.

The inferior school achievement of homeless children stems from a variety of interwoven causes. They change schools more often; they are sick more frequently than other poor children; the crowded conditions in which they live are not conducive to homework, and may even deprive them of sufficient sleep. Their nutrition is inadequate; many go hungry and thus they are not able to focus in class.[22] Their parents may be too distressed or emotionally unbalanced to help them and guide them. Older children may not want to go to school because they fear the ridicule of peers who, even though poor themselves, at least can claim a permanent address. Frequent school changes isolate them socially, lead to disengagement from school, and even to falling in with a crowd of antisocial peers. Moreover, schools are unprepared to address these children's multiple problems (Molnar, Roth, and Klein, 1990).

THE ELDERLY

Poverty has decreased substantially among the elderly. In 1959, 35 percent of the American elderly were poor compared with 10.5 percent in 1995. This is lower than the 13.8 percent overall poverty rate, and substantially lower than children's poverty level. In 1991, 16 percent of the Canadian elderly were poor—15.6 percent of the 65-to-69 age group and 20.8 percent of those 70 and over (Statistics Canada, 1993a). The slightly higher level of poverty among Canadian than American elderly may be attributed to differences in poverty cutoff levels. The official Canadian cutoff, in 1989, was $14,701 for an elderly couple and $10,751 for a single individual.[23]

In 1991, the official American poverty line for an older couple was $8,241 and $7, 086 for individuals (Atchley, 1994:231). The drastic reduction of poverty among the elderly, mainly those between the ages of sixty-five and seventy, has resulted from more generous social security payments, increased Medicare, improved pension plans, and higher educational levels with each succeeding cohort of seniors.

The causes of elderly poverty are different from those of child poverty (Atchley, 1994). The elderly who are poor are in this situation because of inadequate retirement income or pensions, and most of them were not poor when employed, although they generally had low incomes. Once disadvantaged, older individuals do not generally escape from that condition (Coe, 1988). Income, though not wealth, peaks between the ages of thirty-five and fifty-four, after which it usually declines sharply, to the point where the income of the 65-to-74 age group is similar to that of the 15-to-24 age group. The main difference, however, is that those seniors who have benefited from lifelong and well-paid employment have accumulated assets, particularly ownership of a dwelling and a car, which reduce the pressure placed on their current income (Cheal, 1996).

The distribution of the elderly in the population varies by ethnicity, and this demographic reality carries important poverty-related ramifications. In 1990, in the United States, only 5 percent of Hispanics and of Native Americans, 8 percent of blacks, but 13 percent of whites were age sixty-five or older (U.S. Bureau of the Census, 1990b). Despite the preponderance of whites in the elderly population, African Americans constitute 36 percent of the poor elderly. Among the elderly, 33 percent of blacks are impoverished compared with only 10 percent of whites, 14 percent of Asians, 22 percent of Hispanics, and 35 percent of Native Americans (U.S. Senate Special Committee on Aging, 1992). The Native rate, however, may be as high as 50 percent depending on the criteria used.

Although the causes of these racial differences are addressed in the next chapter, suffice it to say here that in 1988, there were sharp educational differences among the elderly by race and ethnicity. Hispanic elderly had a median of 7.5 years of schooling compared with 8.4 years for blacks and 12.2 years for whites.[24] Among all current elderly, the younger cohort is more educated than the older cohort, and it can be expected that future generations of seniors will be even more educated—a factor that should lower the prevalence of poverty among the elderly. Unfortunately, current indications are that the gap between minorities and whites may remain well into the next century. In summary, there are two groups of elderly who suffer from particularly elevated rates of poverty: minorities and women, especially *minority women*. This situation occurs on both sides of the American-Canadian border (Wanner and McDonald, 1986).

ELDERLY WOMEN

Nearly 15 percent of elderly women are poor in the United States and 22 percent in Canada, compared with 8 percent of elderly American men and 11 percent of elderly Canadian men.[25] Single elderly women living alone are even poorer: 25 percent in the United States[26] and 44 percent in Canada.[27] *These rates are higher than children's poverty rates*, and are expected to rise in the near future. Among the elderly, women constitute 70 percent of the poor. Therefore, elderly poverty is synonymous with feminine poverty. Minority group membership exacerbates elderly indigence. Taeuber (1991) indicates that 66 percent of black women and 61 percent of Hispanic elderly women living alone are impoverished. African-American women have traditionally occupied jobs such as house-cleaning that carried low pay and no benefits.

Current cohorts of elderly women are at a particularly elevated risk for poverty because, when younger, they generally were not employed, or were so for only brief periods. They accumulated little wealth, fewer benefits, and smaller pension plans than elderly men. They are widowed earlier than men and thereafter no longer have two incomes in their household. In fact, they may lose their primary source of income upon becoming widowed or divorced. Widowed women obtain an average of about 60 percent of their income from Social Security (Schwenk, 1992). In the United States, low-income women who are divorced or widowed are the least likely group to have private health insurance.

Consequently, older women in general are more vulnerable than men to not receiving proper medical attention. But there are again differences by race, so that in 1993, the life expectancy for African-American men and women was 66 and 74.7 years, respectively, compared with 73.5 and 80.1 years, respectively, for white men and women—a very wide gap (U.S. Bureau of the Census, 1993d). As frailty increases with age, it becomes difficult for many elderly women to visit health providers because they depend on others for transportation. If their children are also indigent, their situation deteriorates further. A Congressional report[28] indicates that half of indigent widowed women have been poor before, and a substantial minority of poor elderly women have been economically disadvantaged all their lives (McLaughlin and Holden, 1993).

Poverty in old age, particularly for women, leads to social isolation, inadequate housing, fear of crime, malnutrition, lack of access to medical care, and the inability to reciprocate for services that relatives or neighbors provide. A feeling of hopelessness and powerlessness may pervade the lives of poor elderly women who have few relatives, and in particular no daughter, to care for them.[29] Indigent elderly women do not have the satisfaction of leaving any form of tangible inheritance to their children. This means that their children, who may have been raised in a disadvantaged family, cannot count on inheriting anything that could lift them out of poverty if they ever become indigent themselves.

This situation is particularly problematic for African-American elderly women who, as discussed previously, are disproportionately disadvantaged, whose poverty predated old age, and whose children and grandchildren are also disproportionately indigent (Perry, 1994). When these generations succeed each other in the flow of time, current middle-aged black women may become elderly women who are particularly vulnerable to having a family network that is too disadvantaged to meet their needs. In fact, there are indications that black mothers already perceive their adult children to be less supportive than do white mothers (Umberson, 1992). Black families with older parents engage less in intergenerational exchanges than do white families (Lawton, Silverstein, and Bengtson, 1994), probably because of lower financial and social capital.

CONCLUSION

There is a continuing and accruing risk for poverty that begins in childhood, persists through adulthood, and results in economic calamity in females' senior years. Children who grow up poor are more likely to beget children during their adolescence and, consequently, to remain disadvantaged or near the poverty level as adults. These adults in turn face an elevated risk of becoming indigent elderly. As shown, current rates of child poverty and single motherhood are unusually high. With rising youth unemployment and criminality, as well as poverty as a result of single parenting, one may justifiably expect that, in the next decades, elderly poverty may increase. This means that recent more favorable trends for these age levels may be reversed, particularly among minority groups.

The national costs of child poverty will cumulate throughout the lives of disadvantaged children (Qvortrup, 1994b; Sgritta, 1994). When they reach their senior years, their health status will often be seriously affected by deficits accrued from early childhood on. Medicare costs will consequently increase at a time when the ratio of employed adults to seniors will have dangerously diminished because of low fertility since the 1960s, hence providing fewer governmental sources of transfer payments for the elderly via the taxation system.

Failure to prevent child poverty because of adverse economic, welfare, and educational policies, as well as the failure to curb dangerously high rates of single parenting, will have long-term detrimental consequences socially, culturally, and economically. Current savings in governmental budgets through cost cuttings will merely increase the necessity for larger and costlier outlays for taxpayers ten years hence.

Chapter 8

Visible Minorities, Discrimination, and Segregation

A great deal of poverty in North America, as well as in many large heterogeneous countries of the world, is caused directly or indirectly by past and/or current discriminatory practices and segregation of groups that are racially or ethnically distinct.[1] In some cases, such as that of African Americans as well as Native Americans and Canadians, current patterns of discrimination and segregation related to poverty are historically rooted. In other instances, such as the various Spanish-speaking ethnic groups, there are causal historical factors stemming from conquest in southwestern states, while recent waves of Hispanic immigration have brought with them their own causes and consequences of poverty. In Canada, except for First Nations, and in some areas Francophones (a linguistic and cultural minority), historical factors related to conquest play no role in segregation and poverty. Rather, poverty among Canada's visible minority groups, when it does exist, is related to recent immigration. It also stems from the ill-fated timing of the new residents who arrived during a period when jobs were scarce and government retrenchment placed a premium on reducing expenditures for employment-generating programs.

In this chapter, the situation of black Americans, that of Natives on both sides of the American-Canadian border, and that of various Latino groups in the United States is examined. The contents of this discussion are complemented by other chapters' material on racial/ethnic differences in specific domains. American rather than Canadian data are emphasized, in part because Canada has been oriented toward studying ethnicity rather than race (Krotki and Reid, 1994). This distinction between the two countries in terms of research focus resides in the Canadian reality which, with the exception of a few black settlements,[2] has been largely Native and Caucasian until this century, with recent concerns aimed at language issues rather than racial ones. In addition, Canada has a long established federal policy promoting multiculturalism (O'Neill and Yelaja, 1994).

RECENT ROOTS OF INEQUALITIES

Between 1910 and 1970,[3] 6.5 million African Americans moved from the south to the north. Of these, 5 million moved after 1940, following the introduction of cotton harvesters that could do the work of fifty men (Lemann, 1991). In 1940, 77 percent of all blacks lived in the south but, after 1960, 50 percent remained in the south, and only 25 percent resided in rural areas. The propitious economic conditions in the north helped African Americans secure well-remunerated employment in steel, rubber, and automobile industries. However, these newcomers were less welcome and were more discriminated against than European immigrants (Lieberson, 1980). Race relations deteriorated because whites felt numerically threatened (Boyd, 1996): European immigration was curtailed during the 1920s, but the northern movement of African Americans continued into the 1960s. As Wilson (1987:142) explains, "Eventually, other whites muffled their dislike of Poles and Italians and Jews and directed their antagonism against blacks."

Wilson also points out that these recent arrivals skewed the age distribution of northern blacks toward youth so that, in 1977, the median age for inner-city whites was 30.3 compared with 23.9 for blacks. International research indicates that large cohorts of youth are less easily integrated and controlled, particularly when economic conditions are changing (Braungart and Braungart, 1989). It would therefore be important to analyze the role played by the comparative size of impoverished youth populations in the disorganization of their neighborhoods.

From the 1940s through the 1960s, black professionals and the black middle class resided in the inner cities near blacks who were poor, albeit on different streets. They sustained the communities' basic institutions so that schools, churches, recreational facilities, commercial establishments, and services strongly anchored the neighborhoods. Thus, this mixture of social classes within the African-American community contributed to its viability and social organization. With the advent of the civil rights changes in the 1960s, many middle-class and stably employed working-class blacks chose to relocate and moved out of the inner cities.[4] So did whites. Their departure initiated the demise of many institutions and commercial establishments; it also coincided, in the 1970s, with the beginning of economic changes which brought with them higher rates of unemployment among African Americans, particularly young males.

As shown in previous chapters, this unemployment resulted from the decline or relocation of industries that had until then provided reasonably paid entry-level jobs in all northeastern cities. These changes were also synchronous with the expansion of industries that required more education. Hence, young blacks with low education were de facto barred from the newly created jobs, while at the same time the occupations that they had traditionally held disappeared (Wilson, 1987:40-41). For instance, New York, Chicago, Philadelphia, and Detroit—cities that contained more than 25 percent of the national inner-city poverty in 1982—lost more than 1 million jobs in retail and manufacturing between 1967 and 1976 (Kasarda, 1983).

As inner-city neighborhoods became poorer, the concentration of poverty further isolated the residents from mainstream American life (Green, Tigges, and Brown, 1995). Although the rates of single motherhood had always been higher among blacks than whites, it is only recently that they have become overwhelmingly prevalent (Billingsley, 1992). *Prior to this, two-parent families had been the norm among African Americans* (Gutman, 1976). In 1940, 17.9 percent of black families were headed by a woman, often following widowhood, compared with 10 percent for whites. The black rates crept up to 21.7 percent in 1960, 28 percent in 1970, 40 percent in 1980, and shot up to over 60 percent in 1995 (versus 17 percent for whites). Among *poor* blacks, 30 percent of families were headed by a woman in 1959 compared with 74 percent twenty years later (Wilson, 1987:27).

Such recent changes point to causative factors related to combined developments in culture and economy, rather than history. Moreover, as Wilson (1987) points out, it is paradoxical that rates of black unemployment, single mothering, and poverty concentration went up drastically *after* the civil rights period rather than before.

His reasoning is that past and current racism alone cannot account for the rapid increase in ghettoization, poverty, and disorganization. Rather, inner-city neighborhoods have become poorer because of the *overall* economic and social situation in the United States. In turn, this situation has affected those who were already economically vulnerable because of historic factors as well as segregation-related variables. To pursue this line of reasoning, the economic vulnerability of African Americans and other minorities in inner cities has evolved over the past two decades and *has taken on a life of its own separate from its historical roots.*

Racism still prevails among individuals and in unwitting institutionalized ways rather than in widespread, purposive institutionalized ways. Racism exists in some geographic areas more than others and towards some groups more than others. However, current economic conditions in general and the current life conditions of the inner cities brought by prior racism may have taken precedence over current racism in the perpetuation of poverty in these districts.[5] *Once poverty has reached a critical mass,* criminality, violence, single motherhood, school dropout, and young male idleness independently produce detrimental effects on neighborhoods and adjacent areas as well as on adults as parents, and on youth and children. These effects of poverty in turn create additional consequences in a feedback loop, each set of consequences reinforcing the other and serving to entrench poverty and segregation. When such a critical point is reached, interventions are necessary both at the global economic and social levels and within the communities themselves.

But there are also factors of a noneconomic nature that influence inequality between blacks and whites, such as national and state-level support of civil rights and affirmative action. Based on the 1980 census, the sociologist Beggs (1995) compared racial inequality in earnings and in the type of occupations people held according to states' support of civil rights. He found less inequality between blacks and whites both in earnings and in access to high-skill jobs in national corporations because they are more subject to federal rules, regulations, and legally accepted practices. Corporations located in states actively supporting civil rights and affirmative action also exhibited lower levels of inequality. Therefore, laws, court rulings, and public opinion can be effective in changing economic organizations and discriminatory practices in employment.

RACIAL AND ETHNIC INEQUALITIES AND POVERTY

Blacks accounted for 12.4 percent of the American population in 1992; however, they constituted 29.3 percent of the poor, and 40 percent of the welfare rolls. While Hispanics in general comprised only 8 percent of the total population, they accounted for 17 percent of the welfare recipients. In 1991, there were 17.7 million poor whites, 10.2 million poor blacks, and 6.3 million poor Latinos (Jennings, 1994:55). Thirty-three percent of all black children and 21 percent of Hispanic children were on welfare compared with 6 percent of white children (Besharov, 1996:16). Furthermore, African Americans tend to be poor for longer periods than whites (Levitan, 1990:9). Nearly 40 percent of black children experience *long-term* poverty versus 5 percent of white children (Sawhill, 1992). In an eighteen-year longitudinal study[6] of households headed by black men (generally two-parent families), 56 percent had been poor, compared with nearly 21 percent of families headed by a white male. Nearly one-third of all black households had been poor for more than ten of the eighteen years of the study versus 4.5 percent of white households (Devine and Wright, 1993:107).

In 1991, black and Hispanic households had a median income equal to 59.8 percent and 71.4 percent, respectively, of the white median income.[7] But income itself does not fully capture racial inequities: assets, or net worth, is also a key indicator (Blau and Graham, 1990). In 1991, white households had, on average, a net worth of $44,408; this compares with $5,345 for Hispanics, and $4,604 for blacks (Eller, 1994). Among low-income households, net worth averaged $10,257, $645, and one dollar, respectively, for whites, Hispanics, and blacks. Among the economically secure, net worth averaged $129,394, $67,435, and $54,449, respectively, for whites, Hispanics, and blacks. Therefore, lack of assets among blacks in particular exacerbates their economic situation above and beyond income inequities.[8] A further indicator of disadvantage is that, despite lower household income and assets, black households pool the earnings of more wage earners than do white households (Dressler, 1993).

The gap in poverty between various ethnic groups remains after education is considered. In 1990, households headed by a person with less than eight years of schooling were poor in 23 percent of the cases for whites, 32 percent for Latinos, and 39 percent for blacks (U.S. Bureau of the Census, 1992b). With a high school diploma, the gap diminishes substantially but does not disappear entirely. Thus, more than years of schooling are involved in the explanation of differential poverty rates among the races. Cruz (1992) has pointed out the anomaly of Hispanics of Puerto Rican origins. They have more years of formal education than Mexican Americans, yet the Mexican-American poverty rate is lower than that of Puerto Ricans. This could in part be explained by the fact that many Puerto Ricans live in high-poverty areas, many are black themselves or are so labeled, and thus suffer from the same type of environments with limited opportunities as do other blacks. Puerto Ricans also experience a higher prevalence of single-parent families than Mexican Americans. Moreover, Puerto Rican political powerlessness has a long colonial history. To this are added hardships occasioned by increased poverty in New York City because of the disappearance of jobs in the needle industries that had initially attracted Puerto Rican immigrants to the mainland.

In both countries, certainly the poorest group is constituted by Natives. In Canada, poverty is endemic among the 189,365 First Nations people who live on reserves, where less than one-third of individuals age fifteen and over have at least a ninth-grade education. In fact, nearly 50 percent of Natives over age fifteen, not currently in school, have less than a ninth-grade education and only 6 percent have a high school diploma (Frideres, 1994). The Native unemployment rate in 1991 was well over twice that of the national rate. Furthermore, there are large differences between Natives who reside on reserves and the more numerous nonreserve Natives: 20.8 percent unemployment for Native males nationally versus 33.9 percent on reserves. Female unemployment stood at 17.7 percent versus 25.8 percent on reserves. Looked at from the opposite angle, 72 percent of Native males were employed versus only 54 percent of those on reserves. For Native women, the figures were 57 percent and 38 percent, respectively. The average levels of income reflect this situation both nationally and on reserves:

- average income of Native males: $20,578; on reserves: $12,071 (versus $29,847 for Canadian males in general);
- average income of Native females: $13,489; on reserves: $8,948 (versus $17,751 for Canadian females in general).

If we divide Native income into its constituting sources, two salient observations emerge:

- 78.3 percent of Native income nationally originates from employment earnings versus 59.8 percent on reserves;

- 17.9 percent is from government transfer payments versus 37.8 percent on reserves.

Thus, the educational, employment, and income levels of Natives, particularly Native men, is far below that of the Canadian average. Inequalities are particularly striking for Natives who live on reserves. First Nations females are also disadvantaged compared with other females, but the gap is not as large as the male one because females tend to be disadvantaged compared with males across all ethnic groups, including whites. What is most striking is that at least 20 percent of Native men are socially assisted, and that percentage rises to well over 33 percent on reserves (Statistics Canada, 1995a). It is estimated that *at least 51 percent of all First Nations children live in poverty* (Kitchen et al., 1991:15). In 1987, 3.2 percent of all Status Native children were in foster care compared with 0.8 percent for Canada overall (Assembly of First Nations, 1989).[9]

SEGREGATION

Segregation can take place on several levels; it can also be voluntary or enforced, whether directly or indirectly. The many levels of enforced segregation involve the neighborhood, workplace, and school. The latter has been examined in Chapter 5. In this chapter, the focus is on neighborhood and employment.

As shown in Chapter 4, racial minorities tend to congregate in separate neighborhoods. For blacks, because of historical factors, this means that they live in areas of concentrated poverty to a far greater extent than do whites. For instance, Wilson (1987:58) well illustrated this point when he showed that in five large American cities in 1980, 85 percent of poor blacks lived in extreme poverty areas compared with 30 percent of poor whites. Moreover, the number of disadvantaged individuals residing in segregated poverty areas in the five largest American cities (New York, Chicago, Los Angeles, Philadelphia, and Detroit) increased by 58 percent from 1970 to 1980. This number grew by 70 percent in the high-poverty areas, and by "a whopping 182 percent in the extreme poverty areas" (Wilson, 1987:46).

The environmental contexts of African Americans in such neighborhoods, at all income levels, is far worse than that of whites with comparable incomes (Sampson, 1993). A majority of poor whites live in neighborhoods that provide them with safety and resources, while nearly all poor blacks live in disadvantaged neighborhoods lacking such advantages (Sullivan, 1989b). For whites, the consequences of poverty can often be mitigated by positive community factors,[10] while for blacks, the disadvantages of personal poverty are usually compounded by detrimental neighborhood circumstances.

Therefore, it is practically impossible to compare the effects of poverty on blacks and whites, because more often than not, white poverty is not shackled to a deprived urban area. In this context, black poverty is worse than white poverty, and current black urban poverty is worse than that of the 1950s. Yet studies looking at poverty and family structure as predictors of negative outcomes in children fail to consider the differentiated environment of poor whites and blacks. When this difference is taken into account, one should expect worse outcomes among black children,[11] or among any other similarly segregated minority group, because familial social capital can easily be canceled by the deficits of the surrounding community. More detrimental outcomes should be expected for young black adults, particularly in terms of employment, because of a lack of job opportunities, as well as a lack of role models that could further the acquisition of employment-related skills and contacts among young African Americans (Wacquant, 1995).

As Wilson (1987:57) points out, in neighborhoods with high concentrations of poverty, "the chances are overwhelming that children will seldom interact on a sustained basis with people who are employed or with families that have a steady breadwinner." The net effect is that joblessness, as a way of life, takes on a different social and cultural meaning; even the relationship between schooling and postschool employment takes on a different meaning. Wilson (1987:57) concludes, "The development of cognitive, linguistic, and other educational and job-related skills necessary for the world of work in the mainstream economy is therefore adversely affected." He goes on to state that teachers become frustrated and stop teaching academic skills to the extent that they should: "A vicious cycle is perpetuated through the family, throughout the community, and through the schools."

Segregation by a combination of race *and* social class, as is currently the situation in most inner cities, is a potent source of problems: among others, various institutions that are generally sustained by a solid block of middle-class residents are lacking. In Chicago, for example, from 1970 to 1980, 151,000 blacks moved out of these areas and left behind a higher concentration of poverty. "These data support the hypothesis that the significant increase in the poverty concentration in these overwhelmingly black communities is related to the large out-migration of nonpoor blacks" (Wilson, 1987:50). Whites and more affluent members of other minorities have also left these areas. Absence of institutions and lack of access to facilities lower individuals' positive identification with their neighborhood; this is accompanied by a lack of vested interest in their physical and social surroundings, and a reduced level of control over aberrant behaviors in the neighborhoods.

WORK DISCRIMINATION

People can be discriminated against in the labor force on the basis of their gender, race, marital status, religion, language, sexual orientation, or even political persuasion, in any or all of the following ways: by being denied employment in certain types of occupations, by not being promoted once employed (job ceiling),[12] by receiving lower salaries or, more subtly, by not being invited to participate in social activities among employees—whether to join in for lunch, play golf after work, or attend parties at co-workers' homes.

In the United States, there is, as discussed earlier, an income disparity by race at all educational levels. Schiller (1995:193) reports that college graduates' median earnings for 1992 were as follows: $37,360 for whites, $30,355 for Hispanics, and $29,392 for blacks. Several analyses of this situation conclude that such income differentials are more the result of prior discrimination in the lives of individuals, such as neighborhood and school segregation and consequent lower quality education, rather than current on-the-job discrimination. Prior discrimination would explain two-thirds of income differentials; one-sixth is explained by past employment discrimination, and one-sixth by current discrimination in the labor market (Maxwell, 1994; O'Neill, 1990).

A study of young adults demonstrated that black employees' lower scores on racially nonbiased tests of work-related skills explained most of the wage differential between whites and blacks. These results led Neal and Johnson (1996:870) to suggest that future research should focus on the obstacles faced by black children in acquiring employment-related skills.[13] The research carried out by Farkas (1996) in Dallas indicates a direct relationship between linguistic culture, reading ability, and social class as well as racial membership. The study illustrates the following sequence of failure. Black children are too frequently unable to acquire first-grade reading skills. In turn, this leads to an inability to assimilate classroom material *at each grade level*, unless intervention occurs (Alexander, Entwisle, and Dauber, 1994; Farkas, 1996). The end result is that black children remain behind white children the equivalent of two grades on average throughout their entire school careers. A similar situation exist for Hispanics. Goldenberg (1996:1) points out that "even when instructed in Spanish, Latino students in U.S. schools still tend to do poorly academically."

Thus, black and Hispanic college graduates are far more likely to possess less advanced literacy and mathematical skills than white graduates because of an entire range of previous discriminatory situations in terms of residence, parental education, quality of schools, and lack of role models. Inadequate skills may explain in part lower employment rates, and particularly income and promotion differentials even after a university degree has been secured (Farkas, 1996). Overall, the research suggests that *quality* of education over the life course of youths may determine wage inequalities (Levy and Murnane, 1992). This conclusion is supported by a study that compared blacks and whites who had similar mathematical skills: their employment rates were the same (Rivera-Batiz, 1992).

Current employment discrimination is often a result of the structure as well as functioning of professions and companies. To fill in vacancies, companies tend to rely on their employees who inform friends or neighbors of opportunities. Unfortunately, this practice bypasses minorities who are underrepresented in the workplace. People who live in ghettos or barrios do not benefit from a network of relatives, friends, or neighbors who are employed in a sufficiently wide spectrum of occupations (Fernandez Kelly, 1995) and who could inform them of job openings (Portes, 1995a:12).[14] Because unemployment is far higher among residents of such areas, it deprives them of opportunities to learn of job openings,[15] even when they occur in their district. Kasinitz and Rosenberg (1996:503) point out that "racial discrimination and the stigma attached to the local area may actually discourage neighborhood employers from hiring local residents." It is also likely that, in the east, employers discriminate indirectly against inner-city blacks and Puerto Ricans because these two groups have accumulated less work experience than whites and Mexicans (Tienda and Stier, 1996). Hence, lack of prior jobs creates current unemployment which, in a year down the road, results in a lack of work experience—a vicious cycle (Holzer, 1996).

Two-thirds of Canadian adults who belong to a visible minority group immigrated to Canada after 1970. The age-standardized unemployment rate of visible minorities, other than First Nations, stood at 13 percent compared with 10 percent for the rest of the population in 1995. Latinos had the highest rate at 19 percent, blacks were at 15 percent, Koreans and Filipinos at 8 percent, and Japanese at 6 percent (Kelly, 1995). Minority adults with a university education are less likely to hold either a professional or managerial position: 52 percent compared with 70 percent of other adults. Controlling for age and education, 1991 census figures indicate that Canadian-born visible minority men earn on average 8.2 percent less than whites, but the income differential is nearly twice as large among minority immigrants.[16] The possible reasons for this gap are multiple and include discriminatory practices, however subtle they may be.[17]

Affirmative action programs are necessary, and the American government's retreat from these programs may have contributed to the widening black/white gap in employment and earnings (Cancio, Evans, and Maume, 1996). However, such programs should be restructured so that they benefit minority individuals who are *poor,* and not merely the already existing middle class (Rasberry, 1980). As Wilson (1987:115) puts it, policies of preferential treatment should not be addressed strictly in terms of race and ethnic membership, but also "in terms of the actual disadvantage suffered by minority individuals."

HEALTH DIFFERENTIALS

Because minority groups are poorer than whites, their health status is generally less favorable. Moreover, it is reasonable to assume that segregation and discrimination exert a toll above and beyond poverty (Krieger and Fee, 1994).[18] In the United States, Native Americans, African Americans, and Puerto Ricans suffer from a shocking incidence of illnesses and chronic conditions (Hooyman and Kiyak, 1996). Diabetes, heart problems, hypertension, and infectious diseases are more common among minorities in general, both for adults and children (Lamberty and Garcia-Coll, 1994). However, some Hispanic groups experience a lower mortality rate from chronic illnesses, such as cancer and cardiovascular disease—even lower than that of whites (Sorlie et al., 1993).

African Americans are in poorer health than whites at all age levels, and for both genders;[19] moreover, their health declines more rapidly as they get older (Ferraro and Farmer, 1996). Even the risk of HIV infection is astronomically higher among blacks than whites (Kochanek, Maurer, and Rosenberg, 1994). It is also greater among Hispanics, although not as much as for blacks (Mendoza et al., 1991). Minorities suffer from elevated rates of substance abuse, including glue sniffing among children and adolescents. However, once quality of census tracts are considered, the large difference in the use of substances between blacks and whites becomes practically nonexistent (Lillie-Blanton, Anthony, and Schuster, 1993). This is yet another indicator that black segregation in deprived neighborhoods adds a tremendous burden on this group in terms of an entire range of health-limiting behaviors.

Furthermore, because of poverty and segregation, members of minority groups suffer from inadequate access to and lower utilization of medical resources, particularly those that are strictly preventive, including dental and prenatal care. Recourse to mammograms and influenza vaccines is less prevalent among blacks, even controlling for income.[20] Medicaid and Medicare neither guarantee adequate services nor utilization. In impoverished areas, hospitals are often difficult to reach, overcrowded, and employ fewer experienced specialists. In addition, private medical offices are scarce so that residents do not benefit from the monitoring of one constant health care provider. Although the differences in health care use between black and white Medicare beneficiaries diminish when income is controlled for, it does not entirely disappear (Gornick et al., 1996). Moreover, blacks and lower-income white Medicare beneficiaries "are at a higher risk for procedures associated with less than optimal management of chronic disease" (Gornick et al., 1996:798).

Discrimination in everyday life based on one's race leads many middle-class blacks to go to great lengths to distance themselves from poor blacks, and to emphasize appearances, whether in terms of "status" cars, the "right" clothes, interior decorating, or proper behavior. This stems from the fact that residential segregation often forces middle-class blacks to live in or near areas of concentrated poverty. In contrast, all of their same-class white counterparts can separate themselves from the poor in "suitable" neighborhoods (Massey and Eggers, 1990).

Moreover, a black person is often automatically "tagged" as poor, unskilled, and unimportant—a particularly needling form of inequity for middle-class blacks who have worked hard to achieve their status, yet are deprived of its social benefits, including professional recognition. The stereotypical media case is of the black lawyer who arrives in court with his white assistant—and the assistant is presumed to be the lawyer. Furthermore, law-abiding black males are often "mistaken" for criminals by the police, in addition to arousing fears among all groups of being mugged or attacked on the streets (Cose, 1993). One can reasonably assume that the constant personal devaluation experienced by African Americans, as well as the mechanisms to counteract it (including demarcating themselves from poor blacks), lead to stress, a diminished sense of well-being, and the eventual possibility of a deteriorated health condition (King and Williams, 1995; Williams and Collins, 1995).[21]

REDUCED LIFE EXPECTANCY

In Canada, the infant death rate average for 1986 to 1988 was 7.3 per 1,000 in the general population compared with 13.8 and 16.3, respectively, among Status Indians and Inuits. The mortality of children due to injuries was higher for Natives than for the rest of Canada at all age levels because of poorer physical environments. Among adolescents, elevated rates of injury were related to substance abuse. For children age one through four, the incidence of death-by-injury stood at 15 nationally per 100,000 population, yet was 83 for Status Indians. For Canadian adolescents age fifteen to nineteen, the incidence of death-by-injury stood at 48, yet was a staggering 176 for Status Indians.[22] Among males age ten to nineteen, the suicide rate was 12 for Canadians in general and 54 for Status Indians.

Although there are technical difficulties in classifying infant mortality by race and ethnicity,[23] American minority infants[24] also have more elevated death rates than white infants. In 1984 and 1985, Hahn, Mulinare, and Teutsch (1992) estimated an infant mortality rate of 18.4 per 1,000 births for non-Hispanic blacks and 13.1 for Puerto Ricans, compared with 8.9 for whites. Life expectancy among African Americans is particularly low. Black males' life expectancy in Harlem is inferior to that of males in Bangladesh (McCord and Freeman, 1990). Mortality rates as a result of cancer have increased three times as much as those of whites (Boring, Squires, and Health, 1992). One shocking element of African Americans' relatively low life expectancy resides in high mortality by homicide, particularly among males age fifteen to twenty-four. In 1985, the lifetime chances of being murdered was 1 in 21 for black males, compared with 1 in 131 for white males[25]—and the situation has since deteriorated furthermore among blacks. In 1993, young African-American males were four times more likely than their white counterparts to be attacked by someone using a firearm (Snyder and Sickmund, 1995).

Mexican Americans residing in California present the paradox of discrimination, segregation, poverty despite employment, and yet a favorable health profile. Their employment rate is similar to that of whites, but because of low earnings, their level of poverty at 22 percent is identical to that of Californian blacks. With little access to mainstream health care, Mexican Americans nevertheless enjoy a higher life expectancy and fewer infant deaths than both blacks and whites. These health advantages may stem from the larger percentages of Mexican children living in two-parent families compared with blacks, from extended family and community social support, or from less blatant discrimination against them than against blacks. Moreover, they constitute an upwardly mobile group and form solid population blocks that have immigrated voluntarily and have left worse conditions back home (Ogbu, 1994). Hence, their level of stress may be less acute. Nutritional factors (more fruits, less fat), and lower incidences of sexually-transmitted diseases and smoking may also be involved. All other indicators of health, family structure, welfare, and child foster care are more favorable for Mexican Americans than for blacks. In 1989, weapons-related deaths per 100,000 population stood at 14.9 for Mexican Americans versus 12 for Anglos, 6.5 for Asians, and 41 for blacks (Hayes-Bautista, 1996). However, at least one study has found that Latinos' health outcomes deteriorate with length of stay in the United States (Vega and Amaro, 1994). This may well imply that documented Mexican immigrants are healthier to begin with, but then the adverse conditions of poverty and segregation, including the stressors of inner-city disorganization, exert their toll. With the passage of time, they may become less hopeful and more powerless in terms of achieving the American dream.

CONCLUSION

In this chapter, authors who propose simplistic explanations for the higher rates of black or Latino poverty, or explanations based on character, or defects in intelligence, and so on, have not been cited. Jennings (1994) provides an excellent summary and rebuttal of these various theories that basically blame the victims. We will return to the topic of alleged inferiority in Chapter 11.

While one cannot deny that visible minorities currently experience a higher incidence of many problems than whites, the explanatory perspective of this book is systemic rather than individual or racial. Systemic forces at the economic and sociocultural levels set in motion individual vulnerabilities to poverty. *These systemic forces bear down on minority groups more inexorably than on white groups.* Whites can, as a group, more easily escape from individual causes of poverty because they are not burdened by discrimination and its devastating effects.

Chapter 9

Health and Illness Differentials

Societies exhibit wide differences in the physical health and life expectancy of their citizens. Although much remains to be researched, the following multiple causality chain has emerged. Societies constitute environments—material, social, and cultural—that provide varying degrees of well-being for their members. A modern society that fosters a narrower gap between the rich and the poor, that encourages social connectivity rather than isolation, equality rather than discrimination, and actively creates opportunities for employment, education, and adequate health care increases well-being and consequently reduces disease. Investment in the primary and secondary education of women raises mothers' levels of knowledge and self-empowerment, which then results in lower fertility as well as healthier and better educated children. In addition to reducing poverty, these factors contribute to a decrease in child mortality and an increase in life expectancy for the entire society.[1]

HEALTH AND SOCIOECONOMIC STATUS

But what is of greater pertinence to us in this text are differences among social groups within a society. Throughout the world, a direct link exists between socioeconomic status and health as well as life expectancy. That is, health and life expectancy decrease at each descending rung of the socioeconomic ladder (Evans, 1994; Marmot et al., 1991).[2] Persons with lower education, unskilled jobs, and/or reduced income are more often ill, suffer from a higher incidence of emotional problems and feel less happy, in addition to dying earlier than persons with more formal education, better incomes, and occupations that require advanced skills. This is not simply a matter of differences between the rich and the poor, but of a gradient or a progression from one socioeconomic level to the next (Adler et al., 1994).[3] However, incomes above and beyond a certain threshold bring diminishing returns on health and mortality (McDonough et al., 1997).

Health differentials are more pronounced when a wide gap between the rich and the poor exists (Wilkinson, 1992a). In countries such as Japan and Sweden, and to a far lesser extent Canada, opportunities are maximized across all social classes so that even relatively unskilled workers benefit (Wilkinson, 1992b). When the gap between the rich and the poor is narrower, as is the case in some nations such as Sweden, well-being can spread more effectively throughout all socioeconomic levels (Vagero and Lundberg, 1989). Nevertheless, even working-class Swedes' life expectancy is not as favorable as that of their upper-class and middle-class counterparts, but this class difference is less pronounced in Sweden than it is in other societies (Andersen, 1991).[4]

Overall, both animals[5] and human beings who are at the bottom of a hierarchical order fare less well in terms of health and well-being (Marmot, 1986). People situated at the lowest socioeconomic level suffer more from chronic and **acute illnesses** and also lead a less healthy lifestyle.[6] For instance, Wolfe and Hill (1993:91) report the following profile for adults in the lowest decile of income for 1980-1981: 21 percent had some physical limitation of activity, and 31 percent reported both limitations and poor health. These figures can be contrasted with 5 percent and 7 percent for middle-income earners and 3 percent to 5 percent among the affluent. In the mid-1980s, only 3.8 percent of employed persons age eighteen to forty-four reported fair to poor health while 12 percent of the unemployed did (Ries, 1990). In 1989, individuals with minimal earnings mentioned an average of 12.2 sick days in bed compared with four days among the more affluent groups (Mayer and Jencks, 1993). Nearly 27 percent complained of a chronic limitation compared with only 8 percent for the higher incomes, and 22.6 percent reported fair or poor health versus 3.8 percent among the affluent.

In a similar vein, in 1991, economically secure Canadians were less likely than their low-income counterparts to suffer from chronic conditions, except for hay fever (Statistics Canada, 1994). Thirty-seven percent of the respondents in the lowest income bracket were satisfied with their health versus 57 percent and 65 percent, respectively, at the middle and upper echelons. Economically disadvantaged Canadians consult various physicians more often for health problems, but they make fewer visits to medical professionals in terms of preventive medicine. For instance, only 33 percent of Canadians who were poor had consulted a dentist in 12 months compared with 76 percent of nonpoor Canadians, perhaps in part a result of lacking access to dental plans (Statistics Canada, 1994).

The living conditions of the working poor and of the unemployed poor often preclude adequate nutrition. Overcrowding, noise, and pollution contribute added insults to their systems (Stokols, 1992; Whitehead, 1990). Low self-esteem, feelings of powerlessness, and social isolation follow. These constitute both **indicators** and causes of a lack of well-being. This absence of well-being in turn burdens the immune system so that individuals under economic and social duress more easily fall prey to illnesses and die younger (Blackburn, 1991). Disadvantaged living conditions may explain why respiratory infections in day-care infants compared with home-care infants may be less frequent among lower SES families but more frequent within those at a higher SES level (Margolis et al., 1992). On average, low-income families provide a less healthy environment for infants than qualified day care does. In contrast, high-income families provide a healthier environment than day care, especially in terms of preventing contagious respiratory infections.

Rural areas experience more illness than metropolitan areas because their poverty and unemployment rates are higher,[7] group health insurance is less available, and medical facilities are more distant geographically (Straub and Walzer, 1992; Frenzen, 1993). Therefore, as in the case of social class, a socioeconomic hierarchy by the location of residence exists that correlates with health status.

LIFE EXPECTANCY

The Differentials

Life expectancy at birth represents the average number of years that a cohort of people born at a given point in time are expected to live. Because **morbidity** is related to mortality, it is not surprising that a direct correlation between life expectancy and SES exists (Pappas et al., 1993). The Black Report (Townsend and Davidson, 1990) documented how mortality in Great Britain occurs earlier in the lower occupational class than in all other classes. This differential holds true for all ages, for both males and females, and for most causes of death (Whitehead, 1990). Furthermore, *the longer individuals suffer from a disadvantage income,* the higher their mortality rate in the 45- to-65 age bracket (McDonough et al., 1997). Interestingly enough, the authors of the Black Report also discovered that homeowners experienced a lower death rate than renters, and this was true at all occupational levels.

Basically, as a society's standards of living improve and as they spread to the entire population via the trickle-down effect or through direct policies targeting the disadvantaged, as has been the case in Cuba, the life expectancy of the poor rises, but not to the level of the more affluent classes. The difference in average life span between those at the top and the bottom of the hierarchy may even increase temporarily as the poor adopt a "luxury" diet too rich in fat or begin to smoke at a time when the more advantaged groups have largely abandoned these health risks (Marmot, 1986).

Once people suffer from a disease such as cancer, chances of survival are more favorable in the higher SES strata[8]—even when adequate medical attention is provided (Kogevinas et al., 1991). It may well be that the general health of cancer patients who are poor undermines their recovery. Moreover, individuals who are beset by money problems may be unable to muster the mental energy necessary to combat deadly diseases (Karasek and Theorell, 1990). These observations illustrate the inability of advanced medical care to counteract health deficits accrued over a long period, a point to which this discussion will soon return (Power et al., 1990).

As indicated in a previous chapter, minority individuals are doubly disadvantaged. They are more frequently poor and socially devalued, and consequently die younger than whites. African Americans' death rates as a result of heart disease, cancer, and strokes are higher by 5 percent, 17 percent, and 24 percent, respectively, than those of whites (National Council for Health Statistics, 1992). Minority individuals segregated in impoverished neighborhoods may be placed at further risk because of the stressors inherent to the environment, independently of their own financial means (Krieger, 1991).[9] For their part, Native Americans and Canadians are the least healthy group, not only because of poverty, substandard housing, and discrimination, but also because their communities are often geographically isolated and devoid of rudimentary medical care (Barresi and Stull, 1993). Hopelessness pervades Native villages. In 1991, the suicide rate for Canada as a whole was 11 per 100,000 population compared with 22 for Natives.[10] Their life expectancy is furthermore reduced by alcoholism and traffic accidents among their younger cohorts, and by a higher prevalence of all diseases in middle and old age (Rhoades, 1990; Kramer, 1992).

Myths About Life Expectancy

As standards of living are raised and as poverty diminishes, life expectancy rises, at times quite dramatically so. In industrial nations, life expectancy has increased by 6.0 years for men and 8.5 years for women since 1950 (Hooyman and Kiyak, 1996:25). Life expectancy is considered one of the key indicators of the level of economic and social development as well as the quality of life of nations. However, it is a concept that is frequently misunderstood.

For instance, contrary to what is often believed, when the life expectancy of a country such as Sierra Leone in Africa is below forty-five years, as was the case in most Western nations a century ago, this does not mean that there are very few elderly persons. It is not the lack of elderly persons but widespread infant and child mortality that has been the main factor reducing life expectancy in most societies of the world and in Western societies until World War II. When 30 percent to 50 percent of a country's children die before the age of five or even one, this mortality reduces the *average* age at time of death for the entire society. Once child mortality is virtually eradicated and there are no murderous wars, life expectancy shoots up dramatically. At the same time, children who would have died in earlier decades now have the opportunity to live into old age; later on, they raise the number of seniors in the population.

Per 1,000 population, Sweden, Japan, and Canada have the lowest infant mortality in the world, at 4, 5, and 6.8, respectively (in 1991).[11] In contrast, at 9.2, the United States has one of the highest rates in the Western world, in part because of a wide gap between the rich and the poor, as well as between whites and blacks. In comparison, less economically developed countries such as Greece, Portugal, and Mexico show rates of 10, 10.8, and 37, respectively, and the poorest nations' rates are at 100 or over.[12] Within Canada and the United States, there are wide differences in infant mortality depending on a group's economic situation (Clarke, 1996:141). For instance, the incidence of infant deaths for Canadian indigenous people in 1991 was approximately 12.5, or nearly double that of the general population (Health and Welfare Canada, 1992:29). Moreover, rural infant mortality is higher, particularly among LBW babies (Clarke, Farmer, and Miller, 1994).[13]

However, in Western societies, infant mortality has a minimal impact on life expectancy. Instead, what counts are other problems that develop later in life, such as cardiac disease (Fuchs, 1992). Indeed, reduced fertility and infant mortality in Western countries mean that a further reduction of infant mortality would affect overall life expectancy only minimally. But targeting smoking, diets saturated with fat, and drug and alcohol abuse would raise the life expectancy of Western nations by perhaps two to four additional years. For minority groups, a combined focus on improving prenatal and neonatal care, on reducing suicides among First Nations' youth, and decreasing heart disease and diabetes among blacks would reduce these groups' disadvantage in terms of their earlier mortality. But these changes can result only from an improvement in the afflicted individuals' socioeconomic conditions, which leads us to the second misconception concerning the sources of a lengthy life expectancy in modern times.

It resides in the myth that progress in medicine[14] is the key reason why child mortality has decreased, why fewer women are dying in childbirth, and consequently why life expectancy shot up this century. Actually, the reasons for an improvement in life expectancy rest first of all in societies' investments in the general health of their citizens by building sewers and water supply facilities, reducing overcrowding when it exists, providing food, and educating women (Blumberg, 1995; Bunker, Frazier, and Mosteller, 1995). Better sanitary, nutritional, and educational conditions eradicate most of the sources of early mortality, even though citizens may never see a medical doctor. Once these sanitary conditions are in place, a further reduction in mortality takes effect, this time with the help of medical technology, when vaccinations and antibiotics become available. After these basic needs are met, added medical technology contributes only marginally to the overall improvement in life expectancy. In fact, the life span or length of time that human beings can live has not increased dramatically in modern industrialized nations, and is not expected to do so for a long time, as it is genetically set.

EXPLANATION FOR DIFFERENTIALS

How can we explain class differences in disease and life expectancy? Particularly, how can we explain the negative health of the poor? Although reduced access to medical care and less qualified medical services are important elements when serious illnesses are involved among the poor, stressors and disadvantaged lifestyles are more salient contributors. These even undermine the efforts of the medical system in trying to cure serious illnesses (Marmot, Bobak, and Davey Smith, 1995). Physiological, psychological, and behavioral processes are at work. To begin with, individuals who live in poverty encounter more numerous biological risks,[15] such as malnutrition, pollution, and accidents caused by degraded housing, not to omit prenatal deprivation. Second, on average, the immune capacity diminishes when animals and human beings lead a stressful life. They catch many of the contagious illnesses they are exposed to, and once ill, have more difficulty recovering; they are also more likely to die, particularly when they are elderly.

Stressful life events, such as loss of a job or daily duress, have been correlated with higher incidences of various illnesses and diseases.[16] In turn, negative life events and daily stressors are more frequently encountered as we descend the SES ladder, and at the same time, social support becomes more inadequate as a buffer against increased environmental duress. Stressors that are prominent among poverty-stricken people include financial insecurity, unemployment,[17] consequent domestic problems, malnutrition, noisy and overcrowded housing, unsafe neighborhoods, and fear of victimization. To this list can be added the availability of illegal drugs, health-risk behaviors such as smoking, and accidents caused by dilapidated housing. Early pregnancies that, because of a lack of prenatal care, result in LBW infants are also a cause of health differentials because these babies are more at risk of being sickly and dying. Moreover, there are indications that lower-SES persons are more adversely affected than are more affluent persons by similar negative events (McLeod and Kessler, 1990). This lack of resilience probably stems from the accumulation of *additional* stressors already evident in their lives, and by the feelings of powerlessness that may accompany them.

Downward social mobility as a result of illness contributes only minimally to class differences in health (Power et al., 1990). While a certain number of people descend into poverty because of illness, emotional problems, disabilities, or a generally deficient health, far more succumb to illness as a result of poverty (Black, 1992). Once poor *and* ill, it becomes more difficult to leave the ranks of the disadvantaged. The chronically poor are the most bereft at the personal level. They benefit from fewer personal resources such as marketable skills, health, and social support—in other words, their social and human capital is not adequate (Coleman, 1990). Thus powerless, they are more vulnerable to succumb to stressors (Hamilton et al., 1990), and once ill their situation often becomes hopeless.

ILLNESS-RELATED PROBLEMS

Individuals who feel in control of their lives may be better able to impact positively on their health (Rodin, 1986). Conversely, persons who are less in control of their destiny are more likely to engage in risky behaviors such as smoking,[18] heavy drinking, and early pregnancies. These behaviors affect their health negatively, either in the short or long run, and some, such as smoking, can also lead to death via cancer and coronary disease. Beginning to smoke is inversely related to SES and stopping is positively related to SES (Pugh et al., 1991). Lower SES persons are less likely to be physically active during their leisure time, and are more frequently obese.[19] As SES declines, health-enhancing behaviors decrease, even among adolescents (Lowry et al., 1996), and risk-enhancing activities increase. Low-income persons are also less knowledgeable in matters of health. For instance, they are less aware of the causes of heart problems or methods to prevent the spread of sexually-transmitted infections (Roberge, Berthelot, and Wolfson, 1995). Therefore, the impoverished segment of the population is more at risk for experiencing a low level of health, a high incidence of illness, and a shorter life.

Habitual, heavy drinking is more common among the lowest income group than among other groups in society (Fitzgerald and Zucker, 1995). It is also more frequent among the most disadvantaged minority group—Natives (Aday, 1993). In Canada, in 1993, 18 percent of young people age fifteen to twenty-four who were poor were experiencing alcohol-related problems, compared with 8 percent to 10 percent in each of the other four income brackets (Statistics Canada, 1995b). In that study, youths who were heavy drinkers were more likely than any other age group to report that their alcohol consumption resulted in complications in terms of finances, health, family relationships, and work. This means that alcohol-related difficulties are more common among youths, particularly males, who are *already* burdened by economic disadvantages. Furthermore, two-thirds of heavy drinkers had experienced problems resulting from other individuals' drinking, probably because heavy drinkers gravitate toward persons with similar proclivities. Low income is implicated in the etiology of heavy drinking, and a circular process takes place between heavy drinking and poverty. Alcoholism becomes financially and socially costly to already-poor persons, and prevents them from leaving their disadvantaged situation.

Low birth weight (LBW) is another health risk more frequently encountered among the disadvantaged than the affluent, particularly among the poor who have no health insurance for prenatal care (Braveman et al., 1989). In turn, LBW is related to a host of vulnerabilities in the affected infants, including illness, learning disabilities, motor coordination deficits, and mortality (Hack et al., 1991; Middle et al., 1996). The Institute of Medicine (1985) has documented that prenatal care is effective in reducing LBW, whatever its source. Unfortunately, women, and especially pregnant adolescents, who live in poor neighborhoods do not seek prenatal care regularly. This is particularly so early on in the pregnancy at a time when the fetus is most vulnerable. In Canada, in 1990, women over forty-five years and those younger than twenty years had the highest incidence of LBW babies: 10.1 and 6.7 respectively. In both cases this represents a sharp drop since 1985, despite the fact that multiple births have substantially increased and nearly always result in LBW infants.[20] LBW is a costly social problem in terms of medical expenditures alone. It is also one where advances in medical technology—sophisticated intensive-care neonatal units—have obviously been beneficial (Office of Technology Assessment, 1987).

PSYCHIATRIC PROBLEMS

Psychiatric problems[21] are disproportionately represented among the poor (Robins and Regier, 1991),[22] the unemployed, and particularly among the homeless. Disadvantaged mothers are especially prone to depression (Bassuk et al., 1996; Coiro, 1997). Poverty is a "pathway to depression" among women (McGrath et al., 1990). In general, a higher incidence of depression occurs as we descend the social ladder. As is the case for physical health and life expectancy, there is an inverse correlation between social class and psychiatric problems as well as cognitive deficits.[23] This gradient applies to both blacks and whites (Williams and Collins, 1995). In 1991, while only 6 percent of affluent Canadians reported an emotional disorder, 17 percent of those in the lowest income category did (Statistics Canada,1994:28). A proportion of persons with **schizophrenia** drift downward in social status and income; in contrast, simple or **unipolar depression** is more likely to be triggered by already existing economic hardships.[24]

An added complication is that the poor who are mentally ill are far more vulnerable to physical diseases, as well as to alcoholism and addictions, than the poor who are mentally robust. The emotionally disturbed possess less adequate coping skills, their levels of stress and anxiety overwhelm them, and they benefit from fewer personal and social resources. Because of the nature of their illness, they often unwittingly create additional complications in their lives and in the lives of those with whom they live (Lefley, 1989). They are rarely employed continuously and are the least likely of all groups to reach for social assistance and medical help. In the past, severely disturbed individuals were institutionalized and were at least sheltered, fed, and given their medications regularly. Now, over two decades after deinstitutionalization, because of a lack of community resources, these individuals are often homeless and unreachable in terms of sustained treatment that could alleviate their symptoms.

Many persons with chronic mental illnesses are never poor because their spouses or relatives shelter them or care for them. As a result, their life opportunities are maximized compared with those of other psychiatrically ill individuals. They may benefit from competent psychiatric care which reduces their symptoms, they may be employed, and they are in better physical health. Individuals who remain dependent and semisheltered rarely reproduce themselves, reducing the chance of creating a permanent intergenerational underclass of psychiatric patients.

This does not imply, however, that people with serious psychiatric disorders do not have children.[25] Among males, schizophrenia and its precursors tend to appear quite early in life (Burke et al., 1990). This early age of dysfunctionality only infrequently allows them to marry and have children (Saugstad, 1989). However, a majority of women with schizophrenia marry, although less frequently so than other women.[26] Currently, women who suffer from one of the serious mental illnesses are nearly as likely to have children as other women,[27] and as many as 60 percent of their pregnancies may be unplanned (Forcier, 1990).

For their part, adolescents who suffer from emotional problems may be more likely to marry than other teenagers (Forthofer et al., 1996), perhaps to escape from stressful home situations (Brown and Harris, 1993). Such premature marriages are predictors of divorce and future poverty. Among adults, the reverse occurs: the mentally ill are less likely to marry (Forthofer et al., 1996). Therefore, single mothers who suffer from serious emotional problems may be at a particularly elevated risk of not marrying, and thus of being unable to exit poverty via marriage. In such families, poverty and emotional problems reinforce each other. Furthermore, both for adolescents living in divorced single-parent families (Aseltine, 1996) and for divorced adults, heightened vulnerability to economic stressors constitutes a major linkage between divorce and depression (Aseltine and Kessler, 1993).

Loss of income, income instability, and unemployment create distress (McLoyd and Wilson, 1991). The constant threat of being unable to make ends meet erodes well-being and contributes to depression. Suicide rates are particularly elevated among unemployed men. Significant improvements in mental health accompany a return to work.[28] In an interesting ethnography of teen mothers, Horowitz (1995) illustrates the extent to which many low-income people, especially those on welfare, try to hide their poverty in order to maintain their pride. Although this was not the object of her study, one nevertheless can ask what effect such face-saving coping mechanisms exert both on the depletion of much needed financial resources and on mental health.

Bradburn's (1969) widely used Affect Balance Scale assesses both positive and negative feelings related to well-being or lack thereof (five questions for each) With this instrument, individuals can be categorized depending not only on their positive and negative affect score but on the balance between the two: those who are more negative than positive, for example, as well as those who are predominantly positive or negative. A 1991 study, based on such self-reports, discovered that only 10 percent of Canadians in the poorest group scored predominantly on the positive side of affect compared with 25 percent among the affluent group (Statistics Canada, 1994). Twenty-two percent of unemployed persons looking for work had a predominantly negative score, and 35 percent of males who had been unemployed for six months or more were predominantly negative (Health Canada, 1994:15).

When contrasting occupational categories, 23 percent of those in professional and important managerial occupations had a very positive balance score, compared with 14 percent of semiskilled workers. Levels of education follow a similar pattern of increased well-being for respondents with more advanced educational credentials. Moreover, 31 percent of women and 24 percent of men who rated life as being stressful had a negative score. The statistical analysis was unfortunately not **multivariate** so that we do not know where these unhappy persons were located in the class system nor whether they were predominantly poor.

COGNITIVE PROBLEMS

Cognitive problems refer here to deficient IQ scores. Low or subnormal IQ can be genetically determined. It can also result from a mother's malnutrition, smoking, or alcohol or drug use during pregnancy. However, one has to be careful lest one reaches hasty conclusions. Indeed, most alcoholic and drug-addicted mothers are also severely malnourished, may be anemic, and suffer from other health problems. Any or all of these problems together may be causally linked to cognitive deficits in children (McCormack, 1997).[29] A child's malnutrition, lack of stimulation, and general neglect in its first two or three years of life are additional sources of intellectual deficiencies. Lower IQ scores occur disproportionately among the poor. Culturally or environmentally caused retardation, as opposed to a hereditary condition, is the type of mental delay that is probably most common in pockets of poverty and segregation.

Undoubtedly, a genetically rooted low IQ may cause a person's downward mobility compared with his or her more intelligent relatives.[30] But a less than average IQ, whatever its origins, need not lead to poverty, and there are great variations in terms of socioeconomic outcomes. Many brilliant individuals do not get far in life and some may even drift into poverty because of other frailties or because of environmental factors, such as the availability of drugs in their milieu. In contrast, many people who are not particularly endowed intellectually are well off. Family and social resources, as well as other personal resources, such as motivation, social skills, and various abilities, enter the equation and can lead to success. Furthermore, some high-paying occupations do not require a great deal of intellectual ability. The worlds of entertainment and sports come readily to mind.

Although individuals with subnormal IQ may not have children due to a lack of attractiveness as companions, when the afflicted person is otherwise attractive or sociable but unable to practice birth control, children likely result. These children who may be genetically at risk may also be environmentally deprived because of inadequate parenting. Thus, the detrimental effect of the environment compounds that of genes so that poverty may be transmitted through three or four generations. And the same danger of transmission of poverty arises on a larger scale from mental retardation caused strictly by cultural and social deprivation. In the latter case, however, genetic risk does not exist, and some or all of the affected person's offspring may rise out of poverty eventually, especially if there are positive elements in their environment, such as early interventions, that can remedy the deprived home situation.

These discussions lead to the drift hypothesis: the conclusion that inadequate mental abilities cause downward mobility, often into

poverty, which may last over several generations. These cases probably constitute only a small segment of poor people. As will be
discussed in the next chapter, inadequate intellectual skills are generally the product of poverty rather than its cause. Poverty is the
reason why deficient IQs are disproportionately located at the bottom of the social class system.

IS MORE MEDICAL CARE THE SOLUTION?

We have already referred to the widespread myth that medical
care is the key ingredient in a society's health status. We have also
discussed the large differences that exist in morbidity and mortality
between the social classes. Undoubtedly, medical care *is* important,
especially, as discussed earlier, for infants,[31] mothers, and seniors.
Lack of medical attention among these groups results in serious
consequences and added costs. But other conditions in society contribute far more to citizens' illnesses, and are subsumed under the
differentials that exist between the rich and the poor (Scheper-
Hughes, 1992). Substandard housing, pollution, malnutrition,
undereducation, unemployment, and discrimination in the workplace and in daily living cannot be compensated for by access to
physicians.

Therefore, while poverty prevents access to health care, particularly in the United States, it is doubtful that, in the larger scheme of
things, better medical technologies and availability of more physicians would completely eliminate class and racial discrepancies in
disease and life expectancy (Williams, 1990). Neither does it eliminate differences between nations at a same technological level (Marmot and Davey Smith, 1989). Beliefs to the contrary are deeply
ingrained because they are supported by a powerful group of professionals and associated industries, such as pharmaceutical companies, and are repeated in the media (Lomas and Contandriopoulos,
1994). All of these industries parrot the same message in favor of
the role of physicians, medication, and medical technology.
Together, they form a powerful lobby.

Health care costs have skyrocketed, both in Canada and the
United States, even though the two systems are totally different. Yet,
medical professionals raise a terrible clamor, invoking the specter of

death, when governments attempt to rein in out-of-control costs. In Canada, whenever their incomes are not raised as frequently as desired, physicians enact a variety of service withdrawals, while others threaten to move to the United States. Their actions are nobly rationalized at press conferences under the guise of "protecting the deteriorating quality of health care." They do not, however, complain much when nurses lose their positions or, better yet, when hospital beds are cut! In 1996, the Canadian Medical Association came near to proposing a two-tiered medical system that would have ensured that *their* interests were well served, but would in fact have destroyed the universality of health care, and thus further diminished the life circumstances of the poor. In the United States, overly-paid managed care executives are at the forefront of the transformation of medicine into gigantic megaprofit corporations. This restructuring may well occur at the expense of quality care and taxpayers, and particularly to the detriment of the poor.

Evans and Stoddart (1994:55) convincingly argue that, after a certain point, *more* medical care and technology have diminishing returns for the population as a whole, and perhaps, we might add, the poor in particular: "A society that spends so much on health [medical] care that it cannot or will not spend adequately on other health-enhancing activities may actually be reducing the health of its population." *Excessive health care costs, created by technological expansion and the proliferation of highly-paid medical experts, divert funds.* These funds could be allocated toward income supplements for the working poor and the indigent elderly, expanded day care and nutrition programs for disadvantaged children, supplementary nutrition for pregnant women, building affordable housing, and providing more personal health services in the guise of nurse practitioners.

Medical care per se achieves none of these goals. In fact, after a certain point, it obstructs these goals and contributes to class differences. What prevents politicians and citizens alike from fully appreciating this reality is that, in the short run, it is obvious to everyone who consults a physician that such an intervention generally improves various acute illnesses. Of course, in this discussion, we are not talking of eliminating these consultations. But what is less obvious and takes longer to appear in vital statistics—often decades—is that balanced nutrition, low levels of stress, stable employment, decent income, and adequate housing create health, reduce the incidence of disease, and raise life expectancy.[32] They also reduce the necessity for frequent visits to physicians.

In fact, early *quality* day care for disadvantaged children has the following results, most of which are long term, *and unfortunately are not immediately visible, thus not influential in voting booths.* Early quality day care raises a mother's ability to be employed, hence to alleviate her poverty. It also enhances a child's capability to learn, to adapt well in school, and to remain in school longer, thus steering that child away from poverty in his or her own adult life (Martin, Ramey, and Ramey, 1990). In turn, the nutritional benefits that day care provides to disadvantaged children constitutes a physiological advantage that may carry beneficial consequences into their old age, and could reduce the level of elderly disability and medical costs in subsequent decades (Hertzman, Frank, and Evans, 1994). "Insults to health may accumulate over the entire life span" and bring a general susceptibility to disease among persons who have spent part of their existence in poverty (Marmot, Bobak, and Davey Smith, 1995:201).[33] Unfortunately, political decisions generally aim at short-term expedients and results which leave the next generations more vulnerable and in no better health (Brenner, 1995).

CONCLUSION

Ill health occurs as a function of genetic predispositions, of socioeconomic factors, and other environmental conditions. Currently, society is willing to pay a hefty price to cure disease after it has occurred. It would be more humane and less expensive to invest in its prevention. Not all diseases, particularly those where there is a genetic factor, can be prevented, but most diseases and illnesses result more from how one lives than from what genes one inherits. And how one lives is in most part determined by one's position in society,[34] rather than by medical sophistication. The latter can only alleviate at great cost what poverty creates.

Chapter 10

Poverty and Delinquency

In this chapter, delinquency is considered a result of poverty, although it can also be a source of poverty. At the individual level, delinquency, and later on adult criminality, can lead to a life of disadvantage. When poverty results from delinquency, it often follows poverty that began within the individual's family of origin. When an already impoverished adolescent breaks the law, conviction and especially incarceration may deepen the youth's detrimental economic situation and that of his family.

The focus of this chapter is on juvenile delinquency rather than on adult criminality. It is not, however, the purpose here to present an in-depth discussion of all the theories and data explaining delinquency. Rather, we review the main ones and emphasize antecedents that are related, directly or indirectly, to poverty. This chapter largely leaves aside juvenile delinquency encountered among the nonpoor.

ASPECTS OF DELINQUENCY

Delinquency officially involves an arrest and therefore an awareness on the part of authorities that a minor has committed a crime. Researchers have access to police statistics for arrests, and these come closer to estimating actual levels of delinquency than court statistics for convictions. More complete and detailed data are gathered with self-reports of delinquency. This involves researchers distributing questionnaires to adolescents in school, for instance. These questionnaires request background information, and ask the youths to place check marks alongside a list of infractions to indicate which they have committed. This method is also used in research with delinquents who have been arrested to determine what other transgressions they have perpetrated in addition to those that are officially known.

After decades of upward trends, neither criminality nor apprehended delinquency has increased in the past few years. In fact, U.S. criminality rates went down in 1996 and 1997, in great part because of the spectacular decrease in New York City. But *violent* delinquency has continued to rise overall (Wethington, 1996), and begins at younger ages than in previous decades. One now routinely hears of boys age six to ten who participate in brutal acts and who carry firearms. The phenomenon of violent youth gangs is especially destructive in American inner cities, creating victims beyond those who are directly hurt or even killed. As delinquency has become more lethal, it has attracted more media attention and spread feelings of fear and insecurity in the population at large—particularly among disadvantaged but law-abiding children who frequently worry about their own safety at school or in their neighborhoods (Sheley and Wright, 1995).

Offending peaks around age seventeen (Wolfgang, Thornberry, and Figlio, 1987). "By the early twenties, the number of active offenders decreases by over 50 percent; by age 28, almost 85 percent of former delinquents desist from offending" (Moffitt, 1994:4). Most delinquents are arrested only once, unless they use drugs regularly, and commit crimes to support their habit. Although offenders who are repeatedly apprehended constitute only a minority of all delinquents, they commit perhaps as many as 60 percent of all recorded offenses, and their crimes tend to be more serious (Farrington, 1987). There is a hard core of juvenile delinquents in our social landscape, and these youngsters usually originate from deprived neighborhoods or families.

PERSONAL PATHWAYS TO DELINQUENCY

There are at least two developmental pathways to delinquency. Delinquents who initiate destructive behaviors very young and graduate to more serious and violent crimes are, on average, different from delinquents who start in mid- to late adolescence (Farrington et al., 1988) This dichotomy is referred to as early-onset versus late-onset delinquency (Simons et al., 1994). Early-onset delinquents generally exhibit more behavioral problems, are diagnosed more frequently with personality disorders, commit a majority of the serious crimes reported, and may come from a dysfunctional or pathological family. Such delinquency is usually accompanied and preceded by conduct disorders[1] that begin early in life.[2] The more antisocial the child is at an early age, the more persistent the problem.

This type of delinquency is also labeled life-course-persistent (Moffitt, 1994). This small group of males[3] "display high rates of antisocial behavior across time and in diverse situations. The professional nomenclature may change, but the faces remain the same as they drift through successive systems aimed at curbing their deviance; schools, juvenile-justice programs, psychiatric-treatment centers, and prisons. The topography of their behavior may change with changing opportunities, but the underlying disposition persists throughout the life course" (Moffitt, 1994:11). These individuals are very costly to society, victimize many, and contribute to the intergenerational transmission of criminality and poverty in their families.

Early-onset delinquency frequently but not unavoidably leads to adult criminality and other deviances if no intervention occurs, especially when the neighborhood is criminogenic (Le Blanc and Fréchette, 1989). It is also from this group of early-onset delinquents that adult psychopathic criminals emerge (Lynam, 1996). Moreover, very few cases of adult antisocial personality emerge that have not been preceded by conduct disorders in childhood (Robins, 1978; White et al., 1990). Although late-onset delinquents include some youngsters who are similar to the aforementioned ones, in general they tend to come from adequate families and to function better in many respects. They are less persistently antisocial, and do not as a rule become recidivists or adult criminals (Moffitt et al., 1996).

For their part, Nagin and Land (1993) divide adolescent offenders into three categories: those who are not convicted beyond late adolescence ("adolescence-limited delinquency"), those who are "low-level chronic" offenders, and those labeled "high-level chronic" offenders. Nagin, Farrington, and Moffitt (1995) pursued this typology and found that, by age thirty-two, the two types of chronic and repeatedly arrested offenders lived in poorer neighborhoods and material conditions than the delinquents whose convictions ended with adolescence. Moreover, compared with the other groups, high-level chronic offenders admitted to more criminality from ages fourteen through thirty-two that had not come to the attention of the authorities. Half of them reported having hit their wives by age thirty-two (Farrington and West, 1990).

In contrast, the adolescence-limited offenders began their delinquency two years older, on average, than the other two categories, and committed far fewer illegal acts. They had, by definition, no convictions after twenty-one, and by age thirty-two, their employment pattern was undistinguishable from that of nondelinquents. However, according to their self-reports, many continued to engage in petty property crime, particularly theft; "they also continued to use illicit drugs, drink heavily, and get into fights" (Nagin, Farrington, and Moffitt, 1995:128). These authors conclude that those adolescence-limited offenders who pursued criminality were better able than the other two types of offenders to restrict themselves to forms of deviant activities that did not lead to arrest, and consequently did not harm their family relationships or necessarily result in poverty.

CAUSES OF DELINQUENCY

The research on the etiology of delinquency has become quite sophisticated in the past two decades, with a diverse and complementary array of theories.[4] The etiological models not only differentiate between personal pathways to delinquency but they implicate a multitude of causal variables. The familial environment continues to be emphasized with a focus on parents' characteristics—including their mental states, personalities, disciplinary practices, and criminality. Other theories emphasize peers, gangs, siblings, opportunities, motivation, beliefs, school performance, maltreatment, and personality. An occasional exploration of genetics and neurology also appears in the literature (Moffitt, 1994),[5] and is generally related to the study of aggressiveness (Miles and Carey, 1997). These explanatory models have been tested mainly on males.

Delinquents who commit serious offenses and are arrested seem to originate predominantly from a background that combines multiple risk factors: family poverty, deprived neighborhood, questionable peers, unstable parenting and inadequate supervision, as well as childhood behavioral problems (Farrington, 1991b). A disproportionate number of delinquents belong to single-parent families, and this finding holds for both black and white, Canadian, American, and British delinquents (see review by Sampson, 1993).[6] Moreover, serious juvenile delinquency originates far more from disadvantaged families, and this finding has also been replicated in several countries.[7]

One familial factor that researchers emphasize is parental monitoring. Poorly supervised youngsters are at greater risk for delinquency, as well as for other problems such as illicit drug use, early sexual involvement, and school underachievement (Patterson, Reid, and Dishion, 1992). However, parental supervision may be more important in early adolescence, while peers may be more influential among older teenagers (Aseltine, 1995). Inadequate supervision, especially at younger ages, occurs more frequently in homes rife with marital conflict, or with only one parent, and/or where one or both parents are emotionally disturbed, use drugs, or have committed crimes. In such families, a detrimental parent-child relationship, poor supervision, and parental example may be proximal causes of delinquency. The report by the Panel on High-Risk Youth (1993:50) states that, "a major part of the explanation for this high rate of adolescent deviance in single-parent families is their propensity to permit adolescents to have early control over their own behavior."

Although proper parental supervision is emphasized as a preventative element, we surmise that there are other salutary processes at work in families that monitor their children. Specifically these families are probably better organized, are headed by stable parents, have children with easier temperaments, and spend more time interacting prosocially than other families, whether single- or two-parent families. Among blacks, however, high parental education and stable two-parent families are less predictive of positive adolescent behaviors and outcomes than among whites. This race differential stems from the fact that African Americans (and other minorities, including Hispanics) live in disadvantaged and disorganized neighborhoods that can outweigh the benefits of parental influence and family structure (Dornbusch and Ritter, 1991).

In an article reporting that Toronto adolescents who are homeless for over a year resort to criminality more than those whose homelessness is transient, McCarthy and Hagan (1991) expose unusually high rates of deviant and delinquent activities that occurred among these youngsters *while they were still at home*, that is, before they became homeless, which for many presumably resulted from running away. While living with their families, over one-third had already "beaten up" someone; 21 percent had stolen from cars; and over one-fourth had taken their parents' cars without permission, had vandalized property, had stolen after a breaking and entering, had used hallucinogens, and had trafficked in drugs—to name only a few of the activities which distinguished this group from transient homeless adolescents. These figures suggest that adolescents leave home prematurely because they do not get along with their parents. This difficult family situation is partly related to their delinquent activities as well as their running away. However, the possibility also exists that some of these adolescents are very difficult and cause discord between themselves and their well-meaning parents (Ambert, 1992 and 1997b). Whatever the etiology, this study is a good example of the fact that delinquency and a deviant lifestyle during adolescence can lead to poverty and homelessness, although a percentage of these youngsters originate from poor homes.

POVERTY AND DELINQUENCY

Poverty and Social Control

In disrupted neighborhoods with a high level of criminality, a substantial transient population, concentration of poverty, and gang supremacy, children do not need a dysfunctional family to become antisocial and delinquent (Sampson, 1993). However, a single parent may have more difficulty than two parents to outweigh the strength of the negative environmental forces (Wilson, 1987).[8] We know that communities that are able to control teenage groups, especially gangs, experience less delinquency (Sampson and Groves, 1989). Participation in gangs, in contrast, facilitates juvenile criminality (Fagan, 1990). In neighborhoods where groups of tough teenagers congregate, particularly at night, adults avoid the area and stay home because of fear of victimization (Kasinitz and Rosenberg, 1996), effectively leaving social control in the hands of delinquent youths and criminal adults.

The school and classroom are included here as part of the environments related to social control.[9] For instance, Kellam (1994:155) shows that there can be a difference even within one school in terms of negative peer influence. He reports that "in one class, being aggressive was deviant, whereas in another not being aggressive was deviant." He is referring here to elementary school children who exert their own form of peer control, albeit in two entirely different directions. One can perhaps push matters further and suggest that it is the combination of classroom, school, and neighborhood influences that often makes these children difficult at an early age, thus at risk for early-onset delinquency, and that *their behavior is then sufficient to disrupt parenting practices*. Such children may constantly escape from family influence and supervision by "hanging around" with their older siblings, cousins, and peers in gangs that take on the role of socialization agents very early in their lives (Hogan and Kitagawa, 1985). Children with vulnerable predispositions or temperaments succumb more easily in these environments.[10] The family may play very little role whatsoever, whether positive or negative, because the environment is too powerful.

Studies indicate that violence rises in areas that have an increasing concentration of poverty[11] and instability (Bursik and Grasmick, 1993). Black children who are poor are more affected than similar white children because they disproportionately reside in such disadvantaged and disorganized areas. In the 1980s, Sullivan (1989b) found that 70 percent of New York City's blacks who were poor lived in neighborhoods with a high concentration of poverty, while 70 percent of whites who were poor lived in neighborhoods that were not particularly disadvantaged. In other words, poor white children live in "superior ecological niches," and this certainly decreases opportunities for delinquency.[12] This ecological reality also increases the likelihood that black children's vulnerable predispositions are actualized, while those of white children stand a better chance of being muted, thus leading to lower delinquency rates.

Impoverished neighborhoods are also prey to a highly visible, lucrative drug trade that undermines traditional sources of authority and of status. As one report states, "The operation of drug markets and the violence associated with them have weakened inhibitions against violence in all neighborhood contexts" (Panel on High-Risk Youth, 1993:68). Not only does this imply a destruction of traditional forms of social control, but it also means the instauration of a new order (or disorder) that provides a deviant context for child socialization as well as deviant employment opportunities for youth (Fagan, 1993).

Poverty and Segregated Minorities

As mentioned earlier, in certain neighborhoods segregated by race and poverty, the level of social disorganization and negative peer influence may be so high that it destroys positive parental influence in many families. In contrast, most poor white families do not live in disorganized and impoverished areas; thus, positive parenting remains of greater consequence for their children. The possibility may well exist that, confronted by walls of insecurity and repeated lack of success, too many of these besieged minority parents may already have lowered their standards of parenting, if only to keep peace with children who have become rapidly intractable as a result of association with deviant peers. For instance, there are indications that African-American parents supervise their children's television viewing less than other parents, thus allowing the negative influence of television to enter into their homes more than is the case among whites who are in addition generally living in less disadvantaged areas (Muller and Kerbow, 1993). Therefore, television violence may reinforce neighborhood violence.

What may happen in disadvantaged minority areas is that the critical mass of efficient parents that would be necessary to wrest the control of children's lives away from detrimental influences no longer exists. In Chapters 4 and 5, it was explained that a critical mass of both "affluent" neighbors and intellectually alert students is necessary for children to do well in school. Segregated minority neighborhoods that are also poor are currently lacking a critical minimum mass of positive sources of influence for children and youth, at levels including the family, adults in general, schools, and peers; however, this was not necessarily so in the past (Wilson,

1987). In other words, there is a lack of social capital that could be utilized to produce human capital among children and youth (Coleman, 1988).

This positive critical mass has been replaced by another critical mass that is both deviant or at least tolerant of deviances, such as vandalism, drugs, prostitution, violence, and teen gangs (Gottfredson and Hirschi, 1990:97). This critical mass is also permissive in terms of school dropout and adolescent pregnancy, two behaviors that in themselves would be harmless in a different context or a different culture but that, in our type of society, present enormous liabilities for the youths involved, their families, neighborhoods, and society at large. In sum, a lack of economic and social capital feeds deviance and, in turn, deviance compounds and perpetuates deficits in economic, human, and social capital, particularly among segregated minority groups.

Because black indigence at the individual level is compounded by segregation in high-poverty districts, the quality of neighborhoods is an important etiological factor in crime and delinquency among blacks,[13] and in racial differences in criminality. Indeed, when quality of neighborhood is controlled for, the percentage of black delinquents is no higher than that of white delinquents.[14] Because a disproportionate number of young African-American males engage in illegal activities, males and females of all ages and races, but particularly blacks, "are more likely to be victimized by young black males than by any other demographic subgroup and by a wide margin" (Devine and Wright,1993:124). Therefore, especially in the northeast and the south, as well as in a few large Canadian cities, where there are substantial groups of blacks, the fear aroused by young black males may not be entirely unjustified under certain circumstances that are actually mainly intraracial, although it is a fear that is largely fueled by prejudices.[15] This situation is unfair to African Americans because it reinforces racist stereotypes that then affect the large majority of law-abiding young black men. In addition, it contributes to police harassment of law-abiding blacks who are "mistaken" for suspected criminals (West, 1993).[16]

Concerns that young African-American males may be discriminated against by being arrested for *similar* offenses more often than their white counterparts have been widely disproved (Tonry, 1995), although, as will soon be discussed, the focus on arrests for crack cocaine produces a result which is tantamount to discrimination. Another concern voiced is that blacks commit a disproportionate number of their crimes against other blacks, and the police do not investigate black-on-black crimes as thoroughly as they do when whites are the victims. This argument may be valid in certain areas. However, when victimization statistics are tabulated by race they correspond quite well with arrest statistics, both currently[17] and in the recent past (Blumstein, 1983; Tonry, 1995:50-51).

The net result is that poverty conditions fostered by discrimination and segregation lead to an overrepresentation of members of disadvantaged minority groups among violent criminals and in the penal system (Reiss and Roth, 1993). For example, in Ontario, Native youths are four times more likely to be in jail than their numbers in the population would predict, and five times more in Manitoba (Kitchen et al., 1991:13). The same situation exists for blacks in both countries and is highly related to the poverty and lower status of visible minority groups in North America. Poverty combined with segregation, whether social or geographic, presents a structure for socialization into deviance and opportunities for delinquency (Jencks, 1992).[18] Moreover, it is quite likely that, once arrested, poor minority adolescents reap more negative life-course trajectories than adolescents from middle-class families who benefit from better social resources (Hagan, 1994).

As Tonry (1995) convincingly argues, crime reforms in the United States, particularly those aimed at the traffic of crack cocaine, have been catastrophic for young black males who, because of poverty, engage in this drug trade. Since 1984, the 211 percent increase in murders committed by black youths is related to their greater involvement in the crack trade compared with white youths whose murder rate increased by 64 percent during the same period (Wethington, 1996). Murders aside, incarcerating and severely punishing certain drug-related offenses has not diminished crime but has only added to the vicious cycle of poverty. As Chambliss (1995:253) points out, the focus on arresting drug users and traffickers on the street de facto discriminates against young African Americans. The result is that "the poor black community is a community of ex-convicts where 50 percent of children may have a parent involved with the law or hiding from it" (Miller, 1992). The national economic costs incurred by this type of law enforcement policy could be more wisely spent with better results and fewer expenses (Tonry, 1995:45) at the preventive level, by providing a more adequate education to black children from age three on, and by creating employment opportunities in disadvantaged neighborhoods.

Poverty and Dysfunctional Opportunity Structure

The social disorganization or disorder[19] of a neighborhood with a high concentration of poverty leads to criminality because effective social controls are no longer in place. Moreover, the inferior quality and episodic nature of jobs available in such an area may also decrease individuals' stakes in conforming to laws (Crutchfield, 1995). In turn, criminality further deepens the negative social and economic conditions of the area,[20] and more residents who can afford to leave do so. The few local employment opportunities are often relocated for fear of crime. Therefore, poverty combined with social disorganization feeds criminality and the latter reinforces the cycle of poverty.

In a longitudinal study, Farrington et al. (1986) have shown that individuals commit more offenses when unemployed. This finding again indicates the salience of socioeconomic factors as triggers for criminality within the life span of each individual. This difference in criminality between periods of employment and unemployment may be due to the individual's need for material resources that unemployment effectively frustrates, as well as to an excess of time which heightens the person's availability for crime. Unemployment can also mean the loss of inhibitions against deviance that may be sustained by having a job and co-workers with whom one interacts within the boundaries of legality. In this sense, unemployment erects barriers to positive social ties and effective social control in a person's life. In contrast, employment leads to social control and inhibitions against crime (Sampson and Laub, 1993).[21] There is a life-course continuity between unemployment, school dropout, and juvenile as well as adult offenses (Farrington, 1992). Individuals who criminally offend are less likely to seek, obtain, and retain jobs and thus are frequently unemployed; this pattern is often initiated during adolescence, beginning with school dropout or truancy.

Freeman (1991) provides the following statistics on the relationship between dropout and criminality: about 18 percent of all former 18-to-24-year-old dropouts and 30 percent of 25-to-34-year-old former dropouts are under the jurisdiction of the criminal justice system. These figures are far higher among blacks: 41 percent of the 18-to-24-year-olds and 75 percent of the 25-to-34-year-olds who did not complete high school are under the supervision of the criminal justice system. These last statistics stem in great part from the insularity from mainstream social controls that exists among young black dropouts who live in high-deviance and high-poverty neighborhoods, as well as from the fact that they thereby have far more acquaintances, friends, and even relatives who engage in criminality than in legal employment.

African-American dropouts are more familiar with illegal activities as alternative sources of income than are white dropouts, particularly when the latter live in a safe district. For instance, Hagan (1994:97) reviews several studies indicating that, in some neighborhoods, probably at least one-third of all black males participate in the drug trade and temporarily earn a far superior income than they would earn in less exciting and poorly remunerated service sector jobs. But any short-term advantages that youth derive from criminal gang participation or illegal activities soon turn into long-term economic and social liabilities, including arrest and incarceration (Padilla, 1992).[22]

Drug use frequently increases the chance that a person will commit crimes. For instance, Horney, Osgood, and Marshall (1995) determined that drug use was related to a 54 percent increase in property crimes and a 100 percent increase in assaults. Overall, drug use raised the odds of committing a crime sixfold. They also found that heavy drinking was related to a surge in property crime. A substantial proportion of crimes are therefore committed as a result of the combination of poverty and drug use—as well as drug transactions. More to the point, the poor, and particularly the minority poor, who suffer from addictions far more than whites, are in a no-win paradox. On the one hand, the economy fails to provide jobs that are accessible to them, yet they are blamed for not being employed. On the other hand, the state has failed to stop the flow of illegal drugs—in fact, provider nations have urged North America to reduce its underground demand for drugs—yet the poor are blamed for their addictions. In both instances, the onus is placed on individuals. Yet one cannot find a job where none exists. Neither can a teenager become addicted where drugs are unavailable. The easy availability of guns and of drugs is a major problem (Zuckerman, 1996).

POVERTY AND THE MEDIA

Poverty in itself, even in concentration, does not entirely explain North American criminality and delinquency. When social disorganization is added to poverty, a more potent explanatory model emerges. However, there is an additional variable which has not been sufficiently considered as a cause of social disorganization, or as Garbarino (1995) puts it, as a cause of the "social toxicity" of our environment—and this is the audiovisual media, particularly television and videos (Seppa, 1997).[23]

On both sides of the American-Canadian border, there are strong political pressures to reduce gratuitous violence on television and in films; in particular, American children watch more television than do children in other industrialized countries (Ceci, 1996). The literature on the negative effects of television viewing in general, and television violence in particular, is extensive (Liebert and Sprafkin, 1988). There are estimates that television has contributed to a doubling of homicides (Centerwall, 1989). Since its introduction, the contents of television have evolved markedly in the depiction of family life, childhood, adolescence, sexuality, and the incidence as well as the magnitude of violence. In particular, programs accessible to children have become more detrimental (Comstock and Strasburger, 1990). This evolution of the contents of the media is often conveniently rationalized by statements such as "Our society has changed; it's only logical that the media reflect this reality." However, *could it not be said instead that it is the media that is changing society?*

Indeed, the media introduces new fashions in clothing, lifestyles, family behaviors, adolescent activities, and even lethal weapons. One can think also of the language heard on television. It is difficult to explain the sudden and widespread lack of civility, the sudden aggressive posturing and acting out of youth, which did not exist twenty years ago, without a modeling impetus (American Psychological Association Commission on Violence and Youth, 1993). *This lack of civility has since taken on a life of its own, but the prevalence of such complex and numerous nasty behaviors cannot be explained other than by a permissive social atmosphere reflected on television.* It cannot be explained by poverty alone because poverty does not in itself necessarily lead to aggressive behaviors. And it certainly did not do so before the advent of television.

At the same time that this evolution in the media was taking place, other changes were occurring. First, the quantity and quality of youths' and children's contacts with caring and responsible adults have diminished at home, in schools, and in neighborhoods. Parents are employed longer hours, teachers spend less time with individual children and often live outside neighborhoods that are poor. Second, children's lives have become much less stable and predictable with the rise in parental divorce, single parenting, courtship, remarriage, cohabitation, and redivorce, as well as economic instability. Third, poor children, particularly those belonging to minority groups, experience insecurity, fear, and danger in their neighborhoods.

Therefore, as the media became more violent, less constructively educational, and more threatening, children's own environments, particularly those of poor children, deteriorated as well. This means that the social disorganization and lack of civility that disadvantaged children are exposed to on television (Waters, 1993) and in videos produce a more negative effect on them because their real environments often mimic what they see, and because their real environments are no longer adequate to protect them, inform them, and guide them in more positive directions.[24] Many poor children lack the presence of parents and other stable older persons who act like mature adults rather than deviant peers. A twelve-year-old child living with a twenty-seven-year-old mother who is acting up in a variety of ways that are identical to those of the child lacks the presence of a mature, stable, and authority-vested parent. These factors coalesce to exacerbate children's opportunities to develop behavioral problems, cognitive deficits, and create opportunities and skills for delinquency.

CONCLUSION

Delinquency and criminality rose spectacularly after 1950 and have since stabilized at a high level—although violent and lethal acts committed by children and young adolescents have continued to increase. All these changes have occurred within four decades—too brief a period for an explanation residing at the genetic level. In other words, although individual criminality may in some cases be partly influenced by genetic factors, it is not possible that our gene pool has created this trend by deteriorating within so short a period of time (Rutter, 1997). The answer therefore lies outside of the realm of genetics. The rise in crime and violence does mean that children and youngsters *now find themselves more often than similar children in the past in an environment that encourages the development of antisocial traits*, promotes related behaviors, and offers opportunities for deviance. This environment does not provide them with the structure nor the social control that would allow them to rein in negative tendencies, to learn prosocial behaviors, and to become conforming adolescents.

Many environments are involved in the development of delinquency. At the global level, we have seen that neighborhoods with a high concentration of poverty generally harbor substantial delinquency and criminality activity. Such areas offer a structure for the development of deviant behaviors because of the examples set by adults, and because there is no effective social control in the streets or in the boarded-up buildings of the area (Sampson, 1997). Moreover, youngsters have too much idle time on their hands, no age-appropriate leisure activities, and no emotional commitment to schooling. Compared with middle-class adolescents, they also stand to lose less by committing serious crimes and are often embedded in a criminal opportunity structure (Hagan and Palloni, 1990). Last but not least, these children and youngsters are entertained by forms of mass media that glorify deviant behaviors such as gratuitous violence, drug use, swearing, fighting, indiscriminatory sex, and what Garbarino (1995) refers to as nastiness. The media also extol materialism, which inflates poor children's expectations of obtaining possessions that are beyond their reach.

Thus, both at the neighborhood and media level, as well as at school, impoverished children and youngsters are presented with a lack of controlling structures and an abundance of negative role models. The adults at home are frequently unable to proactively teach children mainstream social skills and to discourage traits such as aggressiveness, hyperactivity, defiance, or even helplessness. Among what Ogbu (1991) calls involuntary minorities, particularly blacks, defiance may actually be encouraged in some neighborhoods and families. When the children have personal strengths, they are seldom afforded the opportunities to expand their skills and to branch out positively. In many cases the family functions relatively well, but the constant exposure to the media, the effect of aggressive peers, and the discouraging school mentality all coalesce to render otherwise fit children into ones with little motivation and quite a few acquired deviant skills. These deviant skills in turn exacerbate poverty.

At the individual and aggregate levels, serious delinquency that is repeated contributes to poverty because the youngsters generally do not complete school, have few social and marketable competencies, acquire little employment experience, often are incarcerated, and may have police records that will close job opportunities to them in the future. If these delinquent youths beget children, these mothers and their children will almost certainly be poor. Thus, serious delinquency is in great part created by poverty. In a negative feedback loop, it serves to exacerbate poverty, and to lower the quality of life of already socially isolated neighborhoods. It carries enormous monetary costs for society (Wethington, 1996) as well as emotional and interpersonal costs at the individual and familial levels (Lynam, 1996).

Chapter 11

Poverty Undermines Genetic Potential

One of the issues that many people consider and that we have begun to explore indirectly in several of the previous chapters, and more directly in Chapter 10, is whether the poor are somehow inferior. This notion is unwittingly fanned by scientific books such as Herrnstein and Murray's (1994) *The Bell Curve*.[1] Might it be possible that poverty is, if not deserved, at least justified by a certain intellectual, psychological, or moral deficit that is irremediable? This question is centuries old. In many instances, it is racially or politically motivated. But it is an issue that can now be put to rest with the help of science, particularly behavior genetics. In the past, genetics has been used for ideological purposes to prove that certain groups in society were indeed inferior. The consequences have been devastating. Current behavior genetics' focus, however, is radically different from previous emphases and concerns of sociobiology. It is not tainted by racial ideologies. It is a science studying the *combined* effect of genes and environment on personalities *within families* and not between groups, racial or otherwise.[2]

While the nature versus nurture controversy or the role of environment versus genes may still be eagerly discussed elsewhere, behavior geneticists have long replaced this futile dichotomy with a perspective emphasizing the interactional role of genetics and environment together (Wachs, 1983): one cannot exist without the other (Plomin, 1990). Very pertinent to our concerns here is that behavior geneticists themselves point out that the overall environment, and not just the familial one, is a more important influence than genes on most behaviors (Plomin, 1994b and 1995). Behaviors *per se* are not inherited but influenced by traits and abilities that are partly inherited (Pike et al., 1996). In addition, geneticists emphasize personality *change*,[3] the *vari-*

ability of genetic and environmental influences over time,[4] prevention, intervention, and the complexity of the role of genes.

What is at stake in this book are presumed maladaptive behaviors on the part of the poor: were they born like that? In this chapter, this question can be refuted. I will do so by expanding upon data and ideas from the field of behavior genetics. It can be proposed that poverty prevents the actualization of abilities and positive predispositions, that it exacerbates or triggers negative predispositions, and, finally, that it triggers dysfunctional behaviors in people who are genetically sound.

It is important to note that intelligence as measured by IQ tests[5] is only *one* of several abilities that have to be considered when discussing notions such as poverty caused by inferiority (e.g., Gardner, 1995). While intelligence is certainly an important quality—perhaps overemphasized currently—other dimensions of personality are relevant to success in life, and are also affected by genes and environment. Some are physical stamina, appearance, prosociability, ability to concentrate, interpersonal skills, capacity to delay gratification, commitment, motivation, specific talents such as musicality and manual dexterity, to mention only a few. In this perspective, inadequacy in some of these competencies may be compensated by the presence of others and lead to success in life—success as measured by either education, income and/or occupation, as well as specific achievements, whether political, humanitarian, artistic, or manual such as house building. We begin with a presentation of the knowledge garnered via the science of behavior genetics, and apply it to the question at hand in subsequent sections.

GENETICS AND CHILD OUTCOMES

Outline of Behavior Genetics Principles

Poverty affects individual development through deficits in the quality of family life, school, peer, and neighborhood environments. So far, human developmentalists have focused nearly exclusively on the role that parents play in their children's negative outcomes. Thousands of studies have sought to prove that childrearing practices in general are the prime factor that determines a child's personality, mental health, behavior, and achievement. While there is no doubt that parents influence their children, they are far less important in the determination of their offspring's personality, emotionality, abilities, and life choices than hitherto believed (Ambert, 1995 and 1997a). The fallacy of the traditional research findings stems from a neglect of genetic considerations along with environmental ones.

The entire research linking parental practices to various child outcomes is clouded by one fundamental limitation (Scarr, 1993): *it confounds genetic and environmental influences* (Plomin, DeFries, and McClearn, 1990). What is interpreted as cultural transmission[6] or the effect of childrearing is in great part genetic (Kendler, 1995a and 1996). Indeed, in biological families, parenting behaviors and child outcomes have one common factor:[7] the fact that parents and children share genes (Rowe, 1994). These genes in part influence both the parenting behaviors that are assumed to affect their children and the children's personalities and behaviors; this common factor, to which we return later on, is referred to as the **passive genotype-environment correlation.**

Children inherit 50 percent of their genes on average from each of their two parents. This means that biological children are more similar to their parents than they are to randomly selected adults. It also means that as the degree of biological relatedness or **genetic loading** increases, people share more of their genes. Twins who are identical, or **monozygotic,** share 100 percent of their genetic make-up and are similar to each other, even when they have been adopted into different families at birth and have therefore lived entirely separate lives (Plomin, 1994a). In contrast, fraternal twins are **dizygotic** and may share about 50 percent of their genes, while half-siblings share about 25 percent of their genes; adopted siblings and stepsiblings show no genetic similarity other than random ones. Therefore, in order to study the role played by genes and environment, behavior geneticists utilize samples containing siblings, particularly twins, adopted children, and stepsiblings. They also compare twins reared apart in adoptive families with twins reared together in their biological families in order to tease out the differential impact of genes from that of the environment.

If we take two biological siblings, each has inherited 50 percent of his or her genes from the same two parents. It follows that, on average, they will be more similar to each other in personality and abilities than they will be to the other children in the neighborhood or to an adopted sibling. But the two siblings, unless they are identical twins, can also be quite different because the combination of genes each has inherited is not identical. For instance, while Pedro may have inherited his mother's IQ and facial features and his father's artistic nature, his sister Maria may have inherited her father's facial features, so that the two siblings may not even share a physical resemblance. In addition, Maria may have inherited her father's more average IQ and her mother's optimistic disposition. Hence, in some families a child may be different from both siblings and parents.

While siblings share the same gene pool, the *configuration* of genes inherited by each is what determines his or her own genetic make-up. A child may inherit a gene from the mother that cancels the potential effect of another gene inherited from the father, or instead increases the potency of that gene within a given context. The resulting **configuration of traits** may be very different. Thus, in instances of poverty created by a parent's genetically influenced lack of abilities, one or all of the children may inherit a more positive configuration of traits that will lead to remaining in school longer and hence raising them out of poverty *if they live in a favorable environment that allows for such a possible outcome* (Ceci et al., 1997).

A second reason why children are often different from their parents is that parents can be mere *carriers* of genes that do not affect their own personalities or behaviors. They may, for instance, carry genes for mental illness but these genes do not affect them. Unfortunately, some of these genes can be passed on to their children in an active way, particularly when both parents are carriers, so that children will be negatively affected.[8] This principle of genetics thus contributes to explain why some children are different from their parents even though they share so many of their genes.

Genotype-Environment Correlations

Most personality characteristics can be explained by genes as well as by "correlations"[9] between genetic and environmental factors. These correlations form the cornerstone of the dynamics between genetics and environment. They help explain how genes and environment work together to produce results in terms of people's characteristics and then behaviors. The three **genotype-environment correlations** are: passive, reactive, and active (Plomin, DeFries, and Loehlin, 1977).

As discussed earlier, the *passive* genotype-environment correlation occurs because children and parents share both heredity and environment (Plomin, 1994a). When statistical relationships between children's outcomes (e.g., aggression) and parents' childrearing styles (harsh treatment of children, for instance) are found, environmental researchers conclude that the harsh parental treatment has contributed to or even caused the offspring's aggressiveness. While there is some truth to this, the *way* in which this "causality" occurs is actually quite different from explanations provided by a purely environmental conceptualization. In addition to television violence as well as peer and neighborhood influences, it is not only harsh parenting practices that cause children's aggressive behaviors, but the fact that both these practices *and* child aggressiveness are in part explained by genes shared by parents and children—what we could call "aggression" genes for the sake of simplicity. In other words, both parents and children may be genetically predisposed to aggressiveness, and harsh parenting is simply one manifestation of this trait.

In turn, these genetically influenced harsh parental practices become part of the children's environment and may trigger or encourage the children's negative predisposition to aggressiveness.[10] Moreover, when parents are predisposed to being harsh and aggressive, stressors such as poverty may exacerbate this negative style of parenting[11] to further impact detrimentally on the aggressive children's predispositions—particularly when the family lives in a neighborhood where violence is frequent and reinforces the children's predisposition. The passive genotype-environment correlation occurs only among biologically related persons, and does not take place between parents and adoptive children because they do not share the same genes.

The other two types of correlations, while also occurring in the family, manifest themselves in other contexts as well. The **reactive genotype-environment correlation** refers to the fact that parents, siblings, teachers, and peers *react* to a child's behaviors, which, as has been discussed, are in part genetically influenced. For instance, a parent becomes more controlling or more negative with a difficult child, and in turn this negativity may increase the difficult behaviors (Ge et al., 1996). When introduced to a new schoolmate who is shy, outgoing peers may simply ignore the child. The peers react to the child's shyness, a trait that is in part heritable (Kagan, Reznick, and Snidman, 1989). Scarr and McCartney (1983) refer to this as the "evocative" effect: the child evokes a specific reaction. Finally, an example of the **active genotype-environment correlation** would be a musically gifted child who requests music lessons. Or the child buys records and music sheets, thus creating an environment that fosters his or her talent (Plomin, 1994a). What the concepts of reactive and active genotype-environment correlations illustrate is that children coproduce their development (Goldsmith, 1989). As such, behavior geneticists link with the interactional perspectives in child development that began with Bell in 1968 (Bell and Harper, 1977).

GENETICALLY INFLUENCED CHAINS OF EVENTS

The active and reactive genotype-environment correlations can explain in part various chains of events in a person's life (Saudino et al., 1997). Because of their genetic configuration, certain persons "cause" or initiate entire chains of life events (Rutter and Rutter, 1993). Let's illustrate this point with the example of a child with deficient impulse control,[12] hyperactivity, and verbal aggressiveness. Because he does things on impulse, he has had several accidents.[13] He has fallen from a tree, has crashed his skateboard against a moving car, and later on, gambled all the money that his parents had saved for his education. As a young adult, on an impulse, he joins in a bet to see who can drink the most and ends up comatose in the hospital. As a result he loses the job he has just found because his employer judges him to be irresponsible. The scenario is continued into low occupational success and poverty (Caspi, Elder, and Herbener, 1990). This boy/young man operates according to his genetic predispositions. In turn, the latter are pursued or discouraged depending on how the environment reacts to the behaviors they influence.

In short, genes or the characteristics they contribute create various paths in an individual's life course (Henry et al., 1996), as discussed in the previous chapter regarding early onset of serious delinquency. Does this mean that one's life is preordained by genes? No, it means that, once the influence of genes is accepted, *interventions can be devised to change the environments that combine with genes to create negative life courses,* and, hence, prevent these life courses or at least ward off their worst consequences (Sroufe and Rutter, 1984). It would be helpful to be able to identify those persons who are genetically most at risk of suffering from negative environmental impact such as poverty,[14] or most at risk for *creating* an environment that is stressful (Kendler, 1991). Poverty is one stressful environmental factor that needs to be addressed by researchers in this respect.

Let's take the example of a disadvantaged family with six children. Two siblings who are easygoing and less demanding do not feel deprived and make the best out of a bad situation. They may either adapt to poverty or try to escape from it. Two other siblings sharing the same poverty are materialistic, envious, and demanding. They consequently react with stress, behavioral problems, dissatisfaction, lack of respect for their parents, and even delinquency. These reactions further propel them into another cycle of poverty as they drop out of school and engage in theft. The last two siblings are industrious and determined to improve their circumstances. Their reaction in turn creates different and more successful life paths that they do not share with the other four siblings.

ENVIRONMENTALLY INFLUENCED CHAINS OF EVENTS

When children are born into an environment of disadvantage, this disadvantage tends to persist, whether it is family conflict or poverty (Sameroff et al., 1987). It persists because of mechanisms similar to those stemming from deleterious genetic predispositions (Sameroff, 1994). Therefore, a negative environment can also create chains of events in a person's life, although a person's own characteristics or resilience[15] may put a brake on the process, provided the environment is not extreme. And, naturally, the same applies to advantages. They also cumulate.

We have seen that children born into great poverty experience many disadvantages that tend to perpetuate themselves throughout their growth, unless a parent's remarriage or better paying job rescues them. Poverty is often accompanied by crowded and dilapidated housing, low-quality schools, and unsupervised, deviant peers. In such an environment, unless a child is particularly resilient, she may fall behind at school, lose interest, drop out, and even become pregnant to finally have the feeling of getting something out of life. Unfortunately, the pregnancy itself only compounds the disadvantage and is one more link in a chain of unfortunate events initiated by a negative environment—along with negative predisposing characteristics, for not all children are defeated by their detrimental environment (Garmezy and Masten, 1994; Werner, 1990).

In contrast, a child raised in a middle-class environment has greater chances of attending a school that will motivate her to go on even if she is not particularly bright. (As shown in Chapter 4, parents' SES is a better predictor of a youth's completion of high school and college than are his or her abilities.) Depending on her personality, she will get involved in extracurricular activities that will enhance her already existing advantage. With her parents' support, high school leads to college. The home advantages are accompanied by school and recreational advantages (Rutter and Rutter, 1993). It is as if advantage breeds advantage. Or just as genes "choose" their environment, *environments "beget" other similar environments, and enhance or depress genetic potential as the cycle is perpetuated.*[16] This again provides a reason to interrupt the deleterious environmental cycle and intervene socially to create better conditions[17] for children to grow up in—conditions that will prevent the development of negative predispositions and will actualize positive potential (Bronfenbrenner and Ceci, 1994).

ENVIRONMENTAL RATHER THAN PERSONAL DEFICITS

What this summary of and expansion upon behavior genetics indicates is that, although parents may have a relatively low IQ or suffer from serious mental vulnerabilities—factors that may place them in the category of the poor—their children will not necessarily inherit these negative characteristics. They may inherit them to a lesser degree or may simply inherit a different configuration of characteristics altogether. *Given an appropriate environment,* such children can move out of poverty, and as many do so as do not. Therefore, it is quite unlikely that on the basis of genetic "inferiority" alone, multiple generations within a family will remain trapped in poverty. *In fact, multiple generations of the same family are more likely to remain trapped in poverty because of environmental rather than personal inferiority factors.*

For instance, some people live in rural areas and small towns that, for decades and even centuries, have experienced little economic development, in part because their region depends on a single industry with low wages (C.M. Duncan, 1996). Other rural communities are relatively isolated from the rest of the country. Unless these people move away, all members of their families will remain poor for several generations. Moreover, this intergenerational poverty may contribute to innate[18] but not hereditary intellectual deficits via malnutrition of pregnant women and their small children—a phenomenon occurring on a large scale in various parts of the world. Currently, as inner cities become poorer and more socially isolated, there is the reasonable fear that a greater proportion of youth than before will remain locked in the same poverty they were brought up in. This is because there are no opportunities available at the educational and economic levels, and these individuals are cut off from persons who could help them find jobs. Their poverty has little to do with their genes.

Entire societies lack the means, the political will, or even the physical environment to prosper, and 90 percent of their populations may be poor, as described in Chapter 1. It would certainly be foolish to conclude that 90 percent of these societies' citizens are congenitally mentally delayed or genetically inferior. Iraq, for instance, provides a recent and drastic example of a country's rapid descent into poverty among the general population. The sanctions imposed against Iraq by the United Nations, and the fact that Iraqis are cheated by a regime that builds palaces and rebuilds an expensive army instead of feeding its people, have contributed to creating a nation of indigents. It would certainly be preposterous to conclude that Iraqis have suddenly lost their IQ and other abilities and that their genes have deteriorated!

What is important to understand is that *the development of positive characteristics that are partly genetic, such as a normal IQ and a prosocial personality, requires a favorable environment* (see Bronfenbrenner, 1996). An analogy is the proverbial perfect seed falling into barren soil with no rainfall and no fertilizer. Basically, a child's genetic endowment is akin to a seed: it will flower only when there is adequate nutrition, a minimum of social and affective stimulation, opportunities to learn, and a reasonably safe environment. In contrast, poor nutrition, lack of social and learning stimulation, overcrowding, noise, pollution, detrimental media exposure, and a high rate of dangerous incidents and illegal activities in the neighborhood substantially diminish the chances that a child's positive inheritance will be actualized. In fact, such environments, typical of poor neighborhoods, often stunt intellectual, affective, and moral growth.

Poverty as a multifaceted environment severely limits the actualization of abilities, good character, normal IQ, and motivation; it limits the range of available opportunities (O'Connor and Rutter, 1996). Therefore, even though it is not an acceptable situation, it makes sense that the IQs of children who have spent all their lives in poverty are lower than nonpoor children's IQs or than that of disadvantaged children living in a nonpoor neighborhood which provides them with compensatory resources (Crane, 1994; Ogbu, 1978). What is rather amazing is that at least half of the children in poverty environments overcome their disadvantages. But there is more to this line of reasoning than meets the eye. A deprived, unstimulating, and even criminogenic environment produces another negative effect: *it exacerbates a child's negative predispositions*. Let's again take the example of aggressiveness, which is partly genetic, and imagine a child predisposed to aggressiveness born into a family where the parents fight constantly, are irritable and harsh because of daily stressors, are too busy making ends meet and don't supervise him. He is allowed to watch violent television programs, and is left to roam a neighborhood where kids fight and engage in criminal activities. The child also attends school with a large number of aggressive peers. This child, already predisposed to aggression, is "seeded" into an environment that encourages his aggressive tendencies at every turn or, at the very least, does nothing to control them. In fact, such an environment contributes to the development of aggressive behavior even in children who have *no* predisposition to it: they simply learn it or are pressured into it by peers.

What this example illustrates is the principle that a detrimental environment prevents or, at the very least, discourages the development of socially valued characteristics such as academic abilities, good work habits, and prosociability. Instead, it encourages the development of negative traits, such as impulsivity, aggressiveness, low attention span, laziness, and "attitudes" against authority. *The combination of positive characteristics that are never actualized and negative characteristics that are encouraged by the environment* may well result in a low-IQ youth who is impulsive, aggressive, not interested in school, who fights, joins a gang, gets a criminal record, has a child whom he can't support, and so on. And if these negative chains of events are multiplied by the number of inhabitants who may be at risk, we can understand how some poor neighborhoods have a concentration of low IQ persons and school dropouts, as well as elevated rates of teenage childbearing, delinquency, criminality, unemployment, and hostile attitudes against authority and education.

One also has to consider that, at the genetic level, there are children who have inherited a configuration of good genes which makes them resilient to many adversities in their environments and allows them to escape poverty more easily than others (Garmezy and Masten, 1994). A sunny temperament may shield such children from quarrelsome siblings, aggressive peers, and material deprivation (see Tschann et al., 1996). That same easy temperament may even get them to be noticed favorably by one adult, whether a parent, a relative, or a teacher. The relationship then becomes a resource that helps the child overcome some or all of the negative aspects of his or her environment.[19] Traits that are not valued in our society, such as shyness, may also serve a protective function[20] against the development of behavioral problems in criminogenic areas or families.[21] In contrast, an outgoing and independent child (traits that are valued in North America) may be propelled into socializing with criminogenic elements in his or her district, thus placing the child at risk.

In addition, a high IQ, although it might be somewhat dampened by poverty, combined with a curious and sunny predisposition, may help a child cope, solve problems, remain out of trouble, persist in school, and acquire work habits that lead to a well-remunerated job and subsequent exit out of poverty. In contrast, small children who have difficult personality characteristics react more stressfully to noise, overcrowding, and even the birth of a sibling (Wachs, 1987). When older, these same children are more vulnerable to the stressors of poverty (Elder, Caspi, and Nguyen, 1994), thus more likely to remain disadvantaged into adulthood.

There are other environmental reasons why many children do get out of poverty, even though they may never become affluent. For one, not all poor families are dysfunctional and not all live in disadvantaged neighborhoods. Even very dysfunctional families in deprived neighborhoods may have one member who is competent and who nurtures the child. Second, some children may attend an early preschool program that compensates to some extent for the deprived home and neighborhood environments (Campbell and Ramey, 1994). Finally, few children spend their entire lives in poverty; as their family's economic condition improves, so do their lives and family environment. They may, however, if they belong to a minority group, remain locked within inner-city poverty so that their new familial advantage is counterbalanced by the perpetuation of neighborhood deficits.

POVERTY CREATES INFERIORITY

The question that some people may now raise is this: obviously, not all poor people have low IQs, are deviant or criminal, or produce babies at age fourteen. Does this not mean that those who do are inferior? Here as well, the answer is no and lies in the same interaction between environment and genetics described above. To begin with, *the quality of the gene pool in a population does not change within a twenty-five-year span, which is the time it has taken for the spectacular rise in single parenting.*[22] *Nor can the gene pool have deteriorated during the ten to twenty years during which all manners of negative outcomes among the poor have increased, including violent delinquency.* Therefore, one has to look to environmental factors for an answer to this apparent "inferiority."

The point is that poverty creates individuals who think, behave, and even look as if they were genetically inferior. Many may indeed be constitutionally disadvantaged, but the reason lies in poverty-related prenatal risks and early infancy malnutrition, as well as trauma and deprivation. Given a favorable environment, such persons' children will not inherit this constitutional disadvantage because it is not genetic but is environmentally caused. Even though most poor people will never be affluent, some of their children or grandchildren will be. Moreover, subnormal individuals are not as likely to reproduce themselves; therefore their genes are not perpetuated.

One must establish a distinction between (1) poverty that is created or perpetuated by severely flawed genetic characteristics that are transmitted from generation to generation to a certain proportion of children in each generation (but *not* to all); (2) poverty perpetuated by lower abilities resulting from a lack of opportunities to actualize positive potential, and from environmental deficits that encourage the development of negative behaviors; and (3) the learning by each deprived generation of behaviors conducive to remaining in poverty, maintaining abilities at their lowest common denominator, and engaging in deviant behaviors.

As pointed out earlier, outcome (1) above is the least common as there are very few families that are *consistently* inferior genetically over several generations, whether in terms of a subnormal IQ or other severe mental or psychiatric deficits. (At the other end of the spectrum, the correlate is that there are few families that are consistently superior: some of their members may be, but not all.) Despite a great deal of assortative mating, there is too much geographic mobility in a large urban society for the formation of a solid block of inferior genes. This would require that individuals consistently intermarry and remain poor as a result of their inherited deficiencies. Moreover, both at the superior and inferior ends of the spectrum of abilities, including IQ, there are too many genetic permutations possible and too many combinations of competencies possible, as well as too many environmental influences to produce a persistent pattern of intergenerational heredity. The only viable conclusion is that poverty creates inferiority and perpetuates it once it has been created.

THE ABSURDITY OF AFRICAN-AMERICAN INFERIORITY

Most of the literature attempting to prove the genetic inferiority of the poor actually targets African Americans.[23] Previous discussions have shown that a disproportionate number of blacks are poor, uneducated, unemployed, incarcerated, and single parents. Also discussed has been the fact that these are recent developments caused by radical changes in the economy of inner cities and cannot be accounted for by a sudden deterioration of the "black gene pool." But there is also another point, this time related to genes, that is rarely mentioned in the scientific literature and that can be used to argue against the inferiority of blacks as a group. The argument resides in this: blacks in the Americas were originally *selected* by slave traders for profit. They were a merchandise that had to be carefully chosen.

The slave traders' margin of profit was higher when the following conditions were met. First, the slaves survived the dreadful conditions of the long transatlantic trip.[24] Second, upon reaching market, the slaves who fetched the best prices were healthy and well functioning (Burnard, 1996). Consequently, it was all in the *economic* interest of the traders to choose African captives who were healthy, both intellectually and physically, and to disregard the others. A dim-witted slave cannot follow orders. One in ill health cannot survive the trip nor can he or she work. Had a slave trader tried to market intellectually and physically inferior "specimens," potential buyers would have turned to his competition.

Furthermore, this selection process was reinforced at destination and within slavery. Conditions were often heartwrenching, yet the statistics available indicate a similar life expectancy for whites and "Negroes" (Dublin, Lotka, and Spiegelman, 1949). Despite abuses, it was not in the economic interest of owners to starve or mistreat their slaves. Nevertheless, human beings could not remain healthy in slavery conditions if they did not use their heads. Intellectual skills were particularly useful to avert life-threatening situations, to avoid certain particularly detrimental tasks, and to ingratiate themselves with or at least be tolerated by the masters. Moreover, a substantial proportion of slaves were artisans and even managers, another indicator of their abilities (Fogel and Engerman, 1989). For their part, owners would have seen the productivity of their plantations and industries reduced had they been supplied with inferior slaves.[25]

We often speak of the cultural heritage of African Americans: lore brought from Africa and other cultural/social aspects developed during slavery. One other heritage of slavery resides in the fact that the gene pool of blacks could not be, on average, deficient at the intellectual level. That the circumstances of post slavery and particularly the recent living conditions in the ghettos have dulled the intellect of too many is another matter that has been amply discussed earlier in this chapter. *But it has nothing to do with genes.* One can argue, however, that slavery had everything to do with *good* genes: healthy bodies and minds were selected, survived transport, slavery, and postslavery conditions.

CONCLUSION

As a general rule, deprived, insecure, and dangerous environments do not tend to promote superiority. Furthermore, there are *cultural* and *social* factors that combine with a high concentration of poverty to create violence, criminality, drug abuse, familial dislocation, and school dropout, all of which may be erroneously interpreted as signs of innate inferiority. We have already mentioned the effect of the various audiovisual media (television, films, videos, records) that extol questionable values, and which find a fertile ground among the deprived. Other detrimental social factors are the availability of firearms and drugs which establish a deviant set of norms and opportunities.

Once all these variables are combined in a critical mass within an area of poverty, the behavioral and attitudinal modes of youths' adaptation become dysfunctional with respect to integration into mainstream economy and society. In a proportion of poor individuals, inferiority results in a configuration of behaviors and traits that produce the delinquent, criminal, violent, irresponsible, and often drug-addicted elements of the poor neighborhoods. It is among this proportion of the low-income population that the intergenerational transmission of poverty is most likely to occur, mainly as a consequence of detrimental environmental conditions, and in a minority of cases only because of genetic inferiority. However, even genetic inferiority needs a fertile ground to produce detrimental consequences at the *social* level—poverty provides this ground.

Chapter 12

Conclusions, Implications, and Critiques

The acceptance of poverty amidst affluence by societies such as ours is a manifestation of questionable social and political values. At the very least, it is an indication that ideological development has not kept pace with advances in the technological domain, which are by default dictating policy making. Consequently, social and cultural organization is dominated by partly haphazard technological and economic changes. What is needed is social planning so that technology and economy serve our value system and enhance our quality of life.

One of the consequences of recent economic developments is that localized poverty is the price that societies are willing to pay, while at the same time welcoming booming corporate shareholders' dividends and blithely accepting skyrocketing salaries of CEOs who have successfully downsized. The billions spent each year for mergers and takeovers merely subsidize the financial sector to the detriment of job creation at all social class levels. Our society is enthusiastically, and perhaps mindlessly, anticipating the hegemony of an entire superhighway of computers, while this development is precisely what prevents decent people, who do not have the type of competencies necessary to thrive in a technological economy, from earning a living. Many of the unemployed and working poor are so only because of the level of technology that has been reached: the majority of similar persons were employed in previous decades and earned a reasonable income. The term "unemployable" is relative to the economic structure rather than to people's will or ill will. Currently, the economic structure greatly favors perhaps 15 percent or less of the population and advantages at most another 25 percent. The disproportionate benefits and privileges that these affluent groups receive solidify the extant social stratification system.

Corporations enjoy substantial tax advantages that are not available to the rest of the citizenry (Strobel, 1993). It is argued that such policies encourage foreign companies to build subsidiaries in our countries, and prevent our companies from leaving, thus creating and retaining jobs. The counterpart argument is that the tax loopholes and grants siphon off billions of dollars that could be used to help the poor, and to provide assistance to children, the frail, and the elderly. Moreover, corporations who move their assembly lines to low-wage countries and produce goods that the American and Canadian publics then have to import could perhaps be boycotted by these same publics. Such a social movement would encourage a new form of competitiveness: for social responsibility and accountability to the citizens of one's region.

While some economists and financiers see the globalization and the open-door policy of the national economy as a necessity for creating markets and remaining competitive internationally, several negative consequences flow from this situation. The globalization of the economy, including the existence of various free trade agreements, means that a country's control over its destiny becomes more difficult to achieve. Rather, the economies of entire regions or even the world dictate business and governmental policies.[1] With ever larger multinational corporations, investors from other countries de facto exert a certain leverage concerning the direction that these conglomerates take, and this may not be favorable to citizens of one's nation. But, especially, the fact that chief executives of corporations look to their shareholders rather than their employees in decision making means that an economy has been developed that is based strictly on superprofits with little regard for human costs. In global economies, the less powerful individuals in a society—the less educated, the less skilled, and the poor—are lost in the shuffle. They are thrown into the web of poverty. They are expendable.

This having been said, the focus of this concluding chapter rests first on a critical examination of concepts that are taken for granted in the social construction of poverty and wealth. And, second, it is based on a discussion of concepts that are not generally considered. In other words, ideology is in question.[2] Concepts examined are the culture of poverty and its links to ethnic cultures, the new meritocracy, social pathologies, and the overclass. The necessity to reduce the concentration of neighborhood poverty is also discussed.

A SUBCULTURE OF POVERTY?

In some inner-city census tracts, as well as in pockets of rural poverty, a pool of severely economically, socially, and educationally deprived families exists—what is commonly referred to as an "underclass"[3]—who may transmit their poverty from generation to generation to at least a proportion of their children. Their educational deficits, and at times deviant behaviors, isolate them from mainstream society which is the purveyor of employment. What results is the formation of "adaptations" to poverty and insularity that involve early pregnancy, drug addiction, violent crimes, school dropout, devaluation of education, the development of an inner-city language that erects barriers preventing interaction with the rest of society, and a general lifestyle that is antithetical to the adoption of modern work habits. These patterns were not prevalent before the 1960s, that is, before inner cities experienced an increase in segregation, loss of jobs, and a spiralling concentration of poverty. As Devine and Wright (1993:129) point out, the hopeless economic situation of inner-city residents "undermines or prevents individuals from fulfilling social obligations and roles." Lack of job opportunities erodes the motivation to stay in school (Ogbu, 1994).

As a result, the concept of the "culture of poverty" was coined several decades ago, and has since been the source of numerous ideological debates. On one side are theorists and policy makers who define the chronically poor as the cause of their indigence. On the other end of the ideological spectrum, it is pointed out that the poor hold the same values of success as the nonpoor, but suffer from a lack of economic opportunities. I propose here that a term such as "subculture" may be more sociologically accurate. Most individuals placed under the umbrella of the culture of poverty are after all living an American lifestyle and share most of mainstream society's dreams, ideologies, religions, and institutions (Ogbu, 1988). They do partake of the American culture. Subcultures, for their part, both integrate and reinterpret certain aspects of the larger sociocultural landscape. The concept of subculture recognizes that *a segment* of the poor hold different values about *how* to reach American goals, and about what *kind* of success one can realistically wish for in one's own segregated environment, and about what are considered desirable personality characteristics, competencies, behaviors, and even linguistic expression where one lives. A subculture is a far less encompassing term than a culture. Furthermore, it generally arises from the position a group occupies within the legitimate opportunity structure of a society, its consequent segregation, and social insularity. When so defined, there can be a subculture of poverty, but there can also be one of wealth, as will soon be discussed.[4]

The more segregated a group of people becomes because of race and poverty, or because of racial discrimination, and the longer it remains segregated, the more likely its members are to develop a subculture that, in turn, contributes to maintain their poverty. The competencies that have become valued in the subculture are often at odds with success in mainstream society. For instance, the devaluation of educational pursuits among many inner-city youths is accompanied by the valuation of success via organized sports, popular music, drugs, and the infusion of criminality, machismo, and antisocial ideas. This is a subculture which effectively socializes youngsters and prevents their reinsertion into mainstream structures—from which their grandparents or parents had been banished.

Most important in this distinction between a culture and a subculture is the latter's lack of inclusiveness: not all poor individuals and families equally partake of the negative aspects of this subculture of poverty. Most persons, particularly adults and parents, share in the values and goals of the society at large, and are barely touched by the subculture of poverty. Above all, in the perspective of this text, the subculture of poverty is the *result* of segregation and a lack of structural opportunities. It is a creation of social stratification and of the gap that exists between the rich and the poor, the valued and the devalued. It cannot exist without these systemic causes. Its *maintenance,* however, stems from a combination of these same systemic variables interacting with the subcultural elements themselves.

ETHNIC CULTURES AND SUBCULTURES OF POVERTY

Visible minorities may have their own cultures, such as is the case for Mexican Americans and many Native nations. Their culture is constituted of a language and distinct values, including a family orientation, that may greatly differ from those of mainstream America. It may also encompass sharp differences in daily activities and rhythms, arts, and material organization and possessions. Many African Americans also hold certain values, modes of expression, and arts that are grounded both in their different cultural origins and in the history of slavery. Moreover, as immigrants arrive from non-Western societies, their value systems and lifestyles often differ greatly from dominant American values and ways of living. They emphasize interpersonal relations, family orientation, respect for elders, and, for many of Asian origins, education. Interdependence and familism rather than independence and individuality may be stressed (Greenfield, 1994). These values can be constructively used to enrich the North American social and cultural fabric.

Immigrants' cultures of origin inevitably changes over time in their homelands. Therefore, different cohorts of immigrants arriving in subsequent decades from the same country may be quite distinct in some aspects of their culture and patterns of social interaction (Uribe, LeVine, and LeVine, 1994). This consideration carries implications for the schools that educate the succeeding generations of immigrant children. We often tend to think of other societies' cultures as "folkloric" and immutable—as if only our own could change—a rather ethnocentric position.

Ethnic and immigrants' cultures are different from the subculture of poverty. The two entities have to be differentiated. Minority cultures and subcultures are resources that need to be harnessed and utilized by schools to help children's adaptation. Unfortunately, when disadvantaged areas harbor large immigrant minorities, schools, in their battle against the subculture of poverty, often confuse ethnic cultures with the dysfunctional aspects of poverty. In so doing, they fail to capitalize on children's cultural strengths and attempt to eradicate them.

Ethnic cultures constitute social wealth and diversity; in contrast, subcultures of poverty result in social, cultural, and economic inferiority. *An ethnic culture can become diluted by the subculture of poverty.* This occurs when a great proportion of its members are too poor, are segregated, and are barred from the legitimate opportunity structure; as a result they partake of modes of adaptation such as school dropout and criminality that in turn further prevent them either from adapting to mainstream culture or from maintaining their own ethnic culture. To expand upon Portes' (1995a) terminology, an ethnic culture may be "downwardly assimilated" by the subculture of poverty when immigrants settle in deprived and disorganized neighborhoods which assimilate their children. For instance, Wasserman et al. (1990) have found that the longer Puerto Rican adolescents' families have lived in the mainland, the more similar their attitudes and values become to those of blacks whose neighborhoods they share.

An ethnic culture can also be subverted when many of its members achieve social notoriety and reap high incomes through deviant forms of expression that attract and inspire an important segment of its youth. One can think here of "gangsta" rap, which extols violence, racism, drugs, and the exploitation of women, particularly black women. There is nothing, except for a vague resemblance to traditional rhythms, in the long and rich African-American artistic heritage that gives any validity whatsoever for such an art form to be labeled "black." It violates the norms of the black culture because it stems, not from its roots, but strictly from a ghetto subculture that includes criminality. It is yet another example of the dilution of an ethnic culture by a subculture of poverty.

A NEW MERITOCRACY

The type of technology that is evolving is one where cognitive abilities—particularly mathematical, scientific, and technological—are becoming the most salient of all abilities required in order to succeed economically.[5] Educational institutions are pressured and will continue to be pressured to promote these specific skills over and above general knowledge. Currently, for instance, administrators and teachers worry more about the availability of computers at their schools than about their library resources. To use Mundy-Castle's (1974) distinction, technological intelligence is becoming valued over social intelligence. However, the latter is often highly prized by minority groups so that these developments are unwittingly discriminatory. In the rather near future, most of the population will be at the mercy of experts in mathematics, the natural sciences, and computer sciences: a mathematics and computer meritocracy, if you wish. In the very recent past, people who did not possess such skills could find well-remunerated employment in the industrial sector where manual labor predominated. But the downsizing of manufacturing and its technologization mean that qualified jobs involving manual labor have become increasingly less numerous.

Consequently, it may well be that additional training of persons with lower computer and numeracy skills, as well as persons with exceptional manual competencies, will not always land them stable, full-time jobs because they may never meet the new requirements. People can be educated to acquire new skills, but only to a point, because the skills required may not fit within their personal potentials. Moreover, as Deniger et al. (1995:105) put it, "While working on bettering oneself, acquiring new knowledge, and developing skills can be a good thing, it will never create a job." Instead, a socially-conscious society may well want to *preserve* certain occupations that have not yet been technologized.[6] Companies could plan on retaining a proportion of such positions, perhaps with a government subsidy, so that those willing to work but unable to acquire the new competencies could be employed in a productive manner that would not be degrading.

Ideally, a society should be able to refuse certain technological "advances" that add little to quality of life or to request that they be recast so as to be socially useful. One also has to consider that, in a few decades when technology will be rampant, our descendants may well harvest some benefits from basic knowledge and basic skills that have not been computerized. For instance, our ancestors' skills in the wilderness and nature have been lost. Will our grandchildren come to lose the few basic skills we can still practice? The readers who believe that they can detect a bias on the part of this author concerning rampant technologization are correct. This bias does not stem from an inability to adapt to technology, but rather it originates in a particular philosophy concerning quality of life, closeness with the natural environment, a preference for face-to-face human interaction, and a reverence for basic skills and general knowledge. It is a personal philosophy of what one wishes civilization to be.

One also has to consider what activities are valued as worthwhile in our societies. Manual work, except for keyboarding and clicking the mouse, is so devalued that industries have difficulty hiring expert tradespersons. Talented young people are no longer encouraged to take on advanced training in manual work such as toolmaking ("dirty jobs"), particularly if they originate from the upper middle class where many look down on such jobs as proof of social failure. Yet, certain types of trades necessitate very advanced *skills* requiring not only manual dexterity, but creativity and cognitive intelligence. Manual skills without cognitive competencies do not lead far in the occupational hierarchy. The two types of skills combined are necessary for various industries, yet they are no longer valued—thus closing opportunities for youngsters who can think best only when they apply their intellect to concrete material.

Finally, our gene pool will not change as rapidly as technology, if at all. As our modes of production become increasingly foreign to the evolutionary conditions that gave rise to the human species, human adaptation may become less easy to achieve for an ever larger number of individuals. Humanity is not necessarily adaptable to all conditions to which it is submitted and which it creates. For instance, we already know that it cannot adapt to a polluted environment without heavy health penalties. We also know that overcrowding produces stressors. Each technological "advance" creates negative reactions and even deadly consequences, either because of the nature itself of the technology (e.g., arms) or because of the unfortunate ways in which it is utilized. Television violence comes to mind here because there is nothing inherently damaging about television itself. Each technological invention that is sold to the masses or used to control the masses creates victims. As more and more such innovations are released, very few average citizens will be free from negative consequences. Each year, individuals are born who will never have the specific intellectual abilities to acquire enough schooling to meet the new demands of the labor market—although they may have other abilities. Does our changing economy mean that such people, who may be gifted in other but now devalued ways, are less deserving of an occupation?

SOCIAL PATHOLOGIES

A few thoughts on the old concept of social pathologies arise. It is important to critique the emphasis on individual pathologies compared with the silence concerning what are broader economic and technological pathologies. These include the huge incomes of some professionals and managers, the extraordinary profits reaped by companies even as they lay off employees, and the extensive technologization of jobs that, without these "improvements," would employ the less educated (Lubeck and Garrett, 1990). However, as long as these broader economic pathologies benefit a privileged controlling minority, it is difficult to anticipate that they will be addressed, least of all redressed.

One can also critique the fact that the *concept of social pathologies is usually applied only to the poor.* Many individuals at other, more favorable economic levels are pathological—whether one refers here to pedophilia, severe mental illness, alcoholism, or white-collar criminality. But, more to the point, there are other "pathologies" that develop primarily among the rich and powerful as a group, such as abuse of power and control, contempt for one's "inferiors," compulsive accumulation of wealth, and so on. For instance, to expand upon a point made earlier, a pathological need for power can be expressed through technological and scientific advances that allegedly increase consumers' choices, but actually tie them down to technology and its markets. These pathologies may have far more negative effects on *society* than do the pathologies of the poor. In fact, *can one not argue that the social pathologies of the rich create those of the poor?*

These critiques aside, one can argue that poverty breeds individual and social pathologies and these cannot be ignored, nor does avoiding one label or another or skirting the issue help the situation. It is true that some of the pathologies—or, if one prefers, flawed characteristics—such as delinquency and drug abuse constitute in part a response of some of the poor to their hopeless economic and social situation. But these are not *the* modal responses of the entire group of poor and racially segregated persons. *There are indeed several modes of adaptation to poverty,* and while criminality, teenage parenting, and school dropout may be three of them, they are neither helpful, constructive, nor are they unavoidable. Furthermore, these problems are not the preserve of the poor and the segregated because they also occur in groups that are neither poor nor segregated, albeit far less frequently. But, once "pathologies" are installed on a large scale in a neighborhood, they tend to perpetuate themselves and contribute to the reproduction of poverty. They also give rise to additional problems, and make the afflicted individuals' positions even more hopeless than they would otherwise be. Therefore, attempts to eradicate these pathologies are necessary but such attempts can be viable only if the overall economic, social, and cultural situations of the affected individuals and neighborhoods are vastly improved.

A SUBCULTURE OF WEALTH: THE "OVERCLASS"

It has been argued that there is a subculture of poverty and that there are social pathologies that afflict the poor more than others. Poverty is a social problem—the most overpowering of all—but wealth is also a problem, although most people do not include wealth, or, more precisely, the concentration of wealth, as a social pathology. Moreover, while we feverishly discuss the "underclass" and the "culture" of poverty, there is no corresponding ideological inclination toward concepts such as—shall we say—an "overclass"[7] and a "subculture of wealth." Yet, would there be poverty without a mentality favoring the concentration of wealth?

Many writers have asked whether we are in danger of creating an underclass that will be mired in poverty for several generations. Yet one rarely reads the following *and equally worrisome question*: Have a group of people not been created who are going to hold financial, hence political, power for several generations? The existence of this overclass is taken for granted (Arnold and Swadener, 1993). It is *accepted*. The class of the poor is not accepted but that of the rich and the powerful is (the "rich and famous," the "beautiful people"). The rich and famous fascinate the public and grace (or deface) the media. In comparison, the poor are an eyesore better left to their ghettos and pathologies.

For an academic, studying the poor is a veritable door opener in terms of obtaining research grants. Policy makers, the public, and philanthropic organizations all want to see a resolution to the problem of poverty—which actually is a problem of the unjust distribution of resources in North America. Unfortunately, studying the rich is, at best, an esoteric topic. Yet one can argue that it is equally important to study the transmission of attitudes and behaviors that encourage the accumulation and consolidation of privileges. For without such behaviors, widespread poverty would not exist. For the rich, the poor have always largely been an object of philanthropy—thus an object for status enhancement. One certainly does not decry philanthropy because it is much needed, particularly in times of governmental retrenchment in education, welfare, and the arts. But philanthropy can nevertheless be analyzed as a series of gestures that reinforce the status quo for the rich and prevent the stirring of guilt feelings each time they acquire a new Lear jet, a Jaguar, a Cartier diamond watch, or build a $25 million mansion. In a sense, philanthropy is the opiate of the rich.

It is certainly important to research the poor in order to alleviate their situation; but from a critical sociological perspective, there are two caveats. First, the saturation point where enough studies exist may have been reached. More research will not add to the quality of life of the poor. And, second, it would be equally important to research the rich because, after all, the situation of the poor is in their hands. Poverty will never be alleviated if the class system that has evolved is not redressed. The key to the problem of the widening gulf between the rich and the poor, short of a revolution, lies in reducing the accumulation and concentration of wealth. It has long been understood that the key to solving racial discrimination and the problems created by discrimination resides in bringing about changes within the dominant majority. (This, however, does not mean that minorities have no role to play in their self-improvement and harmonious intergroup relations.) Although it is not a new idea for Marxists, it is now necessary to understand in a more fundamental way that the key to solving poverty is found among the powerful and the corporations—not the poor.

REDUCING THE CONCENTRATION OF NEIGHBORHOOD POVERTY

In the meantime, it is urgent to redress the concentration of poverty in particular neighborhoods (Haveman and Wolfe, 1994). By now, the events of the past two decades have made it abundantly clear that building high-density housing complexes to warehouse the poor is a recipe for failure (Bickford and Massey, 1991). So many of these "projects" are now condemned and boarded up in American cities. These sites could provide space to build lower-density units and attractive developments geared for *all* income groups in order to retain the employed and attract the middle class so as to create a mix of social resources in the communities. These developments could include commercial facilities such as food and drug stores, as well as offices, and environmentally safe industries that would provide jobs and services to a more economically diverse community. At the same time, vouchers could substitute for government-subsidized housing in order to desegregate the poor.

In fact, housing vouchers could become downpayments for home ownership for the working poor families.[8] Home ownership by the disadvantaged would result in several societal and personal advantages.[9] First, homeowners are often more conscientious than renters who are more transient. They develop an interest in the quality of their lodging (thus curtailing vandalism) and their entire neighborhood, hence discouraging social disorganization and criminality. Second, home ownership would build a family's assets. Later on in life, this wealth could generate an income and prevent adults from becoming disadvantaged elderly. Home ownership may also create feelings of belongingness and stability, raise the level of social support from neighbors, and contribute to self-esteem and a sense of personal achievement as well as pride (Rohe and Stegman, 1994). In a study including black, white, and Hispanic youth, Hauser (1993) found that parental homeownership had a large effect on school retention and college entry, irrespective of parental social class. Recall here that, as reported in Chapter 7, other studies have established a positive correlation between health and homeownership, even holding income constant.

Thus, with neighborhoods becoming changed for the better, and with the displacment of only those who chose to move, then demands for a higher quality of education would follow. The area's tax base would increase, and so would the school boards' resources. The schools could then attract more qualified staff and raise the motivation level of students. We have already seen that disadvantaged children who attend schools in areas that are economically mixed do better than those in schools where the student body is largely indigent. Other advantages to reducing the concentration of poverty would follow. Not only would crime rates drop in the area but they would decrease for the entire city. A more invested populace would offer more avenues of legitimate activities for youth and would serve as a more effective force of social control. A more functional community would emerge that would supervise its youth more adequately, and in particular prevent the formation of male gangs who engage in illegal and dangerous activities.

Other invaluable approaches to alleviate poverty include more widespread programs offering a subsidy to workers in low-paid jobs so as to maintain them above the poverty level.[10] This might also allow the working poor to accumulate savings that could serve as a cushion in times of unemployment. In the United States, providing continuity of medical care, and universal health insurance, so that illnesses are attended to before they create more costly problems, is another invaluable approach to help the poor. Such programs exist but are not sufficiently widespread and may be in danger of being eliminated. The employed poor are more susceptible to job loss than others. In times of unemployment, these social guarantees would serve as an incentive for finding another job as quickly as possible.

It is worth pointing out, however, that the aspects of the above discussion that may concern employment, particularly that of mothers on welfare, are based on the currently-held notion that parents should be employed, and that caring for and raising children is not in itself a worthwhile occupation. As Risman and Ferree (1995:777) put it, "The core of the problem seems to be that the *society* does not value children and caregiving work enough to ensure the economic and social conditions in which it could be provided."[11] Other researchers correctly point out that forcing mothers to work fails to take into consideration the *children's* perspective and well-being (Wilson, Ellwood, and Brooks-Gunn, 1995). A mother who becomes employed in a frustrating job with a low salary, and who experiences problems with child care as well as with schedules, places her children at risk for not being properly provided for, nurtured, prepared for school, and supervised (Schor and Menaghan, 1995).

Mothers' allowances, as exist in Canada on a modest scale, should be viewed as a woman's salary to care for her children who are a society's future labor force and tax base. In this context, it makes sense to raise rather than lower welfare payments to ensure that children are sufficiently lifted out of poverty and do not repeat their parents' economic failures. It may well be argued that teenage mothers should not be paid to raise their children because, overall, they are not competent to raise any children, period. (No one would actually hire an eleven-to-sixteen-year-old nanny to care full-time for one's own children. This would not even constitute a legally acceptable arrangement.) But one could still seek other ways to prevent early childbearing and additional childbearing by young mothers without penalizing their children. Transfer payments in kind directed to the children themselves rather than the mothers, perhaps via early day care, after-school activities, and community organizations, should be considered.

THE GLOBAL PERSPECTIVE

The problem with most socioeconomic reforms is that results are not always guaranteed or immediately palpable. The investments may produce economic payoffs only later on in the adult lives of the current generations of youngsters—thus too long a delay for a politician's career. Long-term planning is not advantageous for politicians at the polling station as it may offend powerful interest groups vested in short-term gains and benefits. Currently, for several months before general elections, both countries, but even more so the United States, are held hostage to policy-making paralysis. Partisan politics takes over, and fear of losing votes rules the agenda. This is why suggested political reforms restricting a Canadian prime minister and an American president to a single but lengthier term in office are worthwhile proposals. Limiting the number of elected tenures to fewer but longer ones for other officials would similarly reduce the immediate political need to attend to one's reelection. It would increase the odds that elected officials would devote their energies to planning for the long-term interest of the nation. Prime ministers and presidents, limited to one tenure of six years, would be less vulnerable to powerful lobbies of interest groups. They would engage less in politics and more in policy making.

As shown throughout this text, eradicating or substantially reducing poverty can be accomplished only with multipronged reforms and investments. One should be cautious not to interpret the various suggestions discussed to mean that economic dependency can be totally eradicated, for it is the only option for those individuals who will never be able to take care of themselves. Nor is it implied that all individuals and all children would become problem-free were poverty largely eliminated. We are not talking of changing human nature here, but of giving all people a better chance to optimize their life opportunities. Eradicating poverty would not entirely eliminate school dropout, crime, or teenage pregnancy, but it would reduce these problems substantially (Haveman and Wolfe, 1994).

Some of these problems, such as crime and adolescent pregnancy, would further be reduced with the cooperation of the media, particularly television, films, and videos. For, indeed, it is difficult to see how economic factors alone are responsible for the spectacular increase of so many social problems since the 1960s—particularly so because most social problems increased during a period of rapid economic growth (Wethington, 1996). Cultural and social factors enter into play. Some of these social factors no doubt center on the family (Ambert, 1997a). But the family does not function in a vacuum,[12] so that addressing economic, social, cultural, and technological conditions would provide a better structure within which families and their members can function and actualize their potentials.

Glossary

active genotype-environment correlation: This term is used by behavior geneticists to refer to situations whereby individuals choose opportunities and environments that reinforce their predispositions.

acute illness: Consists of one episode that ends by treatment or is self-limited. Examples are the flu or appendicitis. In contrast, a chronic illness persists.

assortative mating: Refers to the theory that people select spouses or mates in a nonrandom fashion. In the case of homogamy, they marry persons who are similar to them on a given characteristic. The characteristic may be physical appearance, IQ, values, one or several personality traits, or even SES. The opposite of homogamy is heterogamy. The opposite of assortative mating is random mating.

authoritarian parenting: Refers to parental behaviors and attitudes that are predominantly controlling and punishing. At the extreme, they can be even harsh and rejecting. The authoritarian approach does not appeal to a child's sense of reasoning or morality. It is a "do-as-I-say or you'll get smacked" type of upbringing. Authoritarian parents may also be inconsistent: they may threaten to punish but do not follow through with the punishment.

authoritative parenting: Combines both warmth and monitoring of children's activities and whereabouts. Authoritative parents make maturity demands on their children. They explain to their children the reasons behind their demands or rules; their method is inductive. Once they have explained the reasons and the consequences, they consistently follow through with enforcement of those rules.

cohort: A group of people who were born around the same time and who therefore go through life experiencing similar sociohistorical conditions. For example, people born during the Great Depression form a cohort.

configuration of traits: The form of personality that several traits take when combined.

correlations: Correlations exist between two factors or variables, such as poverty and violence when, as one increases or decreases, the other also changes. When both change in the same direction (e.g., both increase), this is a positive correlation. A negative correlation exists when one factor increases at the same time that the other decreases, as in the example of an increasing number of cases of delinquency with a decreasing level of socioeconomic status. Correlation is a statistical test.

covariables: Are variables (such as health and visits to the doctor) that vary together, covary, in the presence of another set of variables. Covariables "hang together." *To covary* is the verb form.

cross-pressures: A term used in child development to mean that a child or an adolescent is subjected to influences that oppose each other. This concept applies particularly to parents and peers who may both influence or pressure a child toward opposite goals. Parents may teach the value of hard work while peers may put pressure on a youngster to "party" rather than study.

dizygotic twins: Fraternal twins. Twins that result from two ova fertilized by two spermatozoa.

downard mobility: A type of *social mobility* (which is the passage from one social stratum to another, or from one social class to another). Downward mobility occurs when individuals fall below their parents' stratum (intergenerational mobility) or below the one they have themselves occupied earlier (intragenerational mobility). *Upward mobility* is the opposite.

dysfunctional: This adjective is used in this text to describe both behaviors, persons, and social situations. Dysfunctional behaviors are those that impair a person's functioning and success. They are maladaptive either for society, a particular group, or the person concerned—or all of these. The concept can be applied to social structures and opportunities.

GATT: General Agreement on Tariffs and Trade.

GDP: Gross Domestic Product refers to the dollar value of all final goods and services produced within a country in a given year.

genetic loading: When several relatives share the same personality trait or illness, a high genetic loading exists. When only one person in an extended family suffers from an illness, the genetic loading is low. However, a more appropriate term may be "familial" loading. In this text, this term is used to mean that the greater the number of genes leading to a particular trait that a person has inherited, the greater that person's own genetic loading for that trait.

genotype-environment correlations: See **active, passive,** and **reactive** genotype-environment correlations.

GNP: Gross National Product refers to the dollar value of all final goods and services produced by residents of a country both within the country and abroad. This includes investment income that citizens of a country receive from other countries.

goodness of fit: A concept that is used to describe how a child's personality characteristics fit environmental demands. Or, conversely, how environmental demands, such as family rules and school requirements, agree with a person's temperament. There is a lack of fit when the two do not conform to each other easily; maladjustment is likely to occur. (This term is used with an entirely different meaning in statistics.)

homogamy: See assortative mating.

ideology: Refers to a set of beliefs concerning a social situation and how it should be, or how it should be corrected. These beliefs are generally shared by a group of people and guide their behavior or at least their thinking concerning that particular situation. Groups can hold ideologies pertaining to race relations, welfare, international politics, gender relations, etc.

incidence: Refers to new cases of a specific health problem, illness, emotional disorders, mortality, or criminality within a specific time period, generally a one-year period.

indicator: Indicators are used to measure variables, such as poverty. They are sentences, numbers, or observations that serve to illustrate a variable. Indicators are often coded (or given a number) to derive statistics. An indicator of educational attainment is the number of years of schooling a person has received.

longitudinal studies (or designs): Consist of studying the same people over time. For instance, people may be interviewed at age

18 and restudied again at age 25 and then 35. This research design contrasts with cross-sectional or one-time studies and surveys. A synonym is panel studies.

manic depression (or bipolar depression): A very serious mental illness that is partly hereditary. It involves a loss of contact with reality and shifts over time from a depressed state to a highly excited (manic) state—or the predominance of such a state. In the manic phase, the persons are hyperactive, elated, at times loud and aggressive, and may need to be sedated because they could be dangerous to themselves or to others. In the depressed mode, the persons may feel hopeless, helpless, alone, and have suicidal ideation.

monozygotic twins: Identical twins originating from one ovum fertilized by one sperm, which separates to produce identical embryos.

morbidity: The presence of illness or psychiatric disorder.

multivariate: Refers to a statistical analysis that includes more than two variables. For instance, in studying the effect of poverty on children's school achievement, a researcher may need to include the length of time spent in poverty, the ages of children during poverty, quality of neighborhood, and family conditions.

NAFTA: North American Free Trade Agreement between Canada, the United States, and Mexico.

OPEC: Organization of Petroleum Exporting Countries treaty signed in 1960 by several countries in the Middle East (including Saudi Arabia and Libya), and others elsewhere in the world (including Indonesia, Ecuador, and Venezuela). Their goal was to obtain a better price for their oil products.

passive genotype-environment correlation: A concept used by behavior geneticists to explain the similarity that exists between biological parents and children on certain traits. This similarity leads to childrearing practices that correlate with certain child outcomes, such as aggressiveness or cooperation, because parents and children share both genes and a family environment in part created by these same genes.

prevalence: Refers to the number of cases of a specific health problem, illness, emotional disorder, mortality, or delinquency existing within a specific time period, generally a one-year period. Therefore, prevalence includes new cases as well as cases that had occurred in the previous period and are continuing in the current period. For instance, the prevalence of poor families for the year 1998 includes the number of new cases occurring in 1998 in addition to the number of cases continuing from 1997. As for new cases, it includes both those which last for the rest of the year and those which recover.

prevalent: An adjective that refers to a phenomenon that is widespread.

producer services: Services to producing firms, including manufacturers. These services may be legal, financial, consultative, accounting, and advertising.

reactive genotype-environment correlation: A term used by behavior geneticists for situations where people's (e.g., parents, teachers, peers) reactions to a person are influenced or determined by the person's characteristics, abilities, and behaviors (or misbehaviors).

schizophrenia: A very severe mental illness characterized by various degrees of distancing or withdrawal from reality as it is perceived by others. Interpersonal difficulties are also present. The more severe forms involve hallucinations (hearing voices and seeing things), delusions, loss of contact with one's bodily needs and with external reality, inability to care for oneself, rigid body mannerisms, and inability to initiate or maintain relationships.

social selection: Refers to theories that explain the high rates of mental or physical illness found within low-income groups as a result of individuals being selected into this lower status because of their deficiencies or illnesses. Similarly, these theories explain the higher, average IQ of upper-middle class members as a result of individuals being selected because of their merits or being able to maintain their high-level position because of their merits.

socioeconomic status, or SES: The ranking of people on a scale of prestige for occupation, income, and education. Often used as a synonym or proxy for social class.

systemic: Refers to a problem that is built into a system, an institution, or a society. Solutions to such problems require a restructuring of the institution, a difficult enterprise at best.

unipolar depression or **simple depression:** Contains some elements of hopelessness, helplessness, aloneness, feelings of being
worthless, and, at the extreme, suicidal ideation. Contrary to
manic depression, it does not generally involve a cognitive break
with reality or insanity. People may be depressed off and on in
their lives; others may suffer only one episode and live normally
thereafter. In the latter case, it is a matter of *reactive* depression
caused by severe stressors rather than a consequence of genetic
predisposition. Simple depression, particularly the reactive type,
is far more common than manic depression because it is largely
produced by an accumulation of stressors. It is prevalent among
the poor.

Reference Notes

Chapter 1

1. The average income of residents in the poorest countries was $200 in 1989 or 1 percent of the average income of the dozen richest countries (Vogt, Cameron, and Dolan, 1991).
2. World Bank, 1993; see also Dixon and Drakakis-Smith, 1993.
3. LeVine et al., 1991.
4. Linhares, Round, and Jones, 1986.
5. Sawhill, 1988.
6. U.S. Bureau of the Census, 1995.
7. Duncan, Smeeding, and Rodgers, 1993.
8. Devine and Wright, 1993:50.
9. As reported by Mayer and Jencks, 1993.
10. Statistics Canada, 1993b.
11. Lenski, 1966; Nielsen and Alderson, 1995.
12. See also Margolin and Schor, 1990.
13. U.S. Bureau of the Census, 1991; Haggerty and Johnson, 1996.
14. Canada Year Book, 1993:197.
15. Economic Council of Canada, 1992:6.
16. Economic Council of Canada, 1992.
17. Economic Council of Canada, 1992:22.
18. Colin et al., 1992.
19. Lichter, Johnston, and McLaughlin, 1994. As explained by Flora et al. (1992:8), nonmetropolitan areas are now "broken down into six categories based on size (urbanized, less urbanized, and rural) and location (adjacent or nonadjacent to urban areas)."
20. Also, see Rank and Hirschl, 1993.
21. Gadsden, 1995.

Chapter 2

1. European Union or EEC (European Economic Community).
2. Mercusor, or the Southern Common Market, is a new free-trade zone involving several South American countries. It is not given as much publicity as the other free trade agreements, yet its potential is enormous.
3. Sassen, 1991.
4. See also Canadian Urban Institute, 1993; City of Toronto, 1990.

5. See Romo and Schwartz, 1995.

6. Gottschalk and Moffitt, 1994.

7. Katz and Murphy, 1991.

8. See Sheets, Nord, and Phelps, 1987.

9. See also Devine and Wright, 1993:34.

10. Part-time work that is year round is also related to poverty.

11. *Toronto Star*, Aug. 31, 1996.

12. Devine and Wright, 1993.

13. See also Juhn, Murphy, and Pierce, 1993.

14. The State does invest to some extent in children via schooling, health care, and social assistance. More pertinent is the distinction between society and economy by Wintersberger (1994). He also points out that, "The economy does not invest in but only benefits from children; and families, in contrast, invest in children without benefitting materially. Part of the economic surplus in developed industrial societies is based on the colonization of the family where parents—and in particular, women—work as unpaid volunteers" (1994:234).

15. Statistics from the Canadian Center for Policy Alternatives quoted in the *Toronto Star*, July 20, 1996, p. 1.

16. For the same reasons, several American subsidiaries have relocated to Mexico.

17. U.S. Bureau of the Census, 1994.

18. On the whole, females drop out less than males. When they do, it is often as a result of childbirth which also keeps them from the labor market, hence their higher rates of unemployment.

19. Haines, 1989.

20. Panel on High-Risk Youth, 1993.

21. Abbott and Beach, 1993; Baker and Benjamin, 1994, 1995.

22. The necessity to delimit the contents of this chapter certainly does not allow me to document the extent to which corporations, helped by advanced technology, government subsidies ("corporate welfare"), and economic ideology contribute to social inequality and poverty. The ideology of the necessity of economic growth to resolve poverty merely serves corporations' interests and depletes natural resources the world over. For a complementary text, see Korten, 1995.

Chapter 3

1. See Schiller, 1995, for a discussion and critique of "flawed character" theories.

2. In fact, corporations now resort to legal suits against the media that expose their deficient products or their unethical dealings. This tactic (which only the rich can afford) protects them because the other corporations that are the media's parent companies are growing reluctant to pay the costs of lengthy court procedures and settlements.

3. Statistics Canada, 1992; U.S. Bureau of the Census, 1992b:55. For the United Kingdom, see General Household Survey, 1992.

4. U.S. Bureau of the Census, 1992b. The percentages are nearly identical in the United Kingdom (Roberts, 1995).

5. U.S. Bureau of the Census, 1990a.

6. Bennett, Bloom, and Craig, 1989; Tucker and Mitchell-Kernan, 1995.

7. Stokes and Chevan, 1996; Wilson, 1987.

8. U.S. Bureau of the Census, 1995:D22.

9. The poverty floors are higher in Canada than in the United States, thus producing comparatively higher poverty rates in Canada than if the U.S. cutoffs were used. In the United Kingdom in 1987, 70 percent of children in single-parent families were poor or living at the margin of poverty (Blackburn, 1991).

10. See also Lichter and Landale, 1995; Miranda, 1991.

11. U.S. Bureau of the Census, 1990a.

12. Hernandez (1993:290) concludes that mother-only families contribute to raising the percentage of children living in poverty. However, were the poverty rate of single-mother families no higher than that of two-parent families (as is the case in Holland), children's poverty would diminish.

13. Single mothers are more often unemployed than married mothers, have a lower educational level, on average, and fewer own their homes. In Canada, while 79 percent of two-parent families own their homes, 30 percent of female-headed families do. Moreover, they tend to own homes that are older and in worse condition (Lindsay, 1994). Among renters, 15 percent of single parents have difficulties paying the rent (Lo and Gauthier, 1995).

14. Statistics Canada, 1993.

15. Economic Council of Canada, 1992.

16. See a discussion to the effect that welfare policies have contributed to this increase (Jewell, 1988) and so has the disaggregation of multigenerational female-headed households (Sudarkasa, 1997).

17. Norton and Moorman, 1987.

18. Hoffman, Foster, and Furstenberg, 1993; Maynard, 1995; U.S. Department of Health and Human Services, 1995.

19. See the section titled Mobility Out of and Back into Poverty in Chapter 1 for additional data.

20. Chase-Lansdale, Brooks-Gunn, and Zamsky, 1991.

21. Amato, 1993; Burgoyne, Ormrod, and Richards, 1987; McLanahan and Sandefur, 1994.

22. Le Blanc and Fréchette, 1989; Matsueda and Heimer, 1987; Sampson, 1987.

23. Mulkey, Crain, and Harrington, 1992; Thompson, Alexander, and Entwisle, 1988. The reasons for the lower achievement of children from single-parent families may, however, vary depending on the gender of the custodial parent. Economic factors may be more important in mother-headed families (Downey, 1994).

24. Thornton, 1991.

25. Kahn and Anderson, 1992; Manlove, 1997; McLanahan and Bumpass, 1988; Wu, 1996.

26. Zill, Morrison, and Coiro, 1993.

27. Amato and Keith, 1991.

28. Friedman et al., 1995; Schwartz et al., 1995.

29. For example, for Canada, see Ambert and Saucier, 1984.

30. Hetherington, 1993; Hetherington, Clingempeel et al., 1992; Thomson, McLanahan, and Curtin, 1992.

31. See Bumpass, Martin, and Sweet, 1991.

32. These statements do not apply to home ownership in degraded neighborhoods, where owners may find it more profitable to abandon or burn down their houses than to repair them (Fernandez Kelly, 1995).

33. One of the best studies in this domain was carried out by Jencks et al. (1979). What is particularly innovative in these researchers' approach is their use of samples of brothers, which allowed them to assess the effect of the family background as well as individual effects which geneticists often examine in their studies.

34. See p. 64 of Chapter 3.

35. For a complementary perspective, see Turner, Wheaton, and Lloyd, 1995.

Chapter 4

1. There are indications that rural poverty has worse consequences in some domains, such as health, than urban poverty. Moreover, some of these consequences may differ by race, with poor blacks being more content in rural than in urban areas and the reverse occurring among poor whites (Amato and Zuo, 1992).

2. This methodological problem also exists for rural areas. See Flora et al., 1992.

3. See Bursik and Grasmick (1993) for neighborhood definition.

4. Toronto is the most ethnically and racially diverse city in the world; 50 percent of immigrants to Canada eventually settle in Toronto and its suburbs.

5. This type of minute segregation, in three to five buildings, would make it extremely difficult to test the theories described in this chapter pertaining to high-poverty areas.

6. Panel on High-Risk Youth, 1993:66.

7. See McAdoo, 1997.

8. Dandurand, 1996.

9. Single-parent households are not problematic in themselves. The problem arises when they coreside or corrrelate with poverty and criminality.

10. Gramlich, Laren, and Sealand, 1992; Kasarda, 1990.

11. Safer locations also bring about lower insurance premiums.

12. Wallace and Wallace, 1990.

13. Smith and Jarjoura, 1988; Taylor and Covington, 1988.

14. This section is complemented by sections pertaining to parenting activities in Chapters 6 and 7.

15. See Chapter 5.

16. See Jencks and Mayer, 1990, for a discussion.

17. Brooks-Gunn et al., 1993; Dornbusch, Ritter, and Steinberg, 1991.
18. Rosenbaum et al., 1993
19. See also Connelly et al., 1995; Corcoran et al., 1992; Crane, 1991. However, being poor in a middle-class neighborhood may carry *other* costs such as deficient self-esteem, lower popularity, and feelings of relative deprivation. In fact, being economically disadvantaged is related to peer rejection at school (Pettit et al., 1996). This fairly consistent result, however, occurs in studies that generally do not control for the proportion of children who are disadvantaged in a school or neighborhood, a serious flaw for the purpose of our discussion.
20. Yet the same authors report that there is "not much support for the harmful effect of poor neighborhoods" (Ensminger, Lamkin, and Jacobson, 1996:2412). Obviously, much remains to be studied.
21. One could also argue that, if the parents are otherwise conforming, and children are unaware of their activities, the illicit income could raise the family above the poverty level and thus help children in some ways. This, of course, also assumes that the parents in question are never apprehended.
22. As for many of the theoretical propositions in this chapter, there is no research testing this hypothesis.
23. In this respect, several researchers from different disciplines currently converge, although the terminology they use is somewhat different. One can think here of Steinberg et al.'s (1995) peers' parents' authoritativeness, Sampsons (1997) community social control, Brooks-Gunn et al.'s (1995) collective socialization, and Coleman and Hoffer's (1987) functional community.
24. This also applies to the two largest Canadian cities of Toronto and Montreal. However, because criminal statistics do not include race, one has to depend on an analysis of daily newscasts and visits to jails to compile relevant data.
25. Homelessness is discussed at greater length in Chapter 7.
26. Tessler and Dennis, 1989.
27. Wright, 1989.

Chapter 5

1. This section does not apply equally well to Canada.
2. Hoover-Dempsey, Bassler, and Brissie, 1987.
3. See also Shields and Shaver, 1991.
4. Ashton-Warner, 1963; Grannis, 1994; Lightfoot, 1978; Rumberger and Larson, 1994—all excellent examples of programs that are organized to make the children profit from their own cultural or class background.
5. Boykin, 1994; Carini, 1982.
6. The current debate on Ebonics is relevant to this issue. By "current" is meant as of time of writing completion of this book, that is, July 1997.
7. Hoover-Dempsey, Bassler, and Brissie, 1987.
8. Good et al., 1987.
9. Jackson, 1997; Marotto, 1986.
10. Gartner and Lipsky, 1987; Mitman and Lash, 1988.

11. Mitchell, 1997; Mullis et al., 1991.

12. Finn, 1989.

13. Venezky, Kaestle, and Sum, 1987.

14. Dornbusch et al., 1987; Fehrman, Keith, and Reimer, 1987.

15. Stevenson and Baker, 1987.

16. On the latter point, Sui-Chu and Willms (1996) found no difference by SES.

17. The concept of human capital is found as early as 1961 in the writings of economists such as Schultz (1961) and Becker (1964).

18. David Oldman (1994:54) points out that middle-class children "bring to the school system significant amounts of cultural and economic capital generated within their families of origin. The teachers of middle-class children are, in effect, getting something for nothing."

19. Astone and McLanahan, 1991; Baker and Stevenson, 1986.

20. Canadian Teachers' Federation, 1989.

21. Kohn, Slomczynski, and Schoenbach, 1986.

22. Parents' occupational changes are also accompanied by changes in child-rearing values (Kohn and Schooler, 1983).

23. A more recent study by Orfield (reference unknown) indicates increasing segregation in general.

24. Such a situation could carry long-term or life course disadvantages even when it is accompanied by an increase in test scores while the students are in school.

25. This typology applies not only to the North American situation, but internationally as well.

26. See Portes and MacLeod, 1996.

27. See Knapp and Shields, 1991, among others.

Chapter 6

1. Blake, 1989; Shavit and Pierce, 1991.

2. Dryfoos, 1982; Perlman, Klerman, and Kinard, 1981.

3. However, in 1995 and 1996, single American women's birth rate declined slightly each year.

4. Abrahamse, Morrison, and Waite, 1988.

5. It certainly is not the only adaptation to poverty available; for instance, one could argue that delaying childbearing and remaining in school can also be adaptations to poverty—and very effective ones at that.

6. Sandfort and Hill, 1996.

7. Helm et al., 1990; Lamb and Elster, 1990.

8. This may be especially so for younger compared with older children; Nitz, Ketterlinus, and Brandt, 1995.

9. Borkowski et al. , 1992; Ketterlinus, Henderson, and Lamb, 1991.

10. There is some literature indicating that, at least in the early 1980s, black teen mothers were more likely than older black mothers to seek prenatal care and

to have fewer LBW infants, while the opposite held among whites (Geronimus and Bound, 1990). Although this study is contradicted by larger studies (e.g., Friede et al., 1987), it later led Geronimus (1991) to posit that early pregnancies are a sound reproductive strategy among blacks because the health of women of childbearing age deteriorates very rapidly compared to that of whites (Geronimus, Andersen, and Bound, 1991). Furstenberg (1992:240) argues correctly that this thesis understates the costs of early childbearing.

11. Strobino, 1987. For a review of the literature on some sequelae to very low birth weight, see Zelkowitz et al., 1995.

12. Elder, Caspi, and Burton, 1988: 17 percent in their study.

13. There is a vast literature on adolescence and several journals focus specifically on this topic, for example: *Adolescence, Journal of Adolescence, Journal of Early Adolescence, Journal of Adolescence Research, Journal of Research on Adolescents.* In addition, *Journal of Marriage and the Family,* and *Family Relations* regularly publish on adolescence.

14. See Chapter 10.

15. For an exception, see Elster and Lamb, 1986.

16. Anderson, 1989.

17. However, such correlations do not mean that spousal abuse, particularly wife abuse, does not occur among the rich.

18. See, for example, Patterson, 1988.

19. Corse, Schmidt, and Trickett, 1990.

20. This correlation may, however, stem in part from negative genetic predispositions shared between parents and children.

21. On the intergenerational transmission of abuse, see Ambert, 1997, Chapter 10.

22. See also Minty and Pattinson, 1994.

23. For a presentation and critique of the research on parenting patterns, see Ambert, 1997a, Chapter 3.

24. Belsky, Fish, and Isabella, 1991; Cowan, Cowan, and Kerig, 1992; Gable, Belsky, and Crnic, 1992.

25. McLoyd, 1995.

26. See also Bronfenbrenner and Weiss, 1983.

Chapter 7

1. Starrels, Bould, and Nicholas, 1994.

2. Ehrenreich, Sklar, and Stollard, 1985.

3. See the interesting discussion by Pratto et al., 1997.

4. Lack of respect for impoverished mothers and consequent loss of authority is a phenomenon I observed firsthand in the 1980s in a study comparing poor and affluent custodial mothers: Ambert, 1982.

5. Here as well, during past and recent fieldwork, several mothers have reported being verbally abused and even physically taunted by adolescent children on the basis that "You're just a scum bag" (when they had a boyfriend); or

"No man wants you," or "You're just a poor ugly old bag" (when they did not have a boyfriend).

6. The matter of the *quality* of the peer group is quite important because a part of this literature links "improper" parenting practices with child rejection by peers in school. See Asher and Coie, 1990.

7. The emphasis is on "frequently" as opposed to "always." See Abell et al., 1996; Rosier and Corsaro, 1993.

8. See Alwin, 1986, for instance.

9. Meanwhile, parents' authority and effectiveness, paradoxically enough, are undermined by various media, professionals, and institutions (Ambert, 1992, 1997a; Engelbert, 1994). As Bardy (1994:307) puts it, "The professionals are supposed to support the parents, but the parents may well feel obliged to support the work of the professionals."

10. See also Mitchell, 1991; Smith, 1989. For international data on child poverty, particularly among European countries, consult the various national reports issued from the European Centre in Vienna. Notably, see Saporiti and Sgritta, 1990. For Quebec, see Bouchard et al., 1991.

11. In terms of numbers, this translates into 14 million American children and one million Canadian children who were poor in1994 (Lindsey, 1994).

12. Rural black children, who generally live in the south, are even poorer: 53 percent are (Sherman, 1992).

13. The same situation exists in the United States. In 1991, 40 percent of American poor children belonged to two-parent families (U.S. Bureau of the Census, 1993c).

14. National Council of Welfare, 1993.

15. Bolger, Patterson, and Thompson, 1995; Klerman and Parker, 1991.

16. Elder et al., 1992; Patterson, Reid, and Dishion, 1992; Zill and Coiro, 1992.

17. For a review of the effect of poverty on children, see Chase-Lansdale and Brooks-Gunn, 1995; Zill et al., 1995.

18. Toro et al., 1995; Toro and Wall, 1991.

19. National Coalition for the Homeless, 1989; U.S. Conference of Mayors, 1989.

20. Also cited in Rafferty and Shinn, 1991.

21. Also cited in Rafferty and Shinn, 1991.

22. On child malnourishment in general, see Karp, 1993.

23. National Council of Welfare, 1989.

24. American Association of Retired Persons, 1990.

25. As pointed out earlier, the elevated Canadian rates stem in part from higher poverty lines.

26. Quinn and Smeeding, 1994.

27. National Council of Welfare, 1989.

28. Congressional Research Service, 1987.

29. Studies indicate that daughters more than sons take the responsibility to care for their elderly parents: Spitze and Logan, 1991.

Chapter 8

1. The social classification of people according to their race is a problem in itself. See Gates and Cardozo, 1997.

2. The 1986 data indicated that blacks formed only 0.7 percent of the total Canadian population (Kalbach, 1990). This proportion has since increased markedly in some cities.

3. This section continues and complements sections in Chapter 4. See Marks, 1989.

4. It should be noted, however, that many higher-income blacks moved to fairly racially segregated suburbs with a lower average income than suburbs inhabited by whites or Asians (Logan and Alba, 1993).

5. By this, it is not meant that racism is no longer important but only that, currently, economic conditions in general and in the ghettos may have taken precedence over historical factors.

6. PSID (Panel Study of Income Dynamics) households.

7. U.S. Bureau of the Census, 1992a. See also Browne, 1997.

8. As McAdoo (1997: 146) puts it, "Few Black families have wealth to pass on to their children. Each generation thus must recreate the mobility cycle and generate the effort necessary to succeed and move upward again."

9. Status Indians are those recognized as Natives by the Canadian government. They benefit from certain privileges such as hunting and fishing rights as well as exemptions from most taxes. Status Indians have to be registered and overwhelmingly live on reserves or, after they move, retain their link to their bands. Thus, Native ethnicity does not overlap entirely with being a Status or registered Native.

10. There are many exceptions, particularly in isolated pockets of rural white poverty.

11. However, such a statement may apply to certain outcomes more than others.

12. Ogbu, 1991.

13. Surveys indicate that employers seek employees who can communicate effectively, think critically, can easily be trained, demonstrate positive attitudes and behaviors, are adaptable and responsible, and can work well with others (Conference Board of Canada, 1992; Holzer, 1996).

14. Granovetter, 1985.

15. See also Bound and Freeman (1992) on the erosion of employment among young black men.

16. *Maclean's*, September 2, 1996, p. 10.

17. But see Maxim (1992) concerning visible minorities and self-employment.

18. Krieger, 1990; Krieger et al., 1993.

19. Geronimus, Andersen, and Bound, 1991.

20. Council on Ethical and Judicial Affairs, AMA, 1990.

21. See also Krieger, 1990.

22. Canadian Institute of Child Health, 1994:143.

23. Hahn, Mulinare, and Teutsch, 1992.

24. Except among Mexican Americans, which will be discussed later in this section.

25. U.S. Department of Justice, 1985.

Chapter 9

1. Caldwell, 1986. See also discussion in Tesh, 1988.

2. Marmot et al., 1991.

3. The best and most comprehensive studies have been carried out in Great Britain: Smith and Eggers, 1992. For a critique of this literature on the grounds that it fails to include biologically predetermined conditions, see Marsland and Leoussi, 1996.

4. Townsend and Davidson, 1990; Wilkinson, 1992a, 1992b.

5. Sapolsky, 1990.

6. See Ross and Wu, 1995 and 1996, for a review and new data on education; Linn, Sandifer, and Stein, 1985, for data on employment; Blackburn, 1991, for social class; Ross and Huber, 1985, for income; Ford et al., 1991; Winkleby et al., 1992, for lifestyle. See also Fox, 1989; Power, Manor, and Fox, 1991.

7. Rural Sociological Society Task Force on Persistent Rural Poverty, 1993.

8. Leon and Wilkinson, 1988; Wilkinson, 1992a, 1992b.

9. For similar results in Great Britain, see Carstairs and Morris, 1989.

10. See discussion by Earls, Escobar, and Manson, 1990.

11. Cuba's infant mortality rate also falls within this category as a result of the availability of education, universal prenatal health care, and pediatric care.

12. Canada Year Book, 1993:110.

13. See also Farmer, Clarke, and Miller, 1993.

14. Marmor, 1992.

15. Wachs, 1996.

16. Harris, 1991; Cohen, Tyrell, and Smith, 1993.

17. Unemployment carries differential health consequences depending on the availability of employment in a given district and the person's own capital (Turner, 1995).

18. Winkleby, Fortmann, and Barrett, 1990; Matthews et al., 1989.

19. Ford et al., 1991; Kahn, Williamson, and Stevens, 1991; Statistics Canada, 1994.

20. Canadian Institute of Child Health, 1994:27. Multiple births have increased because of the use of fertility drugs, the implantation of multiple embryos, and the greater number of women who give birth after thirty-five, an age when the risk of releasing more than one ovum increases.

21. Psychiatric problems include, among many others, **manic depression** and schizophrenia, as well as lesser problems such as simple depression and anxiety.

22. Bruce, Takeuchi, and Leaf, 1991; Hamilton et al., 1990; Peirce et al. 1994.

23. Dohrenwend et al., 1980; Hollingshead and Redlich, 1958; Kessler et al., 1984; Srole et al., 1968.

24. Social selection or drift versus social causation theories: Dohrenwend et al., 1992.

25. Nor is it implied that their children will unavoidably become mentally ill. See Ambert, 1997a.

26. National Institute of Mental Health, 1986.

27. Apfel and Handel, 1993.

28. Hawton and Rose, 1986; Kessler, Turner, and House, 1988; Ross and Huber, 1985; Warr, 1985.

29. As McCormack (1997) further points out, the research on fetal alcohol syndrome is quite fragmented and rarely considers the totality of a woman's poverty and health status. Such "syndromes" show that the helping professions sustain "their own status on the backs of vulnerable women—a classic case of having a solution without a problem" (p. 4).

30. Jencks et al., 1979; Waller, 1971.

31. Office of Technology Assessment, 1988.

32. See the discussion by Barker, 1990, compared with Elford, Whincup, and Shaper, 1991.

33. See also Davey Smith and Shipley, 1991.

34. Kitchen et al., 1991.

Chapter 10

1. Caspi and Moffit, 1991; Sampson and Laub, 1993.

2. Farrington, 1991a; Lewis, Robins, and Rice, 1985.

3. Males are generally studied, but there is no reason that this does not apply to females as well, albeit with different profiles of offending perhaps (Moffitt, 1994).

4. For reference to these theories, an introductory text to criminality and juvenile delinquency is suggested. For the theorists themselves, see Agnew and White, 1992; Bursik, 1988; Gottfredson and Hirschi, 1990; Luckenbill and Doyle, 1989; Sampson, 1997; and Warr, 1993, to name only a few.

5. For various etiological perspectives, see Caspi et al., 1994; Grasmick et al., 1993; Kolvin et al., 1988a and 1988b; Loeber and Stouthamer-Loeber, 1986; Moffitt, Lynam, and Silva, 1994; Robins et al.,1996; Rowe and Gulley, 1992; Sampson and Groves, 1989; Warr, 1993; Warr and Stafford, 1991; Zingraff et al., 1994.

6. This finding probably applies to many other Western nations. For instance, it applies to New Zealand and Australia, as well as to Francophones in Quebec.

7. Fergusson, Horwood, and Lynskey, 1994; Wilson and Herrnstein, 1985.

8. Ensminger, Kellam, and Rubin, 1983; Kupersmidt et al., 1995.

9. Werthamer-Larsson, Kellam, and Wheeler, 1991.

10. As they do in families that are conflictual (Tschann et al., 1996).

11. Taylor and Covington, 1988.

12. See Attar, Guerra, and Tolan, 1994; Shakoor and Chalmers, 1991. Wilson, 1987:59.

13. Reiss, 1986.

14. Peeples and Loeber, 1994, quoted in Tonry, 1995:130.

15. Fishman, Rattner, and Weimann, 1987.

16. See review by Hagan, 1994:147-151.

17. Smith, Devine, and Sheley, 1992.

18. With a consideration of the caveats in Cloward and Ohlin's (1960) differential opportunity theory.

19. Skogan, 1990.

20. Schuerman and Kobrin, 1986.

21. See also Laub and Sampson, 1993.

22. See also Hagedorn, 1988.

23. See Ambert, 1997, Chapter 2.

24. Children and adults in the lower-SES group watch television more than among the more educated groups (Wartella, 1995).

Chapter 11

1. For critiques, see Lieberman, 1995; Fraser, 1995. See also Murray, 1995.

2. There are several differences between sociobiology (often with a focus on evolution) and behavior genetics.

3. Goldsmith, 1993.

4. Cairns, McGuire, and Gariepy, 1993; Kendler, 1995a.

5. A long digression would be required to discuss the pros and cons of IQ tests and the several issues surrounding what constitutes intelligence.

6. Cavalli-Sforza and Feldman, 1973.

7. Pike et al., 1996.

8. This is in part related to recessive genes.

9. The term "correlations" used here does not have the same meaning as the one used in statistics. For the latter, see **correlations** in Glossary.

10. It should be recollected from an earlier chapter, however, that harsh parenting practices do not unavoidably lead to aggressiveness in children, even when the children are genetically predisposed to be aggressive. Parents may discipline harshly but be otherwise loving and be perceived as such by their children, hence precluding the actualization of aggressiveness in children. This outcome will be even more likely if they live in a peaceful neighborhood and are not subjected to television violence.

11. Patterson and Capaldi, 1991.

12. Friedman et al. (1995), using the death certificates of the respondents in the longitudinal study initiated by Terman in 1921 (Terman and Oden, 1947) on gifted children, found that those who had been impulsive children had both more often been divorced and had died younger. Adults who had been prudent and conscientious as children had a 30 percent lower likelihood of dying at any year.

13. Accidents may have a genetic component, probably created by physiological and personality characteristics such as motor coordination and risk taking. Phillips and Matheny (1993; referred to in Plomin, 1994a) have found correla-

tions of 0.51 for monozygotic twins in terms of accidents in their first three years, compared with 0.13 for dizygotic (fraternal) twins.

14. Weatherall, 1992.

15. For a review of the research on resilient children, see Luthar, 1991.

16. Elder, 1985; Sampson and Laub, 1992.

17. Laub and Sampson, 1993; Magnusson and Bergman, 1990. See also Pulkkinen and Tremblay, 1992.

18. Innate characteristics are the ones we are born with. Some are genetic, thus hereditary, others are caused by intrauterine environmental factors, and others stem from accidents that occur during the birthing process.

19. Werner and Smith, 1982; Werner, 1990.

20. Kagan, 1994.

21. Farrington et al., 1988; McCord, 1988.

22. A refutation of Herrnstein and Murray's (1994) book, *The Bell Curve.*

23. As a scientific rebuttal of alleged black genetic inferiority, see the clever research article by Scarr et al., 1977; also Crane, 1994.

24. Mortality rates averaged 13 percent to 16 percent (Hagendorn, 1996).

25. The United States imported far fewer slaves than other colonies such as Brazil and the various Caribbean nations. Rather, slaves survived better in the United States than elsewhere because of more adequate treatment, nutrition, and health standards, as well as the absence of diseases that existed in the tropics. Thus, far fewer slaves had to be imported as the years went by, and their numbers increased through reproduction—mainly marital reproduction. Thus, although the United States imported only 6 percent of the slaves transported between 1500 and 1825 (compared with Brazil's proportion of 36 percent and the British Caribbeans' of 17 percent), by 1825, 36 percent of the slaves in the West lived in the United States (Fogel and Engerman, 1989).

Chapter 12

1. According to the World Economic Forum based in Geneva (Serrill, 1996), the ten most economically dynamic nations are all, except for the United States which has dropped to fourth place on the list, relatively small and more easily manageable: Singapore, Hong Kong, New Zealand, Luxembourg, Switzerland, Norway, Canada, Taiwan, and Malaysia.

2. Left aside are prescriptions and suggestions concerning the stimulation of job formation, education and training, as well as welfare reforms because most books on poverty discuss these at great length.

3. See Jencks and Peterson, 1991; Mincy, 1994. For a comprehensive definition of an underclass, see Jargowsky and Bane, 1990b:17. For the initial definition, see Ricketts and Sawhill, 1988.

4. In itself, the term subculture is value neutral: it can describe a negative or a positive phenomenon.

5. Murnane, Willett, and Levy, 1995. This point is also made in *The Bell Curve* by Herrnstein and Murray, 1994.

6. See also Townsend and Davidson, 1990:165.

7. A concept probably first introduced by M. Lind (1995), albeit with somewhat different connotations.

8. This concept is different from that of resident management of public housing. While some of these programs have been very successful, they do not necessarily alleviate the area's concentration of poverty.

9. South and Crowder (1997) point out that home ownership increases the likelihood that people will not leaver their poor neighborhood, which they see as a disadvantage.

10.See Rifkin, 1995, pp. 258 ff for a review. There is unfortunately a danger in government subsidies to the working poor: they provide employers with a rationale to maintain salaries at very low levels.

11. Italics in the original.

12. See Prilleltensky, 1997; also Cheal, 1996.

Bibliography

Abbott, M., and Beach, C. 1993. Immigrant earnings differentials and birth-year effects for men in Canada. *Canadian Journal of Economics*, 26, 505-524.

Abell, E., Clawson, M., Washington, W.N., Bost, K.K., and Vaughn, B.E. 1996. Parenting values, attitudes, behaviors, and goals of African American mothers from a low-income population in relation to social and societal contexts. *Journal of Family Issues*, 17, 593-613.

Abrahamse, A.F., Morrison, P.A., and Waite, L.J. 1988. *Beyond stereotypes: Who becomes a single teenage mother?* Report R-3489-HH5/NICHD. Santa Monica, CA: The Rand Corporation.

Aday, L.A. 1993. *At risk in America*. San Francisco: Jossey-Bass.

Adler, N.E., Boyce, T., Chesney, M.A., Cohen, S., Folkman, S., and Kahn, R. 1994. Socioeconomic status and health. The challenge of the gradient. *American Psychologist*, 49, 15-24.

Agnew, R. and White, H.R. 1992. An empirical test of general strain theory. *Criminology*, 30, 475-499.

Alexander, K.L., Entwisle, D.R., and Dauber, S.L. 1994. *On the success of failure*. Cambridge, UK: Cambridge University Press.

Alwin, D.F. 1986. From obedience to autonomy: Changes in traits desired in children, 1924-1978. *Public Opinion Quarterly*, 52, 33-52.

Amato, P.R. 1993. Children's adjustments to divorce: Theories, hypotheses and empirical support. *Journal of Marriage and the Family*, 55, 23-38.

Amato, P.R., and Keith, B. 1991. Parental divorce and adult well-being. A meta-analysis. *Journal of Marriage and the Family*, 53, 43-58.

Amato, P.R., and Zuo, J. 1992. Rural poverty, urban poverty, and psychological well-being. *Sociological Quarterly*, 33, 229-240.

Ambert, A.-M. 1982. Differences in children's behavior toward custodial mothers and custodial fathers. *Journal of Marriage and the Family*, 44, 73-86.

Ambert, A.-M. 1992. *The effect of children on parents*. Binghamton, NY: The Haworth Press.

Ambert, A.-M. 1994. An international perspective on parenting: Social change and social constructs. *Journal of Marriage and the Family*, 56, 529-543.

Ambert, A.-M. 1995. A critical perspective on the research on parents and adolescents: Implications for research, intervention, and social policy. In D.H. Demo and A.-M. Ambert (Eds.), *Parents and adolescents in changing families* (pp. 291-306). Minneapolis, MN: National Council on Family Relations.

Ambert, A.-M. 1997a. *Parents, children, and adolescents: Interactive relationships and development in context*. Binghamton, NY: The Haworth Press.

Ambert, A.-M. 1997b. The effect of delinquency on parents. *Family and Corrections Network* Report, 13. Palmyra, VA: Family and Corrections Network.

Ambert, A.-M., and Saucier, J.-F. 1984. Adolescents' academic success and aspirations by parental marital status. *Canadian Review of Sociology and Anthropology*, 21, 62-74.

American Association of Retired Persons. 1990. *A portrait of older Americans.* Washington, DC: AARP.

American Psychological Association Commission on Violence and Youth. 1993. *Violence and youth: Psychology's response,* vol. 1. Washington, DC: American Psychological Association.

Andersen, O. 1991. Occupational impacts on mortality declines in the Nordic countries. In W. Lutz (Ed.), *Future demographic trends in Europe and North America.* New York: Academic Press.

Anderson, E. 1990. *Streetwise: Race, class and change in an urban community.* Chicago: University of Chicago Press.

Anderson, E. 1993. Sex codes and family life among poor inner-city youths. In R.I. Lerman and T.J. Ooms (Eds.), *Young unwed fathers* (pp. 74-98). Philadelphia: Temple University Press.

Aneshensel, C.S., and Sucoff, C.A. 1996. The neighborhood context of adolescent mental health. *Journal of Health and Social Behavior,* 37, 293-310.

Apfel, R.J., and Handel, M.H. 1993. *Madness and loss of motherhood.* Washington, DC: American Psychiatric Press.

Aquilino, W.S. 1996. The life course of children born to unmarried mothers: Childhood living arrangements and young adult outcomes. *Journal of Marriage and the Family,* 58, 293-310.

Arber, S., Gilbert, N., and Dale, A. 1995. Paid employment and women's health: A benefit or source of role strain. *Sociology of Health and Illness,* 7, 375-400.

Armey, D. 1994. Public welfare in America. *Journal of Social, Political and Economic Studies,* 19, 245-249.

Arnold, M.S. 1995. Exploding the myths: African-American families at promise. In B.B. Swadener and S. Lubeck (Eds), *Children and families "at promise"* (pp. 143-162). Albany, NY: State University of New York Press.

Arnold, M.S., and Swadener, B.B. 1993. Savage inequalities and the discourse of risk: What of the white children who have so much green grass? *Educational Review,* 15, 261-272.

Aro, H.M., and Palosaari, U.K. 1991. Parental divorce, adolescence, and transition to young adulthood: A follow-up study. *American Journal of Orthopsychiatry,* 62, 421-429.

Aseltine, R.H., Jr. 1995. A reconsideration of parental and peer influences on adolescent deviance. *Journal of Health and Social Behavior,* 36, 103-121.

Aseltine, R.H., Jr. 1996. Pathways linking parental divorce with adolescent depression. *Journal of Health and Social Behavior,* 33, 133-148.

Aseltine, R.H., and Kessler, R.C. 1993. Marital disruption and depression in a community sample. *Journal of Health and Social Behavior,* 34, 237-251.

Asher, S.R., and Coie, J.D. (Eds.). 1990. Peer rejection in childhood. Cambridge: Cambridge University Press.

Ashton-Warner, S. 1963. *Teacher.* New York: Simon and Schuster.

Assembly of First Nations. 1989. *National Inquiry into First Nations Child Care.* Ottawa: AFN.

Astone, N.M., and McLanahan, S.S. 1991. Family structure, parental practice, and high school completion. *American Sociological Review,* 56, 309-320.

Atchley, R.C. 1994. *Social forces & aging.* 7th ed. *Belmont, CA:* Wadsworth.

Attar, B.K., Guerra, N.G., and Tolan, P.H. 1994. Neighborhood disadvantage, stressful life events, and adjustment in urban elementary-school children. *Journal of Clinical Child Psychology,* 23, 391-400.

Baker, D.P., and Stevenson, D.R. 1986. Mothers' strategies for children's school achievement: Managing the transition to high school. *Sociology of Education,* 59, 156-166.

Baker, M., and Benjamin, D. 1994. The performance of immigrants in the Canadian labor market. *Journal of Labor Economics,* 12, 369-405.

Baker, M., and Benjamin, D. 1995. The receipt of transfer payments by immigrants to Canada. *Journal of Human Resources,* 30, 650-676.

Bane, M.J. 1986. Household composition and poverty. In S.H. Danziger and D.H. Weinberg (Eds.), *Fighting poverty* (pp. 209-231). Cambridge, MA: Harvard University Press.

Bane, M.J., and Ellwood, D.T. 1986. Slipping into and out of poverty: The dynamics of spells. *Journal of Human Resources,* 21, 1-23.

Barber, B.K. 1992. Family, personality, and adolescent problem behaviors. *Journal of Marriage and the Family,* 54, 69-79.

Bardy, M. 1994. The manuscript of the 100-year project: Towards a revision. In J. Qvortrup, M. Bardy, G. Sgritta, and H. Wintersberger (Eds.), *Childhood matters: Social theory, practice and politics* (pp. 299-318). Aldershot, UK: Avebury.

Barker, D.J. 1990. The fetal and infant origins of adult disease. *British Medical Journal,* 301, 1111.

Barresi, C., and Stull, D. 1993. Ethnicity and long-term care: An overview. In C. Barresi and D. Stull (Eds.), *Ethnic elderly and long-term care* (pp. 3-22). New York: Springer.

Bassuk, E.L., Weinreb, L.F., Buckner, J.C., Browne, A., Salomon, A., and Bassuk, S.S. 1996. The characteristics and needs of sheltered homeless and low-income housed mothers. *Journal of the American Medical Association,* 276, 640-646.

Baumrind, D. 1994. The social context of child maltreatment. *Family Relations,* 43, 360-368.

Baydar, N., and Brooks-Gunn, J. 1991. Profiles of America's grandmothers: Those who provide care and those who do not. In *Grandmothers' lives, grandchildren's lives: An interdisciplinary approach to multigenerational parenting.* Symposium at the Biennial Meeting of the Society for Research in Child Development, Seattle.

Becker, G. 1964. *Human capital.* New York: Columbia University Press.

Beggs, J.J. 1995. The institutional environment: Implications for race and gender inequality in the U.S. labor market. *American Sociological Review,* 60, 612-633.

Bell, C.C., and Jenkins, E.J. 1991. Community violence and children on Chicago's southside. *Psychiatry,* 56, 46-54.

Bell, R.Q. 1968. A reinterpretation of the direction of effects in studies of socialization. *Psychological Review,* 75, 81-85.

Bell, R.Q., and Harper, L. V. 1977. *Child effects on adults.* Hillsdale, NJ: Lawrence Erlbaum.

Belsky, J., Fish, M., and Isabella, R. 1991. Continuity and discontinuity in infant negative and positive emotionality: Family antecedents and attachment consequences. *Developmental Psychology,* 27, 421-431.

Bennett, N.G., Bloom, D.E., and Craig, P.H. 1989. The divergence of Black and White marriage patterns. *American Journal of Sociology,* 95, 692-722.

Bennett, N.G., Bloom, D.E., and Miller, C.K. 1995. The influence of nonmarital childbearing on the formation of first marriages. *Demography,* 32, 47-62.

Berger, E.H. 1991. *Parents as partners in education.* New York: Merrill.

Besharov, D.J. 1996. Poverty, welfare dependency, and the underclass: Trends and explanations. In M.R. Darby (Ed.), *Reducing poverty in America* (pp. 13-56). Thousand Oaks, CA: Sage.

Biblarz, T.J., and Raftery, A.E. 1993. The effects of family disruption on social mobility. *American Sociological Review,* 58, 97-109.

Bickford, A., and Massey, D. 1991. Segregation in the second ghetto: Racial and ethnic segregation in American public housing. *Social Forces,* 69, 1011-1036.

Billingsley, A. 1992. *Climbing Jacob's ladder.* New York: Simon and Schuster.

Black, D. 1992. Inequalities in health. In D.E. Rogers and E. Ginzberg (Eds.), *Medical care and the health of the poor* (pp. 43-60). Boulder, CO: Westview Press.

Blackburn, C. 1991. *Poverty and health.* Milton Keynes, UK: Open University Press.

Blake, J. 1989. *Family size and achievement.* Berkeley: University of California Press.

Blank, R.M. 1993. Why were poverty rates so high in the 1980s? In D.B. Papadimitriou and E.N. Wolff (Eds.), *Poverty and prosperity in the USA in the late Twentieth Century* (pp. 21-55). New York: St. Martin's Press.

Blau, F.D, and Graham, J.W. 1990. Black-white differences in wealth and asset composition. *Quarterly Journal of Economics,* 105, 321-339.

Bluestone, B., and Harrison, B. 1982. *The deindustrialization of America.* New York: Basic Books.

Blumberg, R.L. 1995. Introduction: Engendering health and wellbeing in an era of economic transformation. In R.L. Blumberg, C.A. Rakowski, I. Tinker, and M. Monteon (Eds.), *Engendering wealth and well-being* (pp. 1-14). Boulder, CO: Westview Press.

Blumstein, A. 1983. On the racial disproportionality of United States' prison population. *Journal of Criminal Law and Criminology*, 73, 1259-1281.

Bolger, K.E., Patterson, C.J., and Thompson, W.M. 1995. Psychosocial adjustment among children experiencing persistent and intermittent family economic hardship. *Child Development*, 66, 1107-1129.

Boring, C.C., Squires, T.S., and Health, C.W., Jr. 1992. Cancer statistics for African Americans. *CA Cancer Journal*, 42, 7-17.

Borjas, G.J. 1993. Immigration policy, national origin and immigrant skills: A comparison of Canada and the United States. In D. Card and R.B. Freeman (Eds.), *Small differences that matter* (pp. 21-43). Chicago: University of Chicago Press.

Borjas, G.J., and Trejo, S.J. 1991. Immigration participation in the welfare system. *Industrial and Labor Relations Review*, 44, 195-201.

Borkowski, J.G., et al. 1992. Understanding the "new morbidity": Adolescent parenting and developmental delay. In N. Bray (Ed.), *International Review of Research in Mental Retardation*, 18, 159-196. New York: Academic Press.

Bouchard, C. et al., 1991. *Un Québec fou de ses enfants* (A Quebec crazy about its children). Québec: Ministère de la santé et des services sociaux.

Bound, J., and Freeman, R. 1992. What went wrong? The erosion of relative earnings and employment among young black men in the 1980s. *Quarterly Journal of Economics*, 107, 201-230.

Bound, J., and Johnson, G. 1992. Changes in the structure of wages during the 1980s: An evaluation of alternative explanations. *American Economic Review*, 82, 371-392.

Bowles, S., and Gintis, S. 1976. *Schooling in capitalist America: Education and the contradictions of economic life*. New York: Basic Books.

Boyd, M., and Norris, D. 1995. Leaving the nest? The impact of family structure. *Canadian Social Trends*, 38, Autumn, 14-19.

Boyd, R.L. 1996. Demographic change and entrepreneurial occupations: African Americans in northern cities. *The American Journal of Economics and Sociology*, 55, 129-144.

Boykin, A.W. 1994. Harvesting talent and culture: African-American children and educational reform. In R.J. Rossi (Ed.), *Schools and students at risk* (pp. 116-138). New York: Teachers College Press.

Bradburn, N.M. 1969. *The structure of psychological well-being*. Chicago: Aldine.

Brantlinger, E.A. 1993. *The politics of social class in secondary schools*. New York: Teachers College Press.

Braungart, R.G., and Braungart, M.M. 1989. Youth status and national development: A global assessment in the 1980s. *Journal of Youth and Adolescence*, 18, 123-141.

Braveman, P., Oliva, G., Miller, M.G., Reiter, R., and Egerter, S. 1989. Adverse outcomes and lack of health insurance among newborns in an eight-county area of California, 1982-1986. *New England Journal of Medicine*, 321, 508-513.

Brenner, M.H. 1995. Political economy and health. In B.C. Amick, S. Levine, A.R. Tarlov, and D.C. Walsh (Eds.), *Society and health* (pp. 211-246). Oxford: Oxford University Press.

Bridges, E. 1992. *The incompetent teacher: Managerial responses.* New York: Falmer Press.

Briggs, V.M., Jr. 1996. Immigration policy and the U.S. economy: An institutional perspective. *Journal of Economic Issues,* 30, 371-389.

Bronfenbrenner, U. 1996. Foreword. In R.B. Cairns, G.H. Elder, Jr., and E.J. Costello (Eds.), *Developmental Science,* (pp. ix-xvii). New York: Cambridge University Press.

Bronfenbrenner, U., and Ceci, S.J. 1994. Nature-nurture reconceptualized in developmental perspective: A bioecological model. *Psychological Review,* 101, 568-586.

Bronfenbrenner, U., and Weiss, H.B. 1983. Ecological perspective on child and family policy. In E.F. Zigler, S.L. Kagan, and E. Klugman (Eds.), *Children, families, and government.* Cambridge: Cambridge University Press.

Brooks-Gunn, J., and Furstenberg, F.F., Jr. 1986. The children of adolescent mothers: Physical, academic, and psychological outcomes. *Developmental Review,* 6, 224-251.

Brooks-Gunn, J., Klebanov, P., and Duncan, G.J. 1996. Ethnic differences in children's intelligence test scores: Role of economic deprivation, home environment, and maternal characteristics. *Child Development,* 67, 396-406.

Brooks-Gunn, J., Duncan, G.J., Klebanov, P.K., and Sealand, N. 1993. Do neighborhoods influence child and adolescent development? *American Journal of Sociology,* 99, 353-395.

Brooks-Gunn, J., Klebanov, P., Liaw, F. and Duncan, G.J. 1995. Towards an understanding of the effects of poverty upon children. In H.E. Fitzgerald, B.M. Lester, and B. Zuckerman (Eds.), *Children of poverty* (pp. 3-36). New York: Garland.

Brown, G.W., and Harris, T.O. 1993. Aetiology of anxiety and depressive disorders in an inner-city population: 1. Early adversity. *Psychological Medicine,* 23, 143-154.

Browne, I. 1997. Explaining the black-white gap in labor force participation among women heading households. *American Sociological Review,* 62, 236-252.

Bruce, M.L., Takeuchi, D.T., and Leaf, P.J. 1991. Poverty and psychiatric status. *Archives of General Psychiatry,* 48, 470-474.

Bumpass, L.L., Martin, T.C., and Sweet, J.A. 1991. The impact of family background and early marital factors on marital disruption. *Journal of Family Issues,* 12, 22-42.

Bumpass, L.L., Raley, R.K., and Sweet, J.A. 1995. The changing character of stepfamilies: Implications of cohabitation and nonmarital childbearing. *Demography,* 32, 425-436.

Bunker, J.P., Frazier, H.S., and Mosteller, F. 1995. The role of medical care in determining health: Creating an inventory of benefits. In B.C. Amick, S. Levine,

A.R. Tarlov, and D.C. Walsh (Eds.), *Society and health* (pp. 172-210). New York: Oxford University Press.

Burgoyne, J., Ormrod, R., and Richards, M.P.M. 1987. *Divorce matters*. London: Penguin Books.

Burke, K.C., Burke, J.D., Regier, D.A., and Rae, D.S. 1990. Age at onset of selected mental disorders in five community populations. *Archives of General Psychiatry*, 47, 511-518.

Burnard, T. 1996. Who bought slaves in early America? Purchasers of slaves from the Royal African Company in Jamaica, 1674-1708. *Slavery and Abolition*, 17, 68-92.

Bursik, R.J., Jr. 1988. Social disorganization and theories of crime and delinquency: Problems and prospects. *Criminology*, 26, 519-552.

Bursik, R.J., Jr., and Grasmick, H.G. 1993. *Neighborhoods and crime*. New York: Lexington Books.

Burton, L.M. 1990. Teenage childbearing as an alternative life-course strategy in multigenerational black families. *Human Nature*, 1, 123-143.

Burton, L.M., and Bengtson, V.L. 1985. Black grandmothers: Issues of timing and continuity of roles. In V.L. Bengtson and J.F. Robertson (Eds.), *Grandparenthood* (pp. 61-80). Beverly Hills, CA: Sage.

Butler, A.C. 1996. The effect of welfare benefit levels on poverty among single-parent families. *Social Problems*, 43, 94-115.

Butler, J.S. 1991. *Entrepreneurship and self-help among black Americans: A reconsideration of race and economics*. Albany: State University of New York Press.

Cairns, R.B., McGuire, A.M., and Gariepy, J.L. 1993. Developmental behavior genetics: Fusion, correlated constraints, and timing. In D.F. Hay and A. Angold (Eds.), *Precursors and causes in development and psychopathology* (pp. 87-122). Chichester, UK: John Wiley and Sons.

Caldwell, J.C. 1986. Routes to low mortality in poor countries. *Population and Development Review*, 12, 171-220.

Campbell, F.A., and Ramey, C.T. 1994. Effects of early intervention on intellectual and academic achievement: A follow-up study of children from low-income families. *Child Development*, 65, 684-698.

Canada Year Book. 1993. Ottawa: Minister of Industry, Science and Technology.

Canadian Council on Social Development. 1993. *Family security in insecure times*. Ottawa: CCSD.

Canadian Institute of Child Health. 1989. *The health of Canada's children: A CICH profile*. Ottawa: Canadian Institute of Child Health.

Canadian Institute of Child Health. 1994. *The health of Canada's children: A CICH profile*. Ottawa: Canadian Institute of Child Health.

Canadian Teachers' Federation. 1989. *Children, schools and poverty*. Ottawa: Canadian Teachers' Federation.

Canadian Urban Institute. 1993. *Disentangling local governmental responsibilities: International comparisons*. Toronto: Canadian Urban Institute, Urban Focus Series, 93-1.

Cancian, M., Danziger, S., and Gottschalk, P. 1993. Working wives and family inequality among married couples. In S. Danzinger and P. Gottschalk (Eds.), *Uneven tides: Rising inequality in America* (pp. 195-221). New York: Russell Sage Foundation.

Cancio, A.S., Evans, T.D., and Maume, D.J., Jr. 1996. Reconsidering the declining significance of race: Racial differences in early career wages. *American Sociological Review*, 61, 541-556.

Capaldi, D.M., and Patterson, G.R. 1991. Relation of parental transitions to boys' adjustment problems: I. A linear hypothesis: II. Mothers at risk for transitions and unskilled parenting. *Developmental Psychology*, 27, 489-521.

Card, D., and Krueger, A. 1992. Does school quality matter? Returns to education and the characteristics of public schools in the United States. *Journal of Political Economy*, 100, 1-40.

Carini, P. 1982. *The school lives of seven children: A five year study.* Grand Forks, ND: University of North Dakota Press.

Carnegie Council on Adolescent Development. 1989. *Turning points: Preparing American youth for the 21st century.* New York: Carnegie Corporation.

Carstairs, V., and Morris, R. 1989. Deprivation and mortality: An alternative to social class? *Community Medicine*, 11, 210-219.

Carta, J.J. 1991. Education for young children in inner-city classrooms. *American Behavioral Scientist*, 34, 440-453.

Caspi, A., and Moffitt, T. 1991. The continuity of maladaptive behavior: From description to understanding in the study of antisocial behavior. In D. Cicchetti and D. Cohen (Eds.), *Manual of developmental psychopathology.* New York: Wiley.

Caspi, A., Elder, G.H., Jr., and Herbener, E.S. 1990. Childhood personality and the prediction of life-course patterns. In M. Rutter and L. Robins (Eds.), *Straight and devious pathways from childhood to adulthood* (pp. 13-35). Cambridge: Cambridge University Press.

Caspi, A., Moffitt, T.E., Silva, P.A., Stouthamer-Loeber, M., Krueger, R.F., and Schmutte, P.S. 1994. Are some people crime-prone? Replications of the personality-crime relationship across countries, genders, races, and methods. *Criminology*, 32, 163-195.

Catterall, J.S. 1987. On the social costs of dropping out of school. *High School Journal*, 71, 19-30.

Cauce, A.M., Gonzales, N.A., and Paradise, M.J. 1997. Parenting under pressure: African American parents and their adolescent children. Paper presented at the Biennial Meeting of the Society for Research in Child Development, Washington, April 5.

Cavalli-Sforza, L.L., and Feldman, M.W. 1973. Cultural versus biological inheritance: Phenotypic transmission from parents to children (a theory of the effect of parental phenotypes on children's phenotypes). *American Journal of Human Genetics*, 25, 618-637.

Ceci, S.J. 1991. How much does schooling influence general intelligence and its cognitive components? A reassessment of the evidence. *Developmental Psychology*, 27, 703-722.

Ceci, S.J. 1996. American education: Looking inward and outward. In U. Bronfenbrenner et al. (Eds.), *The state of Americans* (pp. 185-207). New York: Free Press.

Ceci, S.J., Rosenblum, T., de Bruyn, E., and Lee, D.Y. 1997. A bio-ecological model of intellectual development: Moving beyond h^2. In R.J. Sternberg and E. Grigorenko (Eds.), *Intelligence, heredity, and environment* (pp. 303-322). Cambridge: Cambridge University Press.

Centerwall, B.S. 1989. Exposure to television as a cause of violence. In G. Comstock (Ed.), *Public communication and behavior*, vol. 2 (pp. 1-58). Orlando: Academic Press.

Centerwall, B.S. 1995. Race, socioeconomic status, and domestic homicide. *Journal of the American Medical Association*, 273, 1755-1758.

Cerny, P.G. 1996. International finance and the erosion of state policy capacity. In P. Gummett (Ed.), *Globalization of public policy* (pp. 83-104). Chattenham, UK: Edward Elgar.

Chambliss, W.J. 1995. Crime control and ethnic minorities: Legitimizing racial oppression by creating moral panics. In D.F. Hawkins (Ed.), *Ethnicity, race, and crime* (pp. 235-258). Albany: State University of New York Press.

Chao, R. 1994. Beyond parental control and authoritarian parenting style: Understanding Chinese parenting through the cultural notion of training. *Child Development*, 65, 1111-1119.

Chase-Lansdale, P.L., and Brooks-Gunn, J. 1995. Introduction. In P.L. Chase-Lansdale and J. Brooks-Gunn (Eds.), *Escape from Poverty: What makes a difference for children?* (pp. 1-8). New York: Cambridge University Press.

Chase-Lansdale, P.L., Brooks-Gunn, J., and Zamsky, E.J. 1991. Grandmothers, young mothers, and 3-year-olds: Interrelations among grandmothers' presence, quality of parenting, and child development. In *Grandmothers' lives, grandchildren's lives: An interdisciplinary approach to multigenerational parenting*. Symposium at the Biennial Meeting of the Society for Research in Child Development, Seattle.

Chavkin, W., Kristal, A., Seabron, C., and Guigli, P.E. 1987. Reproductive experience of women living in hostels for the homeless in New York City. *New York State Journal of Medicine*, 87, 10-13.

Cheal, D. 1996. New poverty: Families in postmodern society. Westport, CT: Greenwood Press.

Children's Defense Fund. 1991. Homeless in rural America. *CDF Reports*, 112, 1, 2, 7.

City of Toronto. 1990. *Cityplan '91: Central area trends report*. Toronto: City of Toronto Planning and Development Department.

Clairmont, D. 1974. The development of a deviance service center. In J. Haas and B. Shaffir (Eds.), *Decency and deviance*. Toronto: McLelland and Stewart.

Clark, W. 1997. School leavers revisited. *Canadian Social Trends*, 44, 10-12.

236 THE WEB OF POVERTY

Clarke, J.N. 1996. *Health, illness, and medicine in Canada,* 2nd ed. Toronto: Oxford University Press.

Clarke, L.L., Farmer, F.L., and Miller, M.K. 1994. Structural determinants of infant mortality in metropolitan and nonmetropolitan America. *Rural Sociology,* 59, 84-99.

Cloward, R., and Ohlin, L. 1960. *Delinquency and opportunity: A theory of delinquent gangs.* New York: Free Press of Glencoe.

Coe, R.D. 1988. A longitudinal examination of poverty in the elderly years. *Gerontologist,* 28, 540-544.

Cohen, S., Tyrell, D.A., and Smith, A.P. 1993. Negative life events, perceived stress, negative affect, and susceptibility to the common cold. *Journal of Personality and Social Psychology,* 64, 131-140.

Coiro, M.J. 1997. Maternal depression symptomatology as a risk factor for the development of children in poverty. Paper presented at the Biennial Meeting of the Society for Research in Child Development, Washington, DC, April 3.

Coleman, J.S. 1988. Social capital in the creation of human capital. *American Journal of Sociology,* 94, S95-S120.

Coleman, J.S. 1990. *Foundations of social theory.* Cambridge: Harvard University Press.

Coleman, J.S., and Hoffer, T. 1987. *Public and private schools: The impact of communities.* New York: Basic Books.

Colin, C., Ouellet, F., Boyer, G., and Martin, C. 1992. *Extrême pauvreté, maternité et santé.* Montréal: Saint-Martin.

Comer, J.P. 1988. Educating poor minority children. *Scientific American,* 259, 5, 42-48.

Comstock, G., and Strasburger, V. 1990. Deceptive appearance: Television violence and aggressive behavior. *Journal of Adolescent Health Care,* 11, 31-44.

Conference Board of Canada. 1992. *Employability skill profile.* Ottawa: Conference Board of Canada.

Conger, R.D., Elder, G.H., Jr., Lorenz, F.O., Conger, K.J., Simons, R.L., Whitbeck, L.B., Huck, S., and Melby, J.N. 1990. Linking economic hardship to marital quality and instability. *Journal of Marriage and the Family,* 52, 643-656.

Congress of the United States. 1990. *Sources of support for adolescent mothers.* Washington, DC: Congressional Budget Office.

Congressional Budget Office. 1990. *Sources of support for adolescent mothers.* Washington, DC: U.S. Government Printing Office.

Congressional Research Service. 1987. *Retirement income for an aging population.* Washington, D C: Government Printing Office.

Connell, R.W. 1994. Poverty and education. *Harvard Educational Review,* 64, 125-149.

Connelly, J.P., Halpern-Felsher, B.L., Clifford, E., Crichlow, W., and Usinger, P. 1995. Hanging in there: Behavioral, psychological, and contextual factors affecting whether African-American adolescents stay in high school. *Journal of Adolescent Research,* 10, 41-63.

Cook, D.A., and Fine, M. 1995. "Motherwit": Childrearing lessons from African American mothers of low income. In B.B. Swadener and S. Lubeck (Eds.), *Children and families "at promise"* (pp. 118-142). Albany, NY: State University of New York Press.

Cooksey, E.C. 1997. Consequences of young mothers' marital histories for children's cognitive development. *Journal of Marriage and the Family*, 59, 245-261.

Corcoran, M. 1995. Rags to rags: Poverty and mobility in the United States. *Annual Review of Sociology*, 21, 237-267.

Corcoran, M., Gordon, R., Laren, D., and Solon, G. 1992. The association between men's economic status and community origins. *Journal of Human Resources*, 27, 575-601.

Corse, S.J., Schmidt, K., and Trickett, P.K. 1990. Social network characteristics of mothers in abusing and nonabusing families and their relationship to parenting beliefs. *Journal of Community Psychology*, 18, 44-59.

Cose, E. 1993. *The rage of a privileged class.* New York: HarperCollins.

Council on Ethical and Judicial Affairs, American Medical Association. 1990. Black-white disparities in health care. *Journal of the American Medical Association*, 263, 2344-2346.

Cowan, P.A., Cowan, C.P., and Kerig, P.K. 1992. Mothers, fathers, sons, and daughters: Gender differences in family formation and parenting style. In P.A. Cowan et al. (Eds.), *Family, self, and society: Towards a new agenda for family research* (pp. 165-195). Hillsdale, NJ: Lawrence Erlbaum.

Crane, J. 1991. The epidemic theory of ghetto and neighborhood effects on dropping out and teenage childbearing. *American Journal of Sociology*, 96, 1236-1259.

Crane, J. 1994. Exploding the myth of scientific support for the theory of black inferiority. *Journal of Black Psychology*, 20, 189-209.

Crutchfield, R.D. 1995. Ethnicity, labor markets, and crime. In D.F. Hawkins (Ed.), *Ethnicity, race, and crime* (pp. 194-211). Albany: State University of New York Press.

Cruz, J.E. 1992. *Developing a Puerto Rican agenda for research advocacy.* Washington, DC: National Puerto Rican Coalition.

Dandurand, P. 1996. Ecole et solidarité (school and solidarity). *Lien social et politiques-RIAC*, 35, 185-188.

Dandurand, R.B. 1994. Divorce et nouvelle monoparentalité. In F. Dumont et al. (Eds.), *Traité des problèmes sociaux*. Quebec: Institut québecois de recherche sur la culture.

Danziger, S., and Gottschalk, T. 1988. Increasing inequality in the United States: What we know and what we don't. *Journal of Post-Keynesian Economics*, 11, 174-195.

Danziger, S., Sandefur, G., and Weinberg, D. (Eds.). 1994. *Confronting poverty: Prescriptions for change.* Cambridge, MA: Harvard University Press.

Davey Smith, G., and Shipley, M.J. 1991. Confounding of occupation and smoking: Its magnitude and consequences. *Social Science and Medicine*, 32, 1297-1300.

Dawson, D.A. 1991. Family structure and children's health and well-being. Data from the 1988 National Health Interview Survey on Child Health. *Journal of Marriage and the Family*, 53, 573-584.

Deater-Deckard, K., Dodge, K.A., Bates, J.E., and Pettit, G.S. 1996. Physical discipline among African American and European American mothers: Links to children's externalizing behaviors. *Developmental Psychology*, 32, 1065-1072.

Deniger, M.-A., et al. 1995. *Poverty among young families and their integration into society and the work force: An Ontario-Quebec comparison*. Ottawa: The Canadian Council on Social Development.

DeParlee, J. 1997. *The New York Times*, February 2, pp. 11-12.

Devine, J.A., and Wright, J.D. 1993. *The greatest of evils: Urban poverty and the American underclass*. New York: Aldine de Gruyter.

Diaz, S., Moll, L.C., and Mehan, H. 1986. Sociocultural resources in instruction: A context specific approach. In California State Department of Education (Eds.), *Beyond language: Social and cultural factors in schooling language minority children* (pp. 187-230). Los Angeles, CA: California State University; Evaluation, Dissemination and Assessment Center.

DiLeonardi, J.W. 1993. Families living in poverty and chronic neglect of children. *Families in Society*, 74, 556-562.

DiMaggio, P. 1982. Cultural capital and school success: The impact of status culture participation on the grades of U.S. high school students. *American Sociological Review*, 47, 189-201.

Dixon, C., and Drakakis-Smith, D. (Eds.). 1993. *Economic and social development in Pacific Asia*. London: Routledge.

Dohrenwend, B.P., Dohrenwend, B.S., Gould, M.S., Link, B., Neugebauer, R., and Wunsch-Hitzig, R. 1980. *Mental illness in the United States: Epidemiological estimates*. New York: Praeger.

Dohrenwend, B.P., et al., 1992. Socioeconomic status and psychiatric disorders: The causation-selection issue. *Science*, 255, 946-941.

Dornbusch, S.M., Ritter, L.P., and Steinberg, L. 1991. Community influences on the relation of family statuses to adolescent school performance: Differences between African Americans and Non-Hispanic whites. *American Journal of Education*, 38, 543-567.

Dornbusch, S.M., Ritter, P.L., Leiderman, P.H., Roberts, D.F., and Fraleigh, M.J. 1987. The relation of parenting style to adolescent school performance. *Child Development*, 58, 1244-1257.

Downey, D.B. 1994. The school performance of children from single-mother and single-father families. *Journal of Family Issues*, 15, 129-147.

Downey, D.B. 1995. When bigger is not better: Family size, parental resources, and children's educational performance. *American Sociological Review*, 60, 746-761.

Dreier, P. 1993. America's urban crisis: Symptoms, causes, solutions. *North Carolina Law Review*, 71, 5, 1372-1375.

Dressler, W.W. 1993. Health in the African American community: Accounting for health inequalities. *Medical Anthropology Quarterly*, 7, 325-345.

Driedger, L. 1991. *The urban factor*. Toronto: Oxford University Press.

Dryfoos, J.G. 1982. Contraceptive use, pregnancy intentions and pregnancy outcomes among U.S. women. *Family Planning Perspectives*, March/April.

Dublin, L.I., Lotka, A.J., and Spiegelman, M. 1949. *Length of life*. New York: Ronald Press.

Dubow, E.F., and Ippolito, M.F. 1994. Effects of poverty and quality of the home environment on changes in the academic and behavioral adjustment of elementary school-age children. *Journal of Clinical Child Psychology*, 23, 401-412.

Duncan, C.M. 1996. Understanding persistent poverty: Social class context in rural communities. *Rural Sociology*, 61, 103-124.

Duncan, G.J. 1991. The economic environment of childhood. In A.C. Huston (Ed.), *Children in poverty, child development and public policy* (pp. 23-50). Cambridge, UK: Cambridge University Press.

Duncan, G.J. 1994. Families and neighbors as sources of disadvantage in the schooling decisions of white and black adolescents. *American Journal of Education*, 103, 20-53.

Duncan, G.J. 1996. Understanding persistent poverty: Social class context in rural communities. *Rural Sociology*, 61, 103-124.

Duncan, G.J., and Hoffman, S.D. 1985. Economic consequences of marital instability. In M. David and T. Smeeding (Eds.), *Horizontal equity, uncertainty and well-being* (pp. 427-470). Chicago: University of Chicago Press.

Duncan, G.J., and Rodgers, W.L. 1988. Longitudinal aspects of poverty. *Journal of Marriage and the Family*, 50, 1007-1021.

Duncan, G.J., Smeeding, T.M., and Rodgers, W. 1993. W(h)ither the middle class? A dynamic view. In D.B. Papadimitriou and E.N. Wolff (Eds.), *Poverty and prosperity in the USA in the late Twentieth Century* (pp. 240-271). New York: St. Martin's Press.

Duncan, G.J., and Yeung, W.-J.J. 1995. Extent and consequences of welfare dependence among America's children. *Children and Youth Services Review*, 17, 159-186.

Earls, F., Escobar, J.I., and Manson, S.M. 1990. Suicide in minority groups: Epidemiologic and cultural perspectives. In S.J. Blumenthal and D.J. Kupper (Eds.), *Suicide over the life cycle* (pp. 571-598). Washington, DC: American Psychiatric Press.

Eckenrode, J., Laird, M., and Doris, J. 1993. School performance and disciplinary problems among abused and neglected children. *Developmental Psychology*, 29, 53-62.

Economic Council of Canada. 1990. *Good jobs, bad jobs: Employment in the service economy*. Ottawa: Minister of Supply and Services.

Economic Council of Canada. 1992. *The new face of poverty.* Authored by J. Maxwell. Ottawa: Minister of Supply and Services.

Edin, K., and Lein, L. 1997. Work, welfare, and single mothers' economic survival strategies. *American Sociological Review,* 62, 253-266.

Eggebeen, D.J., Crockett, L.J., and Hawkins, A.J. 1990. Patterns of adult male coresidence among young children of adolescent mothers. *Family Planning Perspectives,* 22, 219-223.

Eggebeen, D.J., and Hogan, D.P. 1990. Giving between generations in American families. *Human Nature,* 1, 211-232.

Ehrenreich, B., Sklar, H., and Stollard, K. 1985. *Poverty and the American dream: Women and children first.* Boston: South End Press.

Elder, G.H., Jr. 1985. Perspectives on the life course. In G.H. Elder Jr. (Ed.), *Life course dynamics* (pp. 23-49). Ithaca: Cornell University Press.

Elder, G., Caspi, A., and Nguyen, T. 1994. Resourceful and vulnerable children: Family influence in hard times. In R.K. Silbereisen, K. Eyferth, and G. Rudinger (Eds.), *Development as action in context* (pp. 167-182). New York: Springer-Verlag.

Elder, G.H., Jr., Caspi, A., and Burton, L.M. 1988. Adolescent transition in developmental perspective: Sociological and historical insights. In M.R. Gunnar and W.A. Collins (Eds.), *Development during the transition to adolescence* (pp. 151-180). Hillsdale, NJ: Lawrence Erlbaum.

Elder, G.H., Jr., Conger, R.D., Foster, E.M., and Ardel, T.M. 1992. Families under economic pressure. *Journal of Family Issues,* 13, 5-37.

Elford, J., Whincup, P., and Shaper, A.G. 1991. Early life experience and adult cardiovascular disease: Longitudinal and case-control studies. *International Journal of Epidemiology,* 20, 833-844.

Elias, M.J. 1989. Schools as a source of stress to children: An analysis of causal and ameliorated influences. *Journal of School Psychology,* 27, 393-407.

Eller, T.J. 1994. Household wealth and asset ownership: 1991. In U.S. Bureau of the Census, *Current Population Reports,* P, 70-34. Washington, DC: U.S. Government Printing Office.

Ellwood, D.T. 1989. The origins of "dependency": Choices, confidence or culture? *Focus,* 12, 6-13.

Elster, A.B., Ketterlinus, R., and Lamb, M.E. 1990. Association between parenthood and problem behavior in a national sample of adolescents. *Pediatrics,* 85, 1044-1050.

Elster, A.B., and Lamb, M.E. (Eds.). 1986. *Adolescent fatherhood.* Hillsdale, NJ: Lawrence Erlbaum.

Engelbert, A. 1994. Worlds of childhood—Differentiated but different: Implications for social policy. In J. Qvortrup, M. Bardy, G. Sgritta, and H. Wintersberger (Eds.), *Childhood matters: Social theory, practice and politics* (pp. 285-298). Aldershot, UK: Avebury.

Ensminger, M.E. 1995. Welfare and psychological distress: A longitudinal study of African American urban mothers. *Journal of Health and Social Behavior,* 36, 346-359.

Ensminger, M.E., and Slusarcick, A.L. 1992. Paths to high school graduation or dropout: A longitudinal study of a first-grade cohort. *Sociology of Education*, 65, 95-113.

Ensminger, M.E., Kellam, S.G., and Rubin, B.R. 1983. School and family origins of delinquency: Comparisons by sex. In K.T. Van Deusen and S.A. Mednick (Eds.), *Prospective studies of crime and delinquency* (pp. 73-97). Boston: Kluwer-Nijhoff.

Ensminger, M.E., Lamkin, R.P., and Jacobson, N. 1996. School leaving: A longitudinal perspective including neighborhood effects. *Child Development*, 67, 2400-2416.

Entwisle, D.R., and Alexander, K.L. 1992. Summer setback: Race, poverty, school composition, and mathematical achievement in the first two years of school. *American Sociological Review*, 57, 72-84.

Entwisle, D.R., and Alexander, K.L. 1996. Family type and children's growth in reading and math over the primary grades. *Journal of Marriage and the Family*, 58, 341-355.

Epstein, J.L. 1987. Toward a theory of family-school connections: Teachers' practices and parental involvement across the school years. In K. Hurrelmann, F. Kaufmann, and F. Losel (Eds.), *Potential and constraints*. New York: de Gruyter.

Escalona, S. 1982. Babies at double hazard: Early development of infants at biological and social risk. *Pediatrics*, 70, 670-676.

Evans, R.G. 1994. Introduction. In R.G. Evans, M.L. Barer, and T.R. Marmor (Eds.), *Why are some people healthy and others not?* (pp. 3-26). New York: Aldine de Gruyter.

Evans, R.G., and Stoddart, G.L. 1994. Producing health, consuming health care. In R.G. Evans, M.L. Barer, and T.R. Marmor (Eds.), *Why are some people healthy and others not?* (pp. 27-65). New York: Aldine de Gruyter.

Fagan, J. 1990. Social processes of delinquency and drug use among urban gangs. In C.R. Huff (Ed.), *Gangs in America* (pp. 183-222). Newbury Park, CA: Sage.

Fagan, J. 1993. Drug selling and licit income in distressed neighborhoods: The economic lives of street-level drug users and dealers. In A. Harrell and G. Peterson (Eds.), *Drugs, crime and social isolation*. Washington, DC: Urban Institute Press.

Farkas, G. 1996. *Human capital or cultural capital? Ethnicity and poverty groups in an urban school district*. New York. Aldine de Gruyter.

Farmer, F.L., Clarke, L.L., and Miller, M.K. 1993. Consequences of a differential residence designation for rural health policy research: The case of infant mortality. *Journal of Rural Health*, 19, 17-26.

Farrington, D.P. 1987. Early precursors of frequent offending. In J.Q. Wilson and G.C. Loury (Eds.), *From children to citizens: Families, schools, and delinquency prevention* (pp. 21-50). New York: Springer-Verlag.

Farrington, D.P. 1991a. Antisocial personality from childhood to adulthood. *The Psychologist*, 4, 389-394.

Farrington, D.P. 1991b. Childhood aggression and adult violence: Early precursors and later life outcomes. In D. Pepler and H. Rubin (Eds.), *The development and treatment of childhood aggression* (pp. 5-29). Hillsdale, NJ: Lawrence Erlbaum.

Farrington, D.P. 1992. Explaining the beginning, progress, and ending of antisocial behavior from birth to adulthood. In J. McCord (Ed.), *Facts, frameworks, and forecasts* (pp. 235-286). New Brunswick, NJ: Transaction.

Farrington, D.P., and West, D.J. 1990. The Cambridge study of delinquent development: A long-term follow-up of 411 London males. In H.J. Kerner and G. Kaiser (Eds.), *Kriminalitat* (pp. 117-138). New York: Springer-Verlag.

Farrington, D.P., Gallagher, B., Morley, L., St. Ledger, R.J., and West, D.J. 1986. Unemployment, school leaving, and crime. *British Journal of Criminology,* 26, 335-356.

Farrington, D.P., Gallagher, B., Morley, L., St. Ledger, R.J., and West, D.J. 1988. Are there any successful men from criminogenic backgrounds? *Psychiatry,* 51, 116-130.

Fehrman, P.G., Keith, T.Z., and Reimer, T.M. 1987. Home influence on school learning: Direct and indirect effects of parental involvement on high school grades. *Journal of Educational Research,* 80, 330-337.

Ferguson, R. 1991. Paying for public education: New evidence on how and why money matters. *Harvard Journal on Legislation,* 28, 465-498.

Fergusson, D.M., Horwood, L.J., and Lynskey, M.T. 1994. Culture makes a difference . . . or does it? A comparison of adolescents in Hong Kong, Australia, and the United States. In R.K. Silbereisen and E. Todt (Eds.), *Adolescence in context* (pp. 99-113). New York: Springer-Verlag.

Fergusson, D.M., and Lynskey, M.T. 1996. Adolescent resiliency to family adversity. *Journal of Child Psychology and Psychiatry,* 37, 282-292.

Fernandez Kelly, M.P. 1995. Social and cultural capital in the urban ghetto: Implications for the economic sociology of immigration. In A. Portes (Ed.), *The economic sociology of immigration* (pp. 213-247). New York: Russell Sage.

Ferraro, K.F., and Farmer, M.M. 1996. Double jeopardy to health hypothesis for African Americans: Analysis and critique. *Journal of Health and Social Behavior,* 37, 27-42.

Fine, M. 1991. *Framing dropouts: Notes on the politics of an urban-public high school.* Albany: State University of New York Press.

Finn, J.D. 1989. Withdrawing from school. *Review of Educational Research,* 59, 117-142.

Finnie, R. 1993. Women, men, and the economic consequences of divorce: Evidence from Canadian longitudinal data. *Canadian Review of Sociology and Anthropology,* 30, 205-241.

Fischer, D.G. 1993. Parental supervision and delinquency. *Perceptual and Motor Skills,* 56, 635-640.

Fishman, G., Rattner, A., and Weimann, G. 1987. The effect of ethnicity on stereotypes. *Criminology,* 25, 507-524.

Fitzgerald, H.E., and Zucker, R.A. 1995. Socioeconomic status and alcoholism: The contextual structure of developmental pathways to addiction. In H.E. Fitzgerald, B.M. Lester, and B. Zuckerman (Eds.), *Children of poverty* (pp. 125-144). New York: Garland.

Fitzgerald, H.E., Lester, B.M., and Zuckerman, B. (Eds.). 1995. *Children of poverty.* New York: Garland.

Flanagan, C.A. 1990. Families and schools in hard times. In V.C. McLoyd and C.A. Flanagan (Eds.), *Economic stress: Effects on family and child development* (pp. 7-26). San Francisco: Jossey-Bass.

Flora, C.B., Flora, J.L., Spears, J.D., Swanson, L.E., Lapping, M.B., and Weinberg, M.L. 1992. *Rural communities: Legacy & change.* Boulder, CO: Westview Press.

Florsheim, P., Tolan, P.H., and Gorman-Smith, D. 1996. Family processes and risk for externaling behavior problems among African American and Hispanic boys. *Journal of Consulting and Clinical Psychology*, 64, 1222-1230.

Fogel, R.W., and Engerman, S.L. 1989. *Time on the cross: The economics of American Negro slavery.* New York: Norton.

Folk, K.F. 1996. Single mothers in various living arrangements: Differences in economic and time resources. *The American Journal of Economics and Sociology*, 55, 277-292.

Forcier, K.I. 1990. Management and care of pregnant psychiatric patients. *Journal of Psychosocial Nursing*, 28, 11-16.

Ford, E.S., et al. 1991. Physical activity behaviors in lower and higher socioeconomic status populations. *American Journal of Epidemiology*, 133, 1246-1256.

Fordham, S., and Ogbu, J. 1986. Black students, school success: Coping with the burden of "acting white." *Urban Review*, 18, 176-206.

Forthofer, M.S., Kessler, R.C., Story, A.L., and Gotlib, I.H. 1996. The effects of psychiatric disorders on the probability and timing of first marriage. *Journal of Health and Social Behavior*, 37, 121-132.

Fox, A.J. (Ed.). 1989. *Health inequalities in European countries.* Aldershot, UK: Gower.

Franklin, D.L., Smith, S.E., and McMiller, W.E.P. 1995. Correlates of marital status among African-American mothers in Chicago neighborhoods of concentrated poverty. *Journal of Marriage and the Family*, 57, 141-152.

Fraser, S. (Ed.). 1995. *The Bell Curve wars.* New York: Basic Books.

Freeman, R. 1991. Unemployment and earnings of disadvantaged youth in a labor shortage economy. In C. Jencks and P. Peterson (Eds.), *The urban underclass.* Washington, DC: Brookings Institution.

Frenzen, P. 1993. Health insurance coverage in U.S. urban and rural areas. *Journal of Rural Health*, 9, 204-214.

Frideres, J.S. 1994. Racism and health: The case of native people. In B.S. Bolaria and H.B. Dickinson (Eds.), *Health, illness and health care in Canada.* Toronto: Harcourt Brace and Co.

Friede, A., et al. 1987. Young maternal age and infant mortality: The role of low birth weight. *Public Health Reports*, 102, 192-199.

Friedman, H.S., Tucker, J.S., Schwartz, J.E., Tomlinson-Keasey, C., Martin, L.R., Wingard, D.L., and Criqui, M.H. 1995. Psychological and behavioral predictors of longevity. The aging and death of the "Termites." *American Psychologist*, 50, 69-78.

Fuchs, V.R. 1992. Poverty and health: Asking the right questions. In D.E. Rogers and E. Ginzberg (Eds.), *Medical care and the health of the poor* (pp. 9-20). Boulder, CO: Westview Press.

Furstenberg, F.F., Jr. 1991. As the pendulum swings: Teenage childbearing and social concern. *Family Relations*, 40, 127-138.

Furstenberg, F.F., Jr. 1992. Teenage childbearing and cultural rationality: A thesis in search of evidence. *Family Relations*, 41, 239-243.

Furstenberg, F.F., Jr., and Cherlin, A. 1991. *Divided families. What happens to children when parents part?* Cambridge, MA: Harvard University Press.

Furstenberg, F.F., Jr., and Weiss, C.C. 1997. Schooling together: Mutual influences on educational success of teenage mothers and their children. Paper presented at the Biennial Meeting of the Society for Research in Child Development, Washington, DC, April 5.

Furstenberg, F.F., Jr., Brooks-Gunn, J., and Morgan, S. P. 1987. *Adolescent mothers in later life*. New York: Cambridge University Press.

Furstenberg, F.F., Jr., Hughes, M.E., and Brooks-Gunn, J. 1992. The next generation: The children of teenage mothers grow up. In M.K. Rosenheim and M.F. Testa (Eds.), *Early parenthood and coming of age in the 1990s* (pp. 113-135). New Brunswick, NJ: Rutgers University Press.

Furstenberg, F.F., Jr., Belzer, A., Davis, C., Levine, J.A., Morrow, K., and Washington, M. 1993. How families manage risk and opportunity in dangerous neighborhoods. In W.J. Wilson (Ed.), *Sociology and the public agenda* (pp. 231-258). Newbury Park, CA: Sage.

Fyfe, A. 1989. *Child labour*. Cambridge, UK: Polity Press.

Gabe, T. 1992. *Demographic trends affecting Aid to Families with Dependent Children (AFDC) caseload growth*. Washington, DC: Congressional Research Service.

Gable, S., Belsky, J., and Crnic, K. 1992. Marriage, parenting, and child development: Progress and prospects. *Journal of Family Psychology*, 5, 276-294.

Gadsden, V.L. 1995. Literacy and poverty: Intergenerational issues within African American families. In H.E. Fitzgerald, B.M. Lester, and B. Zuckerman (Eds.) *Children of poverty* (pp. 85-118). New York: Garland.

Garasky, S. 1995. The effects of family structure on educational attainment: Do the effects vary by the age of the child? *American Journal of Economics and Sociology*, 54, 89-105.

Garbarino, J. 1995. *Raising children in a socially toxic environment*. San Francisco: Jossey-Bass.

Garbarino, J., and Sherman, D. 1980. High-risk neighborhoods and high-risk families: The human ecology of child maltreatment. *Child Development*, 51, 188-198.

Garbarino, J., Kostelny, K., and Dubrow, N. 1991. *No place to be a child: Growing up in a war zone*. Lexington, MA: Lexington Books.

Garcia-Coll, C., and Garcia, H.A.V. 1995. Hispanic children and their families: On a different track from the very beginning. In H.E. Fitzgerald, B.M. Lester, and B. Zuckerman (Eds.), *Children of poverty* (pp. 57-78). New York: Garland.

Gardner, H. 1995. Cracking open the IQ box. In S. Fraser (Ed.), *The Bell Curve wars* (pp. 23-35). New York: Basic Books.

Gardner, M., and Herz, D.E. 1992. Working and poor. *Monthly Labor Review*, December, 20-28.

Garmezy, N., and Masten, A.S. 1994. Chronic adversities. In M. Rutter, E. Taylor, and L. Hersov (Eds.), *Child and adolescent psychiatry*, 3rd ed. (pp. 191-208). Oxford: Blackwell.

Garrett, P., Ng'andu, N., and Ferron, J. 1994. Is rural residency a risk factor for childhood poverty? *Rural Sociology*, 59, 66-83.

Gartley, J. 1994. *Earnings of Canadians*. Ottawa: Statistics Canada; and Toronto: Prentice Hall of Canada.

Gartner, A., and Lipsky, D.K. 1987. Beyond special education: Toward a quality system for all students. *Harvard Educational Review*, 57, 367-395.

Gates, E.N., and Cardozo, B.N. (Eds.). 1997. *Critical race theory: Essays on the social construction and reproduction of "race."* New York: Garland.

Ge, X., Conger, R.D., Cadoret, R.J., and Neiderhiser, J.M. 1996. The developmental interface between nature and nurture: A mutual influence model of child antisocial behavior and parent behaviors. *Developmental Psychology*, 32, 574-589.

General Household Survey. 1992. London, UK. OPCS, HMSO.

Geronimus, A.T. 1991. Teenage childbearing and social and reproductive disadvantage: The evolution of complex questions and the demise of simple answers. *Family Relations*, 40, 463-471.

Geronimus, A.T., and Bound, J. 1990. Black/white differences in women's reproductive-related health status: Evidence from vital statistics. *Demography*, 27, 457-466.

Geronimus, A.T., Andersen, H.F., and Bound, J. 1991. Differences in hypertension prevalence among U.S. black and white women of childbearing age. *Public Health Reports*, 106, 393-399.

Gibson, M.A., and Ogbu, J.U. 1989. *Accommodation without assimilation: Sikh immigrants in an American high school*. New York: Cornell University Press.

Gilbert, S., and Orok, B. 1993. School leavers. *Canadian Social Trends*, 30, 2-7.

Goldenberg, C. 1996. *Latin American immigration and U.S. schools*. Social Policy Report. Society for Research in Child Development, 10, 1.

Goldsmith, H.H. 1989. Behavior-genetic approaches to temperament. In G.A. Kohnstamm, J.E. Bates, and M.K. Rothbart (Eds.), *Temperament in childhood* (pp. 111-132). New York: John Wiley.

Goldsmith, H.H. 1993. Nature-nurture issues in the behavioral genetics context: Overcoming barriers to communication. In R. Plomin and G.E. McLearn (Eds.), *Nature, nurture & psychology* (pp. 325-340). Washington, DC: American Psychological Association.

Goldsmith, W.W., and Blakeley, E.J. 1992. *Separate societies: Poverty and inequality in U.S. cities.* Philadelphia: Temple University Press.

Good, T.L., Slavings, R.L., Harel, K.H., and Emerson, H. 1987. Student passivity: A study of question asking in K-12 classrooms. *Sociology of Education,* 60, 181-199.

Gorman-Smith, D., Tolan, P.H., and Hunt, M. 1997. Family functioning and exposure to community violence among urban youth. Paper presented at the Biennunal Meeting of the Society for Research in Child Development, Washington, DC: April 5.

Gornick, M.E., et al. 1996. Effects of race and income on mortality and use of service among Medicare beneficiaries. *New England Journal of Medicine,* 335, 791-799.

Gottfredson, M.R., and Hirschi, T. 1990. *A general theory of crime.* Stanford, CA: Stanford University Press.

Gottschalk, P. 1992. The intergenerational transmission of welfare participation: Facts and possible causes. *Journal of Policy Analysis and Management,* 11, 254-272.

Gottschalk, P., and Danziger, S. 1993. Family structure, family size and family income. In P. Gottschalk and S. Danziger (Eds.), *Uneven tides* (pp. 167-193). New York: Russell Sage.

Gottschalk, P., and Moffitt, R. 1994. The growth of earnings instability in the U.S. labor market. *Brookings Papers on Economic Activity,* 2, 217-272.

Gougis, R.A. 1986. The effects of prejudice and stress on the academic performance of Black Americans. In U. Neisser (Ed.), *The school achievement of minority children* (pp. 145-158). Hillsdale, NJ: Lawrence Erlbaum.

Gramlich, E., Laren, D., and Sealand, N. 1992. Moving into and out of poor urban areas. *Journal of Policy Analysis and Management,* 11, 273-287.

Grannis, J.C. 1994. The dropout prevention initiative of New York City. In R.J. Rossi (Ed.), *Schools and students at risk* (pp. 182-206). New York: Teachers College Press.

Granovetter, M. 1985. Economic and social structure. The problem of embeddedness. *American Journal of Sociology,* 91, 481-510.

Grant, J.P. 1992. *The state of the world's children 1992.* New York: Oxford University Press.

Grasmick, H.S., Tittle, C.R., Bursik, R.J., Jr., and Arneklev, B.J. 1993. Testing the core empirical implications of Gottfredson and Hirschi's general theory of crime. *Journal of Research in Crime and Delinquency,* 30, 5-29.

Green, B.L., and Schneider, M.J. 1990. Threats to funding for rural schools. *Journal of Education Finance,* 15, 302-318.

Green, G., Tigges, L., and Browne, I. 1995. Social resources, job search, and poverty in Atlanta. *Research in Community Sociology,* 5, 161-182.

Greenfield, P.M. 1994. Independence and interdependence as developmental scripts: Implications for theory, research and practice. In P.M. Greenfield and R.Q. Cocking (Eds.), *Cross-cultural roots of minority child development* (pp. 1-37). Hillsdale, NJ: Lawrence Erlbaum.

Gutman, H.G. 1976. *The black family in slavery and freedom, 1750-1925.* New York: Pantheon.

Hack, M., et al. 1991. Effect of very low birth weight and subnormal head size on cognitive abilities at school age. *New England Journal of Medicine,* 325, 231-237.

Hagan, J. 1994. *Crime and disrepute.* Thousand Oaks, CA: Pine Forge Press.

Hagan, J., and Palloni, A. 1990. The social reproduction of a criminal class in working class London, circa 1950-80. *American Journal of Sociology,* 96, 265-299.

Hagedorn, J.M. 1988. *People and folks: Gangs, crime and the underclass in a rustbelt city.* Chicago: Lake View Press.

Haggerty, M., and Johnson, C. 1996. The social construction of the distribution of income and health. *Journal of Economic Issues,* 30, 525-531.

Hahn, R.A., Mulinare, J., and Teutsch, S.M. 1992. Inconsistencies in coding of race and ethnicity between birth and death in US infants. *Journal of the American Medical Association,* 267, 259-263.

Haines, D.W. (Ed.). 1989. *Refugees as immigrants: Cambodians, Laotians, and Vietnamese in America.* Totowa, NJ: Rowman and Littlefield.

Halpern, R. 1990. Poverty and early childhood parenting: Toward a framework for intervention. *American Journal of Orthopsychiatry* 60, 6-18.

Hamilton, V.L., Broman, C.L., Hoffman, W.S., and Renner, D.S. 1990. Hard times and vulnerable people: Initial effects of plant closing on auto-workers' mental health. *Journal of Health and Social Behavior,* 31, 123-140.

Handler, J.F. 1995. *The poverty of welfare reform.* New Haven: Yale University Press.

Hansen, D.A. 1986. Family-school articulations: The effects of interaction rule mismatch. *American Educational Research Journal,* 23, 643-659.

Hanson, S.L. 1994. Lost talent: Unrealized educational aspirations and expectations among U.S. youths. *Sociology of Education,* 67, 159-183.

Hao, L. 1996. Family structure, private transfers, and the economic well-being of families with children. *Social Forces,* 75, 269-292.

Harris, I.B. 1996. *Children in jeopardy: Can we break the cycle of poverty?* New Haven: Yale University Press.

Harris, K.M., 1993. Work and welfare among single mothers in poverty. *American Journal of Sociology,* 99, 317-352.

Harris, K.M. 1996. Life after welfare: Women, work, and repeat dependency. *American Sociological Review,* 61, 407-426.

Harris, T.O. 1991. Life stress and illness: The question of specificity. *Annals of Behavioral Medicine,* 13, 211-219.

Harrison, B., and Bluestone, B. 1988. *The great U-turn.* New York: Basic Books.

Harrison, B., Tilly, C., and Bluestone, B. 1986. Rising inequality. In D.R. Obey and P. Sarbanes (Eds.), *The changing American economy* (pp. 111-134). New York: Basil Blackwell.

Haskett, M.E., Johnson, C.A., and Miller, J.W. 1994. Individual differences in risk of child abuse by adolescent mothers: Assessment in the perinatal period. *Journal of Child Psychology and Psychiatry*, 35, 461-476.

Haskins, R. 1995. Losing ground or moving ahead? Welfare reform and children. In P.L. Chase-Lansdale and J. Brooks-Gunn (Eds.), *Escape from poverty. What makes a difference for children?* (pp. 241-272). Cambridge: Cambridge University Press.

Hauser, R.M. 1993. Trends in college entry among blacks, Hispanics, and whites. In C. Clotfelter and M. Rothschild (Eds.), *Studies of supply and demand in higher education* (pp. 61-119). Chicago: Chicago University Press.

Haveman, R., and Buron, L. 1993. Who are the truly poor? In D.B. Papadimitriou and E.N. Wolff (Eds.), *Poverty and prosperity in the USA in the late Twentieth Century* (pp. 58-88). New York: St. Martin's Press.

Haveman, R., and Wolfe, B. 1994. *Succeeding generations: On the effects of investments in children*. New York: Russell Sage Foundation.

Hawton, K., and Rose, N. 1986. Unemployment and attempted suicide among men in Oxford. *Health Trends*, 8, 29-32.

Hayes, C.D. 1987. Adolescent pregnancy and childbearing: An emerging research focus. In S.L. Hofferth and C.D. Hayes (Eds.), *Risking the future: Adolescent sexuality, pregnancy, and childbearing,* vol. 2. Washington, DC: National Academy Press.

Hayes-Bautista, D. 1996. Poverty and the underclass: Some Latino crosscurrents. In M.R. Darby (Ed.), *Reducing poverty in America* (pp. 57-66). Thousand Oaks, CA: Sage.

Health and Welfare Canada. 1992. *Aboriginal health in Canada*. Ottawa: Minister of National Health and Welfare.

Health Canada. 1994. *Emotional balance*. Ottawa: Minister of Supply and Services. Cat. no. H39-295/1994E.

Helm, J., Comfort, M., Bailey, D.B., Jr., and Simeonsson, R.J. 1990. Adolescent and adult mothers of handicapped children: Maternal involvement in play. *Family Relations*, 39, 432-437.

Henry, B., Caspi, A., Moffit, T.E., and Silva, P.A. 1996. Temperamental and familial predictors of violent and nonviolent criminal convictions: Age 3 to 18. *Developmental Psychology*, 32, 614-623.

Hernandez, D.J. 1993. *America's children*. New York: Russell Sage.

Herrnstein, R., and Murray, C. 1994. *The bell curve: Intelligence and class structure in America*. New York: Free Press.

Hertzman, C., Frank, J., and Evans, R.G. 1994. Heterogeneities in mental health status and the determinants of population health. In R.G. Evans, M.L. Barer, and T.R. Marmor (Eds.), *Why are some people healthy and others not?* (pp. 67-92). New York: Aldine de Gruyter.

Hetherington, E.M. 1993. An overview of the Virginia longitudinal study of divorce and remarriage with a focus on early adolescence. *Journal of Family Psychology*, 7, 39-56.

Hetherington, E.M., Clingempeel, W.G., et al. 1992. Coping with marital transitions. *Monographs of the Society for Research in Child Development*, 57, nos. 2-3.

Heyns, B. 1988. Schooling and cognitive development: Is there a season for learning? *Child Development*, 58, 1151-1160.

Heyns, B. 1991. *Childhood as a social phenomenon: National report—USA.* Vienna: European Centre.

Higgins, A., Pencharz, P., Mikolainis, D., and Dubois, S. 1989. Impact of the Higgins nutrition intervention program in birth weight: A within-mother analysis. *Journal of the American Dietetic Association*.

Hilgartner, S., and Bosk, C.L. 1988. The rise and fall of social problems: A public arenas model. *American Journal of Sociology*, 94, 53-78.

Hill, M.S., and Duncan, G.J. 1987. Parental family income and the socioeconomic attainment of children. *Social Science Research*, 16, 39-73.

Hill, P.T., Wise, A.W., and Shapiro, L. 1989. *Educational progress: Cities mobilize to improve their schools.* Santa Monica, CA: Rand.

Hoffman, S., Foster, E.M., and Furstenberg, F.F., Jr., 1993. Reevaluating the costs of teenage childbearing. *Demography*, 30, 1-13.

Hogan, D.P., and Kitagawa, E.M. 1985. The impact of social status, family structure, and neighborhood on the fertility of black adolescents. *American Journal of Sociology*, 90, 825-855.

Hogendorm, J.S. 1996. Economic modelling of price differences in the slave trade between the Central Sudan and the coast. *Slavery and Abolition*, 17, 209-222.

Hollingshead, A.B., and Redlich, F.C. 1958. *Social class and mental illness.* New York: Wiley.

Holm, M. 1995. The impact of structural adjustment on intermediate towns and urban migrants: An example from Tanzania. In D. Simon, W. van Spengen, C. Dixon, and A. Narman (Eds.), *Structurally adjusted Africa* (pp. 91-108). London: Pluto Press.

Holzer, H.J. 1996. *What employers want.* New York: Russell Sage.

Hoover-Dempsey, V., Bassler, O.C., and Brissie, J.S. 1987. Parent-involvement: Contributions to teacher efficacy, school socio-economic status, and other school characteristics. *American Educational Research Journal*, 24, 417-435.

Hooyman, N., and Kiyak, H.A. 1996. *Social gerontology*, 4th ed. Boston: Allyn and Bacon.

Horney, J., Osgood, D.W., and Marshall, I.H. 1995. Criminal careers in the short-term: Intra-individual variability in crime and its relation to local life circumstances. *American Sociological Review*, 60, 655-673.

Horowitz, R. 1995. *Teen mothers—Citizens or dependents?* Chicago: University of Chicago Press.

Huesmann, L.R., Eron, L.D., Lefkowitz, M.M., and Walder, L.O. 1984. Stability of aggression over time and generations. *Developmental Psychology*, 20, 1120-1134.

Huston, A.C. 1995. Policies for children: Social obligation, not handout. In H.E. Fitzgerald, B.M. Lester, and D. Zuckerman (Eds.), *Children of poverty* (pp. 305-321). New York: Garland.

Institute of Medicine. 1985. *Preventing low birthweight.* Washington, DC: National Academy Press.

Jackson, J.F. 1997. Primary grade public schooling: A risk factor for African-American children? Paper presented at the Biennial Meeting of the Society of Research for Child Development, Washington, DC, April 4.

Jackson, S.A. 1993. Opportunity to learn: The health connection. *Journal of Negro Education,* 62, 377-393.

Jargowsky, P., and Bane, M.J. 1990a. Ghetto poverty in the United States, 1970-1980. In C. Jencks and P.E. Peterson (Eds.), *The urban underclass* (pp. 235-273). Washington, DC: The Brookings Institution.

Jargowsky, P., and Bane, M.J. 1990b. Ghetto poverty: Basic questions. In L.E. Lynn, Jr. and M.G.H. McGeary (Eds.), *Inner-city poverty in the United States* (pp. 16-67). Washington, DC: National Academy Press.

Jarrett, R.L. 1996. Welfare stigma among low-income, African American single mothers. *Family Relations,* 45, 368-374.

Jencks, C. 1992. *Rethinking social policy: Race, poverty, and the underclass.* Cambridge, MA: Harvard University Press.

Jencks, C., and Mayer, S.E. 1990. The social consequences of growing up in a poor neighborhood. In L. E. Lynn, Jr. and G.H. McGeary (Eds.), *Inner city poverty in the United States* (pp. 111-186). Washington, DC: National Academy Press.

Jencks, C., and Peterson, P. (Eds.). 1991. *The urban underclass.* Washington, DC: The Brookings Institution.

Jencks, C., et al. 1979. *Who gets ahead? The determinants of economic success in America.* New York: Basic Books.

Jennings, J. 1994. *Understanding the nature of poverty in urban America.* Westport, CT: Praeger.

Jensen, A.R. 1977. Cumulative deficit in IQ of Blacks in the rural South. *Developmental Psychology,* 13, 184-191.

Jensen, L., and Eggebeen, J. 1994. Nonmetropolitan poor children and reliance on public assistance. *Rural Sociology,* 59, 45-65.

Jewell, K. S. 1988. *Survival of the Black family: The institutional impact of U.S. social policy.* New York: Praeger.

Juhn, C., Murphy, K., and Pierce, B. 1993. Wage inequality and the rise in returns to skill. *Journal of Political Economy,* 101, 410-442.

Julian, T. W., and McKenry, P. C. 1993. Mediators of male violence toward female intimates. *Journal of Family Violence,* 8, 39-56.

Kagan, J. 1994. *Galen's prophecy: Temperament in human nature.* New York: Basic Books.

Kagan, J., Reznick, J.S., and Snidman, N. 1989. Issues in the study of temperament. In G.A. Kohnstamm, J.E. Bates, and M.K. Rothbart (Eds.), *Temperament in childhood* (pp. 133-152). New York: John Wiley.

Kagan, S., et al., 1985. Classroom structural bias: Impact of cooperative and competitive classroom structures on cooperative and competitive individuals and groups. In R.E. Slavin et al. (Eds.), *Learning to cooperate, cooperating to learn*. New York: Plenum.

Kahn, H.S., Williamson, D.F., and Stevens, J.A. 1991. Race and weight change in U.S. women: The roles of socioeconomic and marital status. *American Journal of Public Health*, 81, 319-323.

Kahn, J.R., and Anderson, K.E. 1992. Intergenerational patterns of teenage fertility. *Demography*, 29, 39-57.

Kalbach, W.E. 1990. A demographic overview of racial and ethnic groups in Canada. In P.S. Li (Ed.), *Race and ethnic relations in Canada* (pp. 18-47). Toronto: Oxford University Press.

Karakker, K.H., and Evans, S.L. 1996. Adolescent mothers' knowledge of child development and expectations of their own infants. *Journal of Youth and Adolescence*, 25, 651-666.

Karasek, R., and Theorell, T. 1990. *Healthy work: Stress, productivity, and the reconstruction of working life*. New York: Basic Books.

Karp, R.J. (Ed.). 1993. *Malnourished children in the United States*. New York: Springer.

Kasarda, J.D. 1983. Caught in the web of change. *Society*, 21, 4-7.

Kasarda, J.D. 1990. City jobs and residents on a collision course: The urban underclass dilemma. *Economic Development Quarterly*, 4, 313-319.

Kasarda, J.D. 1993. The severely distressed in economically transforming cities. In A.V. Harrell and G.E. Peterson (Eds.), *Drugs, crime, and social isolation* (pp. 45-98). Washington, DC: The Urban Institute.

Kasinitz, P., and Rosenberg, J. 1996. Missing the connection: Social isolation and employment on the Brooklyn waterfront. *Social Problems*, 43, 501-519.

Katz, L.F., and Murphy, K. 1991. Change in relative wages, 1963-1987: The role of supply and demand factors. *Quarterly Journal of Economics*, 107, 35-78.

Kellam, S.G. 1994. The social adaptation of children in classrooms: A measure of family childrearing effectiveness. In R.D. Parke and S.G. Kellam (Eds.), *Exploring family relationships with other social contexts* (pp. 147-168). Hillsdale, NJ: Lawrence Erlbaum.

Kelly, K. 1995. Visible minorities: A diverse group. *Canadian Social Trends*, 37, 2-8.

Kendler, K.S. 1991. A psychiatric perspective on the "nature of nurture." *Behavioral and Brain Sciences*, 14, 398-399.

Kendler, K.S. 1995a. Genetic epidemiology in psychiatry. Taking both genes and environment seriously. *Archives of General Psychiatry*, 52, 595-599.

Kendler, K.S. 1995b. Stressful life events, genetic liability, and onset of an episode of major depression in women. *American Journal of Psychiatry*, 152, 833-842.

Kendler, K.S. 1996. Parenting: A genetic-epidemiologic perspective. *American Journal of Psychiatry*, 153, 11-20.

Kerbow, D., and Bernhardt, A. 1993. Parental intervention in the school: The context of minority involvement. In B. Schneider and J.S. Coleman (Eds.), *Parents, their children, and schools* (pp. 115-146). San Francisco: Westview Press.

Kerr, D., Larrivée, D., and Greenhalgh, P. 1994. *Children and youth: An overview.* Ottawa: Statistics Canada; and Toronto: Prentice Hall of Canada.

Kessler, R.C., Turner, J.B., and House, J.S. 1988. Effects of unemployment on health in a community survey: Main, modifying, and mediating effects. *Journal of Social Issues,* 44, 69-85.

Kessler, R.C., et al. 1994. Lifetime and 12-month prevalence of DSM-III-R psychiatric disorders in the United States: Results from the National Comorbidity Survey. *Archives of General Psychiatry,* 51, 8-19.

Ketterlinus, R.D., Henderson, S., and Lamb, M.E. 1991. The effects of maternal age-at-birth on children's cognitive development. *Journal of Research on Adolescence,* 1, 173-188.

Kim, U., and Choi, S.H. 1994. Individualism, collectivism, and child development: A Korean perspective. In P.M. Greenfield and R.R. Cocking (Eds.), *Cross-cultural roots of minority child development* (pp. 227-257). Hillsdale, NJ: Lawrence Erlbaum.

King, G., and Williams, D.R. 1995. Race and health: A multi-dimensional approach to African American health. In S. Levine, D.C. Walsh, B.C. Amick, and A.R. Tarlov (Eds.), *Society and health: Foundations for a nation.* New York: Oxford University Press.

Kingue, M.D. 1996. Prospects for Africa's economic recovery and development. In A.Y. Yansane (Ed.), *Prospects for recovery and sustainable development in Africa* (pp. 37-50). Wesport, CT: Greenwood Press.

Kitchen, B., Mitchell, A., Clutterbuck, P., and Novick, M. 1991. *Unequal futures: The legacies of child poverty in Canada.* Toronto: Social Planning Council of Metropolitan Toronto.

Klerman, L.V., and Parker, M.D. 1991. *Alive and well: A research and policy review of health programs for poor young children.* New York: Columbia University, National Center for Children in Poverty.

Knapp, M.S., and Shields, P.M. (Eds.). 1991. *Better schooling for the children of poverty.* Berkeley, CA: McCutchan.

Knapp, M.S., and Turnbull, B.J. 1991. Alternative to conventional wisdom. In M.S. Knapp and P.M. Shields (Eds.), *Better schooling for the children of poverty* (pp. 329-353). Berkeley, CA: McCutchan.

Kochanek, K.D., Maurer, J.D., and Rosenberg, H.M. 1994. Why did black life expectancy decline from 1984 through 1989 in the United States? *American Journal of Public Health,* 84, 938-944.

Kogevinas, M., Marmot, M.G., Fox, A.J., and Goldblatt, P.O. 1991. Socioeconomic differences in cancer survival. *Journal of Epidemiology and Community Health,* 45, 216-219.

Kohn, M.L. 1969. *Class and conformity: A study in values.* Homewood, IL: Dorsey Press.

Kohn, M.L., and Schooler, C. 1983. *Work and personality: An inquiry into the impact of social stratification.* Norwood, NJ: Ablex.

Kohn, M.L., Slomczynski, K.M., and Schoenbach, C. 1986. Social stratification and the transmission of values in the family: A cross-national assessment. *Sociological Forum*, 1, 73-101.

Kolvin, I., et al. 1988a. Risk/protective factors for offending with particular reference to deprivation. In M. Rutter (Ed.), *Studies of psychosocial risk: The power of longitudinal data* (pp. 77-95). Cambridge: Cambridge University Press.

Kolvin, I., et al. 1988b. Social and parenting factors affecting criminal offence rates (findings from the Newcastle Thousand Families Study, 1947-1980). *British Journal of Psychiatry*, 152, 80-90.

Korten, D.C. 1995. *When corporations rule the world*. San Francisco: Berrett-Koehler.

Kotlowitz, A. 1991. *There are no children here*. New York: Anchor/Doubleday.

Kozol, J. 1991. *Savage inequalities. Children in America's schools*. New York: Crown.

Kramer, B.J. 1992. Cross-cultural medicine a decade later: Health and aging in urban American Indians. *Western Journal of Medicine*, 157, 281-285.

Krieger, N. 1990. Racial and gender discrimination: Risk factors for high blood pressure? *Social Science and Medicine*, 30, 1273-1281.

Krieger, N. 1991. Women and social class: A methodological study comparing individual household, and census measures as predictors of black/white differences in reproductive history. *Journal of Epidemiology and Community Health*, 45, 35-42.

Krieger, N., and Fee, E. 1994. Social class: The missing link in U.S. health data. *Journal of Health Services*, 24, 25-44.

Krieger, N., Rowley, D.L., Herman, A.A., Avery, B., and Phillips, M.T. 1993. Racism, sexism, and social class: Implications for studies of health, disease, and well-being. *American Journal of Preventive Medicine*, 9, S82-S122.

Krotki, K.J., and Reid, C. 1994. Demography of Canadian population by ethnic group. In J.W. Berry and J.A. Laponce (Eds.), *Ethnicity and culture in Canada* (pp. 17-59). Toronto: University of Toronto Press.

Krugman, P. 1995. Does Third World growth hurt First World prosperity? In K. Ohmae (Ed.), *The evolving global economy* (pp. 113-128). Boston: Harvard Business Review Books.

Kupersmidt, J.B., Griesler, P.C., DeRosier, M.E., Patterson, C.J., and Davis, P.W. 1995. Childhood aggression and peer relations in the context of family and neighborhood factors. *Child Development*, 66, 360-375.

Lamb, M.E., and Elster, A.B. 1990. Adolescent parenthood. In G.H. Brody and I. E. Sigel (Eds.), *Methods of family research: Biographies of research projects* (pp. 159-190). Hillsdale, NJ: Lawrence Erlbaum.

Lamb, M.E., and Teti, D.M. 1991. Parenthood and marriage in adolescence: Associations with educational and occupational attainment. In R.M. Lerner, A.C. Peterson, and J. Brooks-Gunn (Eds.), *Encyclopedia of Adolescence*, vol. 2 (pp. 742-745). New York: Garland.

Lamberty, J.H., and Garcia-Coll, G. (Eds.). 1994. *Puerto Rican women and children: Issues in health, growth and development*. New York: Plenum.

Lamborn, S.D., Dornbusch, S.M., and Steinberg, L. 1996. Ethnicity and community context as moderators of the relations between family decision making and adolescent adjustment. *Child Development*, 67, 283-301.

Land, K., McCall, P., and Cohen, L. 1990. Structural covariates of homicide rates: Are there any invariances across time and space? *American Journal of Sociology*, 95, 922-963.

Landale, N.S., and Fennelly, K. 1992. Informal unions among Mainland Puerto Ricans: Cohabitation or an alternative to legal marriage? *Journal of Marriage and the Family*, 54, 269-280.

Landale, N.S., and Forste, R. 1991. Patterns of entry into cohabitation and marriage among Mainland Puerto Rican women. *Demography*, 28, 587-607.

Lareau, A. 1989. *Home advantage: Social class and parental intervention in elementary education.* New York: Falmer Press.

Larzelere, R.E., Klein, M., Schumm, W.A., and Alibrando, S., Jr. 1989. Relations of spanking and other parenting characteristics to self-esteem and perceived fairness of parental discipline. *Psychological Reports*, 64, 1140-1142.

Laub, J.H., and Sampson, R.J. 1993. Turning points in the life course: Why change matters to the study of crime. *Criminology*, 31, 301-325.

Lawton, L., Silverstein, M., and Bengtson, V. 1994. Affection, social contact, and geographic distance between adult children and their parents. *Journal of Marriage and the Family*, 56, 57-68.

Lazure, J. 1990. Mouvance des générations: Condition féminine et masculine. In F. Dumont (Ed.), *La société québécoise après 30 ans de changements.* Quebec: Institut québécois de recherche sur la culture.

Le Blanc, M., and Fréchette, M. 1989. *Male criminal activity from childhood through youth: Multilevel and developmental perspectives.* New York: Springer-Verlag.

Lee, E.S. 1951. Negro intelligence and selective migration: A Philadelphia test of the Klineberg hypothesis. *American Sociological Review*, 16, 227-232.

Lefley, H.P. 1989. Family burden and family stigma in major mental illness. *American Psychologist*, 44, 556-560.

Lemann, N. 1991. *The promised land: The great Black migration and how it changed America.* New York: Knopf.

Lenski, G. 1966. *Power and privilege: A theory of social stratification.* Chapel Hill, NC: University of North Carolina Press.

Leon, D., and Wilkinson, R.G. 1988. Inequalities in prognosis: Socio-economic differences in cancer and heart disease survival. In A.J. Fox (Ed.), *Inequalities in health within Europe.* Aldershot, UK: Gower Press.

Lerman, R.I. 1993. A national profile of young unwed fathers. In R.I. Lerman and T.J. Ooms (Eds.), *Young unwed fathers* (pp. 27-51). Philadelphia: Temple University Press.

Lester, B.M., McGrath, M.M., Garcia-Coll, C., Brem, F.S., Sullivan, M.C., and Mattis, S.G. 1995. Relationship between risk and protective factors, developmental outcome, and the home environment at four years of age in term and preterm infants. In H.E. Fitzgerald, B.M. Lester, and B. Zuckerman (Eds.), *Children of poverty* (pp. 197-226). New York: Garland.

LeVine, R.A., et al. 1991. Women's schooling and child care in demographic transition: A Mexican case study. *Population and Development Review*, 17, 459-496.

Levitan, S.A. 1988. Part-timers: Living on half-rations. *Challenge*, May-June.

Levitan, S.A. 1990. *Programs in aid of poor*. Baltimore, MD: Johns Hopkins University Press.

Levy, F., and Murnane, R.J. 1992. U.S. earnings levels and earnings inequality: A review of recent trends and proposed explanations. *Journal of Economic Literature*, 30, 1333-1381.

Lewis, C.E., Robins, L.N., and Rice, J. 1985. Association of alcoholism with antisocial personality in urban men. *Journal of Nervous and Mental Disease*, 173, 166-174.

Lichter, D.T., and Eggebeen, D.J. 1994. The effect of parental employment on child poverty. *Journal of Marriage and the Family*, 56, 633-645.

Lichter, D.T., and Landale, N.S. 1995. Parental work, family structure, and poverty among Latino children. *Journal of Marriage and the Family*, 57, 346-354.

Lichter, D.T., Johnston, G.M., and McLaughlin, D. 1994. Changing linkages between work and poverty in rural America. *Rural Sociology*, 59, 395-415.

Lieberman, L. 1995. Herrnstein and Murray Inc.: "IQs 'R US." *American Behavioral Scientist*, 39, 25-34.

Lieberson, S. 1980. *A piece of the pie: Black and white immigrants since 1980*. Berkeley: University of California Press.

Liebert, R.M., and Sprafkin, J. 1988. *The early window*, 3rd ed. New York: Pergamon.

Liem, J.H., and Liem, G.R. 1990. Understanding the individual and family effects of unemployment. In J. Eckenrode and S. Gore (Eds.), *Stress between work and family* (pp. 175-204). New York: Plenum.

Lightfoot, S.L. 1978. *Worlds apart*. New York: Basic Books.

Lillie-Blanton, M., Anthony, J.C., and Schuster, C.R. 1993. Probing the meaning of racial or ethnic group comparisons in crack cocaine smoking. *Journal of the American Medical Association*, 269, 993-997.

Lim, L.Y.C. 1990. Women's work in export factories: The politics of a cause. In I. Tinker (Ed.), *Persistent inequalities: Women and world development* (pp. 101-119). New York: Oxford University Press.

Lind, M. 1995. *The next American nation: The new nationalism and the fourth American revolution*. New York: Free Press.

Lindsay, C. 1994. *Lone-parent families in Canada;* Ottawa: Statistics Canada; Housing, Family and Social Statistics Division, cat. no. 89-522E.

Lindsay, C., Devereaux, M.S., and Bergob, M. 1994. *Youth in Canada*. Ottawa: Statistics Canada; Housing, Family and Social Statistics Division, cat no. 89-511E.

Lindsey, D. 1994. *The welfare of children*. New York: Oxford University Press.

Linhares, E.D.R., Round, J.M., and Jones, D.A. 1986. Growth, bone maturation, and biochemical changes in Brazilian children from two different socioeconomic groups. *American Journal of Clinical Nutrition*, 44, 552-558.

Link, B.G., Susser, E., Steve, A., Phelan, J., Moore, R., and Struening, E. 1994. Life-time and five-year prevalence of homelessness in the United States. *American Journal of Public Health*, 84, 1907-1912.

Linn, M.W., Sandifer, R., and Stein, S. 1985. Effects of unemployment on mental and physical health. *American Journal of Public Health*, 75, 502-506.

Lo, O., and Gauthier, P. 1995. Housing affordability among mothers. *Canadian Social Trends*, 36, 14-17.

Loeber, R., and Stouthamer-Loeber, M. 1986. Family factors as correlates and predictors of juvenile conduct problems and delinquency. In M. Tonry and N. Morris (Eds.), *Crime and justice*, vol. 7. Chicago: University of Chicago, Press.

Logan, J.R., and Alba, R.D. 1993. Locational returns to human capital: Minority access to suburban community resources. *Demography*, 30, 243-268.

Lomas, J., and Contandriopoulos, A.P. 1994. Regulating limits to medicine: Towards harmony in public- and self-regulation. In R.G. Evans, M.L. Barer, and T.R. Marmor (Eds.), *Why are some people healthy and others not?* (pp. 253-286). New York: Aldine de Gruyter.

London, R.A. 1996. The difference between divorced and never-married mothers' participation in the Aid to Families with Dependent Children program. *Journal of Family Issues*, 17, 170-185.

Lorion, R., and Saltzman, W. 1993. Children's exposure to community violence: Following a path from concern to research to action. In D. Reiss et al. (Eds.), *Children and violence* (pp. 55-65). New York: Guilford Press.

Lowry, R., Kann, L., Collins, J.L., and Kolbe, L.J. 1996. The effect of socioeconomic status on chronic disease risk behaviors among US adolescents. *Journal of the American Medical Association*, 276, 792-797.

Lubeck, S., and Garrett, P. 1990. The social construction of the "at risk" child. *British Journal of Sociology and Education*, 11, 327-340.

Luckenbill, D.F., and Doyle, D.P. 1989. Structural position and violence: Developing a cultural explanation. *Criminology*, 27, 419-435.

Luthar, S.S. 1991. Vulnerability and resilience: A study of high-risk adolescents. *Child Development*, 62, 600-616.

Lynam, D.R. 1996. Early identification of chronic offenders: Who is the fledgling psychopath? *Psychological Bulletin*, 120, 209-234.

Maclean's. 1996. September 2, p. 10.

Magnusson, D., and Bergman, L.R. 1990. A pattern approach to the study of pathways from childhood to adulthood. In L.N. Robins and M. Rutter (Eds.), *Straight and devious pathways from childhood to adulthood* (pp. 101-115). Cambridge, UK: Cambridge University Press.

Manlove, J. 1997. Early motherhood in an intergenerational perspective: The experiences of a British cohort. *Journal of Marriage and the Family*, 59, 263-279.

Manning, W.D., and Lichter, D.T. 1996. Parental cohabitation and children's economic well-being. *Journal of Marriage and the Family*, 58, 998-1010.

Margolin, S., and Schor, J. 1990. *The end of the Golden Age*. Oxford, UK: Clarendon Press.

Margolis, P.A., et al. 1992. Lower respiratory illness in infants and low socioeconomic status. *American Journal of Public Health*, 82, 1119-1126.

Marks, C. 1989. *Farewell—We're good and gone: The Great Black Migration*. Bloomington, IN: Indiana University Press.

Marmor, T.R. 1992. Japan: A sobering lesson. *Health Management Quarterly*, 14, 10-14.

Marmot, M.G. 1986. Social inequalities in mortality: The social environment. In R.G. Wilkinson (Ed.), *Class and health: Research and longitudinal data* (pp. 21-33). London: Tavistock.

Marmot, M.G., and Davey Smith, G. 1989. Why are the Japanese living longer? *British Medical Journal*, 299, 1547-1551.

Marmot, M.G., Bobak, M., and Davey Smith, G. 1995. Explanations for social inequalities in health. In B.C. Amick, S. Levine, A.R. Tarlov, and D.C. Walsh (Eds.), *Society and health* (pp. 172- 210). New York: Oxford University Press.

Marmot, M.G., Davey Smith, G., Stansfield, S., Patel, C., North, F., Head, J., White, I., Brunner, E.J., and Feeney, A. 1991. Health inequalities among British civil servants: The Whitehall II study. *Lancet*, 337, 1387-1393.

Marotto, R.A. 1986. "Posin to be chosen": An ethnographical study of inschool truancy. In D.M. Fetterman and M.A. Pitman (Eds.), *Educational evaluation: Ethnography in theory, practice, and politics* (pp. 193-211). Beverly Hills: Sage.

Marsden, L., et al. 1991. *Children in poverty: Better future*. Ottawa: Standing Senate Committee on Social Affairs, Science and Technology.

Marsland, D., and Leoussi, A. 1996. Social misconstruction: Neglect of biology in contemporary British sociology. *American Sociologist*, 27, 42-51.

Martin, S.L., Ramey, C.T., and Ramey, S. 1990. The prevention of intellectual impairment in children of impoverished families: Findings of a randomized trial of educational day care. *American Journal of Public Health*, 80, 844-847.

Mason, C.A., Cauce, A.M., Gonzales, N., and Hiraga, Y. 1996. Neither too sweet nor too sour: Problem peers, maternal control, and problem behavior in African American adolescents. *Child Development*, 67, 2115-2130.

Mason, C.A., Cauce, A.M., Gonzales, N., Hiraga, Y., and Grove, K. 1994. An ecological model of externalizing in African American adolescents: No family is an island. *Journal of Research on Adolescents*, 4, 639-655.

Massat, C.R. 1995. Is older better? Adolescent parenthood and maltreatment. *Child Welfare*, 74, 325-336.

Massey, D., and Denton, N. 1993. *American apartheid: Segregation and the making of the underclass*. Cambridge, MA: Harvard University Press.

Massey, D.S., and Eggers, M.L. 1990. The ecology of inequality: Minorities and the concentration of poverty, 1970-1980. *American Journal of Sociology*, 95, 1153-1188.

Matsueda, R.L., and Heimer, K. 1987. Race, family structure and delinquency: A test of differential association and social control theories. *American Sociological Review*, 52, 826-840.

Matthews, K., et al. 1989. Educational attainment and behavioral and biologic risk factors for coronary heart disease in middle-age women. *American Journal of Epidemiology*, 129, 1132-1144.

Maxim, P.S. 1992. Immigrants, visible minorities, and self-employment. *Demography*, 29,181-198.

Maxwell, N. 1994. The effect of black-white wage differences in the quantity and quality of education. *Industrial and Labor Relations Review*, 47, 249-264.

Mayer, S.E., and Jencks, C. 1993. Recent trends in economic inequality in the United States: Income versus expenditures versus material well-being. In D.B. Papadimitriou and E.N. Wolff (Eds.), *Poverty and prosperity in the USA in the late Twentieth Century* (pp. 121-203). New York: St. Martin's Press.

Maynard, R. 1995. Teenage childbearing and welfare reform: Lessons from a decade of demonstration and evaluation research. *Children and Youth Services Review*, 17, 309-332.

McAdoo, H.P. 1997. Upward mobility across generations in African American families. In H. P. McAdoo (Ed.), *Black families*, 3rd ed. (pp. 139-162). Thousand Oaks, CA: Sage.

McCarthy, B., and Hagan, J. 1991. Homelessness: A criminogenic situation? *British Journal of Criminology*, 31, 393-410.

McClelland, P. 1996. Economic developments. In U. Bronfenbrenner et al. (Eds.), *The state of Americans* (pp. 51-89). New York: Free Press.

McCloskey, L.A., Figueredo, A.J., and Koss, M.P. 1995. The effect of systemic family violence on children's mental health. *Child Development*, 66, 1239-1261.

McCord, C., and Freeman, H.P. 1990. Excess mortality in Harlem. *New England Journal of Medicine*, 322, 173-177.

McCord, J. 1988. Identifying developmental paradigms leading to alcoholism. *Journal of Studies on Alcohol*, 49, 357-362.

McCormack, T. 1997. Fetal glue syndrome. *Newsletter*, 12, Winter, 3-4. Toronto: York University, Institute for Social Research.

McDonough, P., Duncan, G.J., Williams, N., and House, J. 1997. Income dynamics and adult mortality in the U.S., 1972-1989. *American Journal of Mental Health*, in press.

McGrath, E., Keita, G.P., Strickland, B., and Russo, N.F. 1990. *Women and depression: Risk factors and treatment issues*. Washington, DC: American Psychological Association.

McLanahan, S., and Bumpass, L. 1988. Intergenerational consequences of family disruption. *American Journal of Sociology*, 94, 130-152.

McLanahan, S., and Sandefur, F. 1994. *Growing up with a single parent*. Cambridge, MA: Harvard University Press.

McLaughlin, D., and Holden, K.C. 1993. Nonmetropolitan elderly women: A portrait of economic vulnerability. *Journal of Applied Gerontology*, 320-334.

McLeod, J.D., and Kessler, R.C. 1990. Socioeconomic status differences in vulnerability to undesirable life events. *Journal of Health and Social Behavior*, 31, 162-172.

McLeod, J.D., and Shanahan, M.J. 1993. Poverty, parenting, and children's mental health. *American Sociological Review*, 58, 351-366.

McLeod, J.D., and Shanahan, M.J. 1996. Trajectories of poverty and children's mental health. *Journal of Health and Social Behavior*, 37, 207-220.

McLoyd, V.C. 1989. Socialization and development in a changing economy: The effects of paternal job and income loss on children. *American Psychologist*, 44, 293-302.

McLoyd, V.C. 1995. Poverty, parenting, and policy: Meeting the support needs of poor parents. In H.E. Fitzgerald, B.M. Lester, and B. Zuckerman (Eds.), *Children of poverty* (pp. 269-298). New York: Garland.

McLoyd, V.C., and Wilson, L. 1990. Maternal behavior, social support, and economic conditions as predictors of distress in children. In V. C. McLoyd and C.A. Flanagan (Eds.), *Economic stress: Effects on family life and child development* (pp. 49-70). San Francisco: Jossey-Bass.

McLoyd, V.C., and Wilson L. 1991. The strain of living poor: Parenting, social support, and child mental health. In A.C. Huston (Ed.), *Children in poverty: Child development and public policy* (pp. 105-135). Cambridge: Cambridge University Press.

McPartland, J.M. 1994. Dropout prevention in theory and practice. In R.J. Rossi (Ed.), *Schools and students at risk* (pp. 255-276). New York: Teachers College Press.

Mehan, H. 1992. Understanding inequality in schools: The contribution of interpretive studies. *Sociology of Education*, 65, 1-20.

Menaghan, E.G. 1994. The daily grind: Work stressors, family patterns, and intergenerational outcomes. In W. Avison and I. Gotlib (Eds.), *Stress and mental health: Contemporary issues and future prospects* (pp. 115-147). New York: Plenum.

Menaghan, E.G., and Parcel, T.L. 1990. Parental employment and family life: Research in the 1980s. *Journal of Marriage and the Family*, 52, 1079-1098.

Menaghan, E.G., and Parcel, T.L. 1995. Social sources of change in children's home environments: The effects of parental occupational experiences and family conditions. *Journal of Marriage and the Family*, 57, 69-84.

Mendoza, F.S., et al. 1991. Selected measures of health status for Mexican-American, mainland Puerto Rican, and Cuban-American children. *Journal of the American Medical Association*, 265, 227-232.

Menzies, H. 1996. *Whose brave new world?* Toronto: Between the Lines.

Meyer, D.R., and Garasky, S. 1993. Custodial fathers: Myths, realities, and child support policy. *Journal of Marriage and the Family*, 55, 73-89.

Middle, C., Johnson, A., Alderdice, F., Petty, T., and Macfarlane, A. 1996. Birthweight and health and development at the age of 7 years. *Child: Care, Health and Development*, 22, 55-71.

Miles, D.R., and Carey, G. 1997. Genetic and environmental architecture of human aggression. *Journal of Personality and Social Psychology*, 72, 207-217.

Miller, J.M. 1992. *Search and destroy: The plight of African American males in the criminal justice system*. Alexandria, VA: National Center on Institutions and Alternatives.

Mincy, R.B. 1994. The underclass: Concept, controversy, and evidence. In S. Danziger, G. Sandefur, and D. Weinberg (Eds.), *Confronting poverty* (pp. 109-146). Cambridge: Harvard University Press.

Mines, R., and Avina, J. 1992. Immigrants and labor standards: The case of California. In J.A. Bustamonte, C.W. Reynolds, and R.A.H. Ojeda (Eds.), *U.S. Mexico relations: Labor market interdependence* (pp. 429-448). Stanford: Stanford University Press.

Minty, B., and Pattinson, G. 1994. The nature of child neglect. *British Journal of Social Work*, 24, 733-747.

Miranda, L.C. 1991. *Latino child poverty in the United States*. Washington, DC: Children's Defense Fund.

Mishel, L., and Simon, J. 1988. *The state of working America*. Washington, DC: Economic Policy Institute.

Mitchell, A. 1991. The economic circumstances of Ontario's families and children. In R. Barnhorst and L.C. Johnson (Eds.), *The state of the child in Ontario*. Toronto: Oxford University Press.

Mitchell, A. 1997. The poor fare worst in schools. *Globe and Mail*, Toronto, April 18, p. 1.

Mitman, A.L., and Lash, A.A. 1988. Students' perceptions of their academic standing and classroom behavior. *The Elementary School Journal*, 89, 55-68.

Moffitt, T. E. 1994. Natural histories of delinquency. In E.G.M. Weitekamp and H.-J. Kerner (Eds.), *Cross-national longitudinal research on human development and criminal behavior* (pp. 3-61). Dordrecht, Germany: Kluwer.

Moffitt, T.E., Lynam, D.R., and Silva, P.A. 1994. Neuropsychological tests predicting persistent male delinquency. *Criminology*, 32, 277-300.

Moffitt, T.E., Caspi, A., Dickson, N., Silva, P., and Stanton, W. 1996. Childhood-onset versus adolescent-onset antisocial conduct problems in males: Natural history from ages 3 to 18 years. *Development and Psychopathology*, 8, 399-424.

Molnar, J.M., Roth, W.R., and Klein, T.P. 1990. Constantly compromised: The impact of homelessness on children. *Journal of Social Issues*, 46, 109-124.

Montgomery, A.F., and Rossi, R.J. 1994. Becoming at risk of failure in America's schools. In R.J. Rossi (Ed.), *Schools and students at risk* (pp. 3-22). New York: Teachers College Press.

Moore, K. 1992. *Facts at a glance*. Washington, DC: Childtrends.

Morris, P.A., Hembrooke, H., Gelbwasser, A.S., and Bronfenbrenner, U. 1996. American families: Today and tomorrow. In U. Bronfenbrenner et al. (Eds.), *The state of Americans* (pp. 90-145). New York: Free Press.

Mott, F.L. 1991. Developmental effects of infant care: The mediating role of gender and health. *Journal of Social Issues*, 47, 139-158.

Mulkey, L.M., Crain, R.L., and Harrington, A.J.C. 1992. One-parent households and achievement: Economic and behavioral explanations of a small effect. *Sociology of Education*, 65, 48-65.

Muller, C. 1993. Parental involvement and academic achievement. In B.S. Coleman and J.S. Coleman (Eds.), *Parents, their children and schools* (pp. 77-113). Boulder, CO: Westview.

Muller, C. 1995. Maternal employment, parental involvement, and mathematics achievement among adolescents. *Journal of Marriage and the Family*, 57, 85-100.

Muller, C., and Kerbow, D. 1993. Parent involvement in the home, school, and community. In B. Schneider and J.S. Coleman (Eds.), *Parents, their children and schools* (pp. 13-42). San Francisco: Westview.

Mullis, I., et al. 1991. *Trends in academic progress*. Washington, DC: National Center for Educational Statistics, U.S. Department of Education.

Mundy-Castle, A.C. 1974. Social and technological intelligence in Western and non-Western cultures. *Universitas*, 4, 46-52.

Murnane, R.J., Willett, J.B., and Levy, F. 1995. The growing importance of cognitive skills in wage determination. *Review of Economics and Statistics*, 77, 251-265.

Murphy, K., and Welch, F. 1993. Industrial change and the rising importance of skill. In S. Danziger and P. Gottschalk (Eds.), *Uneven tides*. New York: Russell Sage.

Murray, C. 1995. The Bell Curve and its critics. *Commentary*, 99, May, 23-30.

Nagin, D.S., and Land, K.C. 1993. Age, criminal careers, and population heterogeneity: Specification and estimation of nonparametric, mixed Poisson model. *Criminology*, 31, 327-362.

Nagin, D.S., Farrington, D.P., and Moffitt, T.E. 1995. Life-course trajectories of different types of offenders. *Criminology*, 33, 111-139.

National Center for Children in Poverty. 1990. *Five million children: A statistical profile of our poorest young citizens*. New York: Columbia University School of Public Health.

National Coalition for the Homeless. 1989. *American nightmare: A decade of homelessness in the United States*. Washington, DC: National Coalition for the Homeless.

National Commission on Children. 1991. *Speaking of kids: A national survey of children and parents*. Washington DC: National Commission on Children.

National Council for Health Statistics. 1992. *Health: United States, 1990*. Hyattsville, MD: National Council for Health Statistics.

National Council of Welfare. 1989. *A pension primer*. Ottawa: Minister of Supply and Services.

National Council of Welfare. 1992. *Poverty profile update for 1991*. Ottawa: Minister of Supply and Services.

National Council of Welfare. 1993. *Women and poverty revisited*. Cat. no. H68-24/1990E. Ottawa: Minister of Supply and Services.

National Institute of Mental Health. 1986. *Client/patient sample survey of inpatient, outpatient, and partial care programs.* Rockville, MD: Department of Health and Human Services; NIMH, Survey & Reports Branch, Division of Biometry.

Neal, D.A., and Johnson, W.R. 1996. The role of premarket factors in black-white wage differences. *Journal of Political Economy,* 104, 869-895.

Nelson, J.L. 1995. *Post-industrial capitalism. Exploring economic inequality in America.* Thousand Oaks, CA: Sage.

Nielsen, F., and Alderson, A.S. 1995. Income inequality, development, and dualism: Results from an unbalanced cross-national panel. *American Sociological Review,* 60, 674-701.

Nielsen, F., and Alderson, A.S. 1997. The Kuznets curve and the great U-turn. Income inequality in U.S. counties, 1970 to 1990. *American Sociological Review,* 62, 12-33.

Nitz, K., Ketterlinus, R.D., and Brandt, L.J. 1995. The role of stress, social support, and family environment in adolescent mothers' parenting. *Journal of Adolescence Research,* 10, 358-382.

Noble, D.F. 1995. *Progress without people.* Toronto: Between the Lines.

Norton, A.J., and Moorman, J. 1987. Current trends in marriage and divorce among American women. *Journal of Marriage and the Family,* 49, 3-14.

O'Connor, C. 1991. *Sustainable development and poverty alleviation in Sub-Saharan Africa.* London: Macmillan.

O'Connor, T.G., and Rutter, M. 1996. Risk mechanisms in development: Some conceptual and methodological considerations. *Developmental Psychology,* 32, 787-795.

Oderkirk, J. 1992. Parents and children living with low incomes. *Canadian Social Trends,* 27, 11-15.

Office of Technology Assessment; Congress of the United States. 1987. *Neonatal intensive care for low birthweight infants: Costs and effectiveness.* Health Technology Case Study No. 38.

Office of Technology Assessment; Congress of the United States. 1988. *Appropriate care for cataract surgery patients before and after surgery: Issues of medical safety and appropriateness.*

Offord, D.B., Boyle, M., and Racine, Y. 1989. *Ontario Child Health Study: Children at risk.* Toronto: Ontario Ministry of Community and Social Services.

Ogbu, J.U. 1978. *Minority education and caste: The American system in cross-cultural perspective.* New York: Academic Press.

Ogbu, J.U. 1988. Cultural diversity and human development. In D.T. Slaughter (Ed.), *Black children and poverty: A developmental perspective* (pp. 11-28). San Francisco: Jossey-Bass.

Ogbu, J.U. 1991. Immigrant and involuntary minorities in comparative perspective. In M.A. Gibson and J.U. Ogbu (Eds.), *Minority status and schooling* (pp. 3-33). New York: Garland.

Ogbu, J.U. 1994. From culture differences to differences in cultural frames of reference. In P.M. Greenfield and R.R. Cocking (Eds.), *Cross-cultural roots of minority child development* (pp. 365-392). Hillsdale, NJ: Lawrence Erlbaum.

Oldman, D. 1994. Adult-child relations as class relations. In J. Qvortrup, M. Bardy, G. Sgritta, and H. Wintersberger (Eds.), *Childhood matters: Social theory, practice and politics* (pp. 43-58). Aldershot, UK: Avebury.

O'Neill, B.J., and Yelaja, S.A. 1994. Multiculturalism in postsecondary education: 1970-1991. In J.W. Berry and J.A. Laponce (Eds.), *Ethnicity and culture in Canada* (pp. 483-506). Toronto: University of Toronto Press.

O'Neill, J. 1990. The role of human capital in earnings differences between black and white men. *Journal of Economic Perspectives*, 25-45.

Orfield, G. 1993. *The growth of segregation in American schools: Changing patterns of separation and poverty since 1968*. Alexandria, VA: National School Boards Association.

Padilla, F. 1992. T*he gang as an American enterprise.* New Brunswick, NJ: Rutgers University Press.

Panel on High-Risk Youth. 1993. *Losing generations: Adolescents in high-risk settings*. Washington, DC: National Academy Press.

Pappas, G., Queen, S., Hadden, W., and Fisher, G. 1993. The increasing disparity in mortality between socioeconomic groups in the United States, 1960 and 1986. *New England Journal of Medicine*, 328, 538-545.

Patterson, G.R. 1988. Stress: A change agent for family process. In N. Garmezy and M. Rutter (Eds.), *Stress, coping and development in children* (pp. 235-264). Baltimore: Johns Hopkins University Press.

Patterson, G.R., and Capaldi, D.M. 1991. Antisocial parents: Unskilled and vulnerable. In P.A. Cowan and M. Hetherington (Eds.), *Family transitions* (pp. 195-218). Hillsdale, NJ: Lawrence Erlbaum.

Patterson, G.R., Reid, J.B., and Dishion, T.J. 1992. *Antisocial boys*. Eugene, OR: Castalia.

Payne, S. 1991. *Women, health and poverty.* London: Harvester/Wheatsheaf.

Peirce, R.S., Frone, M.R., Russell, M., and Cooper, M.L. 1994. Relationship of financial strain and psychosocial resources to alcohol use and abuse: The mediating role of negative effect and drinking motives. *Journal of Health and Social Behavior*, 35, 291-308.

Pelton, L. 1991. Poverty and child protection. *Protecting Children,* 7, 3-5.

Perlman, S.B., Klerman, L., and Kinard, E.M. 1981. The use of socioeconomic data to predict teenage birth rates. *Public Health Reports*, July-August.

Perry, C. 1994. Extended family support among older Black females. In R. Staples (Ed.), *The Black family* (pp. 75-81). Belmont, CA: Wadsworth.

Persky, J., Sclar, E., and Wiewel, W. 1991. *Does America need cities?* Washington, DC: Economic Policy Institute.

Pettit, G.S., Clawson, M.A., Dodge, K.A., and Bates, J.E. 1996. Stability and change in peer-rejected status: The role of child behavior, parenting, and family ecology. *Merril-Palmer Quarterly*, 42, 267-294.

Pike, A., McGuire, S., Hetherington, E.M., Reiss, D., and Plomin, R. 1996. Family environment and adolescent depressive symptoms and antisocial behavior: A multivariate genetic analysis. *Developmental Psychology*, 32, 590-603.

Pillemer, K. 1985. The dangers of dependency: New findings on domestic violence against the elderly. *Social Problems*, 33, 147-158.

Plomin, R. 1994a. *Genetics and experience: The interplay between nature and nurture.* Thousand Oaks, CA: Sage.

Plomin, R. 1994b. Interface of nature and nurture in the family. In W.B. Carey and S.C. McDevitt (Eds.), *Prevention and early intervention: Individual differences as risk factors for the mental health of children* (pp. 179-189). New York: Brunner/Mazel.

Plomin, R. 1995. Genetics and children's experiences in the family. *Journal of Child Psychology and Psychiatry*, 36, 33-68.

Plomin, R., DeFries, J.C., and Loehlin, J.C. 1977. Genotype-environment interaction and correlation in the analysis of human behavior. *Psychological Bulletin*, 84, 309-322.

Plomin, R., DeFries, J.C., and McClearn, G.E. 1990. *Behavioral genetics: A primer,* 2nd ed. New York: Freeman.

Polakow, V. 1993. *Lives on the edge.* Chicago: The University of Chicago Press.

Portes, A. 1995a. Economic sociology and the sociology of immigration: A conceptual overview. In A. Portes (Ed.), *The economic sociology of immigration* (pp. 1-41). New York: Russell Sage.

Portes, A. 1995b. Children of immigrants: Segmented assimilation and its determinants. In A. Portes (Ed.), *The economic sociology of immigration* (pp. 248-279). New York: Russell Sage.

Portes, A., and McLeod, D. 1996. Educational progress of children of immigrants: The roles of class, ethnicity, and school context. *Sociology of Education*, 69, 255-275.

Portes, A., and Rumbaut, R.G. 1990. *Immigrant America: A portrait.* Berkeley, CA: University of California Press.

Powell, B., and Steelman, L.C. 1993. The educational benefits of being spaced out: Sibship density and educational progress. *American Sociological Review*, 58, 367-381.

Power, C., Manor, O., and Fox, J. 1991. *Health and class: The early years.* London: Chapman & Hall.

Power, C., Manor, O., Fox, A.J., and Fogelman, K. 1990. Health in childhood and social inequalities in health in young adults. *Journal of the Royal Statistical Society*, 153, 17-28.

Pratto, F., Stallworth, L.M., Sidanius, J., and Siers, B. 1997. The gender gap in occupational role attainment: A social dominance approach. *Journal of Personality and Social Psychology*, 72, 37-53.

Prilleltensky, I. 1997. Values, assumptions, and practices: Assessing the moral implications of psychological discourse and action. *American Psychologist*, 52, 517-535.

Pugh, H., Power, C., Goldblatt, P., and Arber, S. 1991. Women's lung cancer mortality, socio-economic status and changing smoking patterns. *Social Science and Medicine*, 32, 1105-1110.

Pulkkinen, L., and Tremblay, R.E. 1992. Pattern of social adjustment in two cultures and at different ages: A longitudinal perspective. *International Journal of Behavioral Development*, 15, 527-553.

Quinn, J.F., and Smeeding, T.M. 1994. Defying the averages: Poverty and well-being among older Americans. *Aging Today*, September/October, 15, 9.

Quinton, D., Pickles, A., Maughan, B., and Rutter, M. 1993. Partners, peers and pathways: Assortative pairing and continuities in conduct disorders. *Development and Psychopathology*, 5, 763-783.

Qvortrup, J. 1994a. Childhood matters: An introduction. In J. Qvortrup, M. Bardy, G. Sgritta, and H. Wintersberger (Eds.), *Childhood matters: Social theory, practice and politics* (pp. 1-23). Aldershot, UK: Avebury.

Qvortrup, J. 1994b. A new solidarity contract? The significance of a demographic balance for the welfare of both children and the elderly. In J. Qvortrup, M. Bardy, G. Sgritta, and H. Wintersberger (Eds.), *Childhood matters: Social theory, practice and politics* (pp. 319-334). Aldershot, UK: Avebury.

Qvortrup, J. 1995. From useful to useful: The historical continuity of children's constructive participation. *Sociological Studies of Children*, 7, 49-76.

Radwanski, G. 1987. *Ontario study of the relevance of education and the issue of dropouts*. Toronto: Ontario Ministry of Education.

Rafferty, Y., and Rollins, N. 1989. *Learning in limbo: The educational deprivation of homeless children*. New York: Advocates for Children. ERIC Document Reproduction No. ED 312-363.

Rafferty, Y., and Shinn, M. 1991. The impact of homelessness on children. *American Psychologist*, 46, 1170-1179.

Raley, R.K. 1996. A shortage of marriageable men? A note on the role of cohabitation in black-white differences in marriage rates. *American Sociological Review*, 61, 973-983.

Ram, B., Norris, M.J., and Skof, K. 1989. *The inner city in transition: Focus on Canada*. Cat no. 98-123. Ottawa: Minister of Supply and Services.

Ramey, C.T., and Ramey, S.L. 1990. Intensive education intervention for children of poverty. *Intelligence*, 14, 1-9.

Rank, M.R., and Hirschl, T. A. 1993. Welfare and the rural poor: Reasons for nonparticipation. *Demography*, 30, 607-622.

Rasberry, W. 1980. Illusion of black progress. *The Washington Post*, May 28, A19.

Rashid, A. 1994. *Family income in Canada*. Ottawa: Statistics Canada, cat. no. 96-318E; and Toronto: Prentice Hall.

Reed, R.J. 1988. Education and achievement of young black males. In J. T. Gibbs et al. (Eds.), *Young, black, and male in America* (pp. 37-96). Dover, MA: Auburn House.

Reiss, A., and Roth, J. 1993. *Understanding and preventing violence*. Washington, DC: National Academy Press.

Reiss, A.J., Jr. 1986. Why are communities important in understanding crime? In A.J. Reiss, Jr. and M. Tonry (Eds.), *Communities and crime* (pp. 1-33). Chicago: University of Chicago Press.

Rhoades, E. 1990. Profile of American Indians and Alaska Natives. In M.S. Harper (Ed.), *Minority aging.* DHHS Publication #HRS (P-DV-90-4). Washington, DC: U.S. Government Printing Office.

Rhodes, M. 1996. Globalization, the State and the restructuring of regional economies. In P. Gurnmett (Ed.), *Globalization and public policy* (pp. 161-180). Cheltenham, UK: Edward Elgar.

Rhodes, R.A.W. 1994. The hollowing out of the state: The changing nature of the public service in Britain. *Political Quarterly*, 65, 138-151.

Richters, J., and Weintraub, S. 1990. Beyond diathesis: Toward an understanding of high-risk environments. In J. Rolf et al. (Eds.), *Risk and protective factors in the development of psychopathology* (pp. 67-96). New York: University of Cambridge Press.

Ricketts, E. R., and Sawhill, I.V. 1988. Defining and measuring the underclass. *Journal of Policy Analysis and Management*, 7, 316-325.

Ries, P. 1990. *Americans assess their health: United States 1987.* Hyattsville, MD: National Center for Health Statistics.

Rifkin, J. 1995. *The end of work.* New York: Putnam's Sons.

Risman, B.J., and Ferree, M.M. 1995. Making gender visible. *American Sociological Review*, 60, 775-782.

Rivera-Batiz, F.L. 1992. Quantitative literacy and the likelihood of employment among young adults in the United States. *Journal of Human Resources*, 27, 313-328.

Rivkin, S.G. 1994. Residential segregation and school integration. *Sociology of Education*, 67, 279-292.

Roberge, R., Berthelot, J.-M., and Wolfson, M. 1995. Health and socioeconomic inequalities. *Canadian Social Trends*, 37, 15-19.

Roberts, J. 1995. Lone mothers and their children. *British Journal of Psychiatry*, 167, 263-277.

Robins, L.N. 1978. Sturdy childhood predictors of adult antisocial behavior: Replications from longitudinal studies. *Psychological Medicine*, 8, 611-622.

Robins, L.N., and Regier, D.A. (Eds.) 1991. *Psychiatric disorders in America: The epidemiologic catchment area study.* New York: Free Press.

Robins, L.N., Locke, B.Z., and Regier, D.A. 1991. An overview of psychiatric disorders in America. In L.N. Robins and D.A. Regier (Eds.), *Psychiatric disorders in America: The epidemiological catchment area study* (pp. 328-366). New York: Free Press.

Robins, R.W., John, O.P., Caspi, A., Moffitt, T.E., and Stouthamer-Loeber, M. 1996. Resilient, overcontrolled, and undercontrolled boys: Three replicable personality types. *Journal of Personality and Social Psychology*, 70, 157-171.

Rodgers, H.R., Jr. 1996. *Poor women, poor children,* 3rd ed. Armonk, NY: M.E. Sharpe.

Rodin, J. 1986. Aging and health: Effects of the sense of control. *Science*, 233, 1271-1276.

Rohe, W.M., and Stegman, M. 1994. The effects of homeownership on the self-esteem, perceived self-control and life satisfaction of low-income people. *Journal of the American Planning Association*, 60, 173-184.

Rohner, R.P., Bourque, S.L., and Elordi, C.A. 1996. Children's perceptions of corporal punishment, caretaker acceptance, and psychological adjustment in a poor, biracial Southern community. *Journal of Marriage and the Family*, 58, 842-852.

Romo, F.P., and Schwartz, M. 1995. The structural embeddedness of business decisions: The migration of manufacturing plants in New York State, 1960 to 1985. *American Sociological Review*, 60, 874-907.

Roosa, M.W., and Vaughan, L. 1984. A comparison of teenage and older mothers with preschool children. *Family Relations*, 33, 259-265.

Rose, H., and McClain, P. 1990. *Race, place and risk: Black homicide in urban America*. Albany, NY: State University of New York Press.

Rosenbaum, J., et al. 1993. Can the Kerner Commission's housing strategy improve employment, education, and social integration for low-income blacks? *North Carolina Law Review*, 71, 1521-1556.

Rosenbaum, J.E. 1991. Black pioneers—do their moves to the suburbs increase economic opportunity for mothers and children? *Housing Policy Debate*, 2, 179-213.

Rosier, K.B., and Corsaro, W.A. 1993. Competent parents, complex lives: Managing parenthood in poverty. *Journal of Contemporary Ethnography*, 22, 171-204.

Ross, C.E., and Huber, J. 1985. Hardship and depression. *Journal of Health and Social Behavior*, 26, 312-327.

Ross, C.E., and Wu, C. 1995. The links between education and health. *American Sociological Review*, 60, 719-745.

Ross, C.E., and Wu, C. 1996. Education, age, and the cumulative advantage in health. *Journal of Health and Social Behavior*, 37, 104-120.

Ross, D.P., Shillington, E.R., and Lockhead, C. 1994. *The Canadian fact book on poverty*. Ottawa: The Canadian Council on Social Development.

Rossi, P.H. 1990. *Down and out in America*. Chicago: University of Chicago Press.

Rossi, P.H., and Wright, J.D. 1993. The urban homeless: A portrait of urban dislocation. In W.J. Wilson (Ed.), *The ghetto underclass* (pp. 149-159). Newbury Park, CA: Sage.

Rowe, D.C. 1994. *The limits of family influence: Genes, experience, and behavior*. New York: Guilford Press.

Rowe, D.C., and Gulley, B.L. 1992. Sibling effects on substance use and delinquency. *Criminology*, 30, 217-233.

Rumberger, R.W. 1990. Second chance for high school dropouts: The costs and benefits of dropout recovery programs in the United States. In D. Inbar (Ed.),

Second chance in education: An interdisciplinary and international perspective (pp. 227-250). Philadelphia: Falmer Press.

Rumberger, R.W., and Larson, K.A. 1994. Keeping high-risk Chicano students in school. In R.J. Rossi (Ed.), *Schools and students at risk* (pp. 141-162). New York: Teachers College Press.

Rumberger, R.W., et al. 1990. Family influences on dropout behavior in one California high school. *Sociology of Education*, 63, 283-299.

Rural Sociological Society Task Force on Persistent Rural Poverty. 1993. *Persistent poverty in rural America.* Boulder, CO: Westview Press.

Rutter, M.L. 1997. Nature-nurture integration. The example of antisocial behavior. *American Psychologist*, 52, 390-398.

Rutter, M., and Rutter, M. 1993. *Developing minds: Challenge and continuity across the life span.* New York: Basic Books.

Rutter, M., Maughan, B., and Ouston, J. 1979. *Fifteen thousand hours.* Cambridge, MA: Harvard University Press.

Samerof, A.J. 1994. Developmental systems and family functioning. In R.D. Parke and S.G. Kellam (Eds.), *Exploring family relationships with other social contexts* (pp. 199-214). Hillsdale, NJ: Lawrence Erlbaum.

Sameroff, A.J., and Seifer, R. 1995. Accumulation of environmental risk and child mental health. In H.E. Fitzgerald, B.M. Lester, and B. Zuckerman (Eds.), *Children of poverty* (pp. 223-253). New York: Garland.

Sameroff, A.J., et al. 1987. Intelligence quotient scores of 4-year-old children: Social environmental risk factors. *Pediatrics*, 79, 343-350.

Sampson, R.J. 1987. Urban black violence: The effect of male joblessness and family disruption. *American Journal of Sociology*, 93, 348-405.

Sampson, R.J. 1992. Family management and child development: Insights from social disorganization theory. In J. McCord (Ed.), *Facts, frameworks, and forecasts* (pp. 63-94). New Brunswick, NJ: Transaction.

Sampson, R.J. 1993. The community context of violent crime. In W.J. Wilson (Ed.), *Sociology and the public agenda* (pp. 259-286). Newbury Park, CA: Sage.

Sampson, R.J. 1997. Collective regulation of adolescent misbehavior: Validation results from eighty Chicago neighborhoods. *Journal of Adolescent Research*, 12, 227-244.

Sampson, R.J., and Groves, W.B. 1989. Community structure and crime: Testing social disorganization theory. *American Journal of Sociology*, 94, 774-802.

Sampson, R.J., and Laub, J.H. 1992. Crime and deviance in the life course. *Annual Review of Sociology*, 18, 63-84.

Sampson, R.J., and Laub, J.H. 1993. *Crime in the making: Pathways and turning points through life.* Cambridge, MA: Harvard University Press.

Sampson, R.J., and Laub, J.H. 1994. Urban poverty and the context of delinquency: A new look at structure and process in a classic study. *Child Development*, 65, 523-540.

Sandfort, J.R., and Hill, M.S. 1996. Assisting young, unmarried mothers to become self-sufficient: The effects of different types of early economic support. *Journal of Marriage and the Family*, 58, 311-326.

Sapolsky, R.M. 1990. Stress in the wild. *Scientific American*, 262, 1, 116-123.

Saporiti, A., and Sgritta, G.B. 1990. *Childhood as a social phenomenon— National report: Italy*. Vienna: European Centre.

Sassen, S. 1991. *The global city: New York, London, Tokyo*. Princeton, NJ: Princeton University Press.

Sassen, S. 1994. *Cities in a world economy*. Thousand Oaks, CA: Pine Forge Press.

Saudino, K.J., Pedersen, N.L., Lichtenstein, P., McClearn, G.E., and Plomin, R. 1997. Can personality explain genetic influences on life events? *Journal of Personality and Social Psychology*, 72, 196-206.

Saugstad, L.F. 1989. Social class, marriage, and fertility in schizophrenia. *Schizophrenia Bulletin*, 15, 9-43.

Sawhill, I.V. 1988. Poverty and the underclass. In *Challenges to leadership: Economic and social issues for the next decade*. Washington, DC: Urban Institute Press.

Sawhill, I.V. 1992. Young children and families. In H.J. Aaron and C.L. Schultze (Eds.), *Setting domestic priorities: What can governments do?* Washington, DC: The Brookings Institution.

Scarr, S. 1985. Constructing psychology: Making facts and fables for our times. *American Psychologist*, 40, 499-512.

Scarr, S. 1993. Biological and cultural diversity: The legacy of Darwin for development. *Child Development*, 64, 1333-1353.

Scarr, S., and McCartney, K. 1983. How people make their own environments: A theory of genotype-environment effects. *Child Development*, 54, 424-435.

Scarr, S., Pakstis, A., Katz, S.H., and Barber, W.B. 1977. The absence of a relationship between degree of White ancestry and intellectual skills within the Black population. *Human Genetics*, 39, 69-86.

Scheper-Hughes, N. (Ed.). 1987. *Child survival*. Dordrecht, Germany: D. Reidel.

Scheper-Hughes, N. 1992. *Death without weeping*. Berkeley, CA: University of California Press.

Schiller, B.R. 1995. *The economics of poverty and discrimination*, 6th ed. Englewood Cliffs, NJ: Prentice-Hall.

Schor, E.L., and Menaghan, E.G. 1995. Family pathways to child health. In B.C. Amick, S. Levine, A.R. Tarlov, and D.C. Walsh (Eds.), *Society and health* (pp. 18-45). New York: Oxford University Press.

Schteingart, J.S., Molnar, J., Klein, T.P., Lowe, C.B., and Hartmann, A.H. 1995. Homelessness and child functioning in the context of risks and protective factors moderating child outcomes. *Journal of Clinical Child Development*, 24, 320-331.

Schuerman, L.A., and Kobrin, S. 1986. Community careers and crime. In A. Reiss and M. Tonry (Eds.), *Communities and crime* (pp. 67-100). Chicago: University of Chicago Press.

Schultz, T. 1961. Investment in human capital. *American Economic. Review*, 51, 1-17.

Schwab-Stone, M.E., Ayers, T.S., Kasprow, W., Voyce, C., Barone, C., Shriver, T., and Weissberg, R.P. 1995. No safe haven: A study of violence exposure in an urban community. *Journal of the American Academy of Child and Adolescent Psychiatry*, 34, 1343-1352.

Schwartz, J.E., Friedman, H.S., Tucker, J.S., Tomlinson-Keasey, C., Wingard, D.L., and Criqui, M.H. 1995. Sociodemographic and psychological factors in childhood as predictors of adult mortality. *American Journal of Public Health*, 85, 1237-1245.

Schwenk, F.N. 1992. Income and expenditures of older, widowed, divorced, and never-married women who live alone. *Family Economics Review*, 5, 2-8.

Seppa, N. 1997. Children's TV remains steeped in violence. APA *Monitor,* June, p. 36.

Serrill, M.S. 1996. Unlock the shackles. *Time*, June 10, p. 37.

Sgritta, G.B. 1994. The generational division of welfare: Equity and conflict. In J. Qvortrup, M. Bardy, G. Sgritta, and H. Wintersberger (Eds.), *Childhood matters: Social theory, practice and politics* (pp. 335-361). Aldershot, UK: Avebury.

Shakoor, B., and Chalmers, D. 1991. Co-victimization of African American children who witness violence: Effects on cognitive, emotional, and behavioral development. *Journal of the National Medical Association*, 83, 233-237.

Shavit, Y., and Pierce, J.L. 1991. Sibship size and educational attainment in nuclear and extended families. *American Sociological Review*, 56, 321-330.

Sheets, R.G., Nord, S., and Phelps, J.J. 1987. *The impact of service industries on underemployment in metropolitan economies.* Lexington, MA: D.C. Heath.

Sheley, J.F., and Wright, J.D. 1995. *In the line of fire: Youth, guns, and violence in urban America.* Hawthorne, NY: Aldine de Gruyter.

Sherman, A. 1992. *Falling by the wayside: Children in rural America.* Washington, DC: Children's Defense Fund.

Shields, P.M., and Shaver, D.M. 1991. School and community influences on effective academic instruction. In M.S. Knapp and P.M. Shields (Eds.), *Better schooling for the children of poverty* (pp. 313-328). Berkeley, CA: McCutchan.

Shihadeh, E.S., and Steffensmeier, D.J. 1994. Economic inequality, family disruption, and urban Black violence: Cities as units of stratification and social control. *Social Forces*, 73, 729-751.

Shinn, M., Knickman, J., and Weitzman, B.C. 1991. Social relationships and vulnerability to becoming homeless among poor families. *American Psychologist*, 46, 1180-1187.

Simon, D. 1995. Debt, democracy and development: Sub-Saharan Africa in the 1990s. In D. Simon, W. van Spengen, C. Dixon, and A. Narman (Eds.), *Structurally adjusted Africa* (pp. 17-44). London: Pluto Press.

Simons, L.M. 1996. High-tech jobs for sale. *Time,* July 22, p. 23.

Simons, R.L., Johnson, C., and Conger, R.D. 1994. Harsh corporal punishment versus quality of parental involvement as an explanation of adolescent maladjustment. *Journal of Marriage and the Family*, 56, 591-607.

Simons, R.L., Wu, C.I., Conger, R.D., and Lorenz, F.O. 1994. Two routes to delinquency: Differences between early and late starters on the impact of parenting and deviant peers. *Criminology*, 32, 247-276.

Skogan, W.G. 1990. *Disorder and decline: Crime and the spiral of decay in American neighborhoods*. New York: Free Press.

Slavin, R.E. 1994. *Educational psychology: Theory and practice*, 4th ed. Needham Heights, MA: Allyn and Bacon.

Smeeding, T., and Rainwater, L. 1995. Cross-national trends in income, poverty, and dependence: The evidence of young adults in the eighties. In K. McFate (Ed.), *Poverty, inequality, and the future of social policy*. New York: Russell Sage.

Smith, D.R., and Jarjoura, G.R. 1988. Social structure and criminal victimization. *Journal of Research in Crime and Delinquency*, 25, 27-52.

Smith, G.D., and Eggers, M. 1992. Socioeconomic differences in mortality in Britain and the U.S. *American Journal of Public Health*, 82, 1079-1080.

Smith, J. 1989. Children among the poor. *Demography*, 26, 235-248.

Smith, M.D., Devine, J.A., and Sheley, J.F. 1992. Unemployment and crime: Age and race effects. *Sociological Perspectives*, 35, 551-572.

SmithBattle, L. 1996. Intergenerational ethics of caring for adolescent mothers and their children. *Family Relations*, 45, 56-64.

Smock, P. 1994. Gender and short-run economic consequences of marital disruption. *Social Forces*, 74, 243-262.

Snyder, H.N., and Sickmund, M. 1995. *Juvenile offenders and victims: A national report*. Washington, DC: Office of Juvenile Justice and Delinquent Prevention.

Solon, G., Corcoran, M., Gordon, R., and Laren, D. 1988. Sibling and intergenerational correlations in welfare program participation. *Journal of Human Resources*, 23, 388-396.

Sorlie, P.D., Backlund, E., Johnson, N.J., and Rogot, E. 1993. Mortality by Hispanic status in the United States. *Journal of the American Medical Association*, 270, 2464-2468.

South, S.J. 1996. Mate availability and the transition to unwed motherhood: A paradox of population structure. *Journal of Marriage and the Family*, 58, 265-280.

South, S.J., and Crowder, K.D. 1997. Escaping distressed neighborhoods: Individual, community, and metropolitan influences. *American Journal of Sociology*, 102, 1040-1084.

South, S.J., and Spitze, G. 1986. Determinants of divorce over the marital life course. *American Sociological Review*, 51, 583-590.

Spitze, G., and Logan, J.R. 1991. Sibling structure and intergenerational relations. *Journal of Marriage and the Family*, 53, 871-884.

Srole, L., Langner, T.S., Michael, S.T., Opler, M.K., and Rennie, T.A.C. 1968. *Mental health in the metropolis: The Midtown Manhattan Study*. New York: McGraw-Hill.

Sroufe, L.A., and Rutter, M. 1984. The domain of developmental psychopathology. *Child Development*, 55, 17-29.

Starrels, M.E., Bould, S., and Nicholas, L.J. 1994. The femininization of poverty in the United States: Gender, race, ethnicity, and family factors. *Journal of Family Issues*, 15, 590-607.

Statistics Canada. 1991a. *School leavers survey.* Ottawa: Employment and Immigration Canada.

Statistics Canada. 1991b. *Ethnic origin: The nation.* Ottawa: Census, Cat. no. 93-315.

Statistics Canada. 1992. *Lone-parent families in* Canada. Ottawa: Housing, Family and Social Statistics Division. Cat no. 89-522E.

Statistics Canada. 1993a. *Selected income statistics.* Ottawa: Minister of Industry, Science and Technology. Cat. no. 93-331.

Statistics Canada. 1993b. *Housing costs and other characteristics of Canadian households.* Ottawa: Minister of Industry, Science and Technology.

Statistics Canada. 1994. *Health status of Canadians.* Ottawa: Minister of Industry, Science and Technology. Cat. no. 11-612E.

Statistics Canada. 1995a. *Profile of Canada's Aboriginal population.* Ottawa: Minister of Industry, Science and Technology. Cat. no. 94-325.

Statistics Canada. 1995b. Alcohol use and its consequences. *Canadian Social Trends*, 38, 18-23.

Steinberg, L., and Darling, N.E. 1994. The broader context of social influence in adolescence. In R.K. Silbereisen and E. Todt (Eds.), *Adolescence in context* (pp. 25-45). New York: Springer-Verlag.

Steinberg, L., Darling, N.E., Fletcher, A.C., Brown, B.B., and Dornbusch, S.F. 1995. Authoritative parenting and adolescent adjustment: An ecological journey. In P. Moen, G.H. Elder, Jr., and K. Luscher (Eds.), *Examining lives in context* (pp. 432-446). Washington, DC: American Psychological Association.

Sternberg, K.J., Lamb, M.E., Greenbaum, C., Cicchetti, D., Dawud, S., Cortes, R.M., Krispin, O., and Lorey, F. 1993. Effects of domestic violence on children's behavior problems and depression. *Developmental Psychology*, 29, 44-52.

Stevenson, D.L., and Baker, D.P. 1987. The family-school relation and the child's school performance. *Child Development*, 58, 1348-1357.

Stevenson, H.W., and Stigler, J.W. 1992. *The learning gap: Why our schools are failing and what we learn from Japanese and Chinese education.* Ciba Foundation Symposium 89. London: Pitman.

Stokes, R., and Chevan, A. 1996. Female-headed families: Social and economic context of racial differences. *Journal of Urban Affairs*, 18, 245-268.

Stokols, D. 1992. Establishing and maintaining healthy environments: Toward a social ecology of health promotion. *American Psychologist*, 47, 6-22.

St. Peter, R.F., Newacheck, P.W., and Halfon, N. 1992. Access to care for poor children. Separate and unequal? *Journal of the American Medical Association*, 267, 2760-2764.

Straub, L.A., and Walzer, N. 1992. *Rural health care: Innovation in a changing environment.* Westport, CT: Praeger.

Straus, M.A. 1994. *Beating the devil out of them: Corporal punishment in American families.* New York: Lexington Books.

Strawn, J. 1992. *The states and the poor: Child poverty rises as the social safety net shrinks.* Social Policy Report. Ann Arbor, MI: Society for Research in Child Development.

Strobel, F.R. 1993. *Upward dreams, downward mobility. The economic decline of the American middle class.* Boston: Rowman Littlefield.

Strobino, D.M. 1987. The health and medical consequences of adolescent sexuality and pregnancy: A review of the literature. In S. Hofferth and C.D. Hayes (Eds.), *Risking the future*, vol. 2 (pp. 93-122). National Research Council. Washington, DC: National Academy Press.

Suarez-Orozco, M.M. 1991. Immigrant adaptation to schooling: A Hispanic case. In M.A. Gibson and J.U. Ogbu (Eds.), *Minority status and schooling* (pp. 37-61). New York: Garland.

Sudarkasa, N. 1997. African American families and family values. In H.P. McAdoo (Ed.), *Black families*, 3rd ed. (pp. 9-40) Thousand Oaks, CA: Sage.

Sui-Chu, E.H., and Willms, J.D. 1996. Effects of parental involvement on eighth-grade achievement. *Sociology of Education*, 69, 126-141.

Sullivan, M. 1989a. Absent fathers in the inner city. *Annals*, 501, 48-58.

Sullivan, M. 1989b. *Getting paid: Youth crime and work in the inner city.* Ithaca, NY: Cornell University.

Swadener, B.B. 1995. Children and families "at promise": Deconstructing the discourse of risk. In B.B. Swadener and S. Lubeck (Eds.), *Children and families "at promise"* (pp. 17-49). Albany: State University of New York Press.

Taeuber, C. 1991. Diversity: The dramatic reality. In S. Bass, E. Kutza, and F. M. Torres-Gil (Eds.), *Diversity in aging* (pp. 1-47). Glenview, IL.: Scott, Foresman.

Taylor, R., and Covington, J. 1988. Neighborhood changes in ecology and violence. *Criminology*, 26, 553-590.

Terman, L.M., and Oden, M.H. 1947. *Genetic studies of genius: The gifted child grows up*, vol. 4. Stanford, CA: Stanford University Press.

Tesh, S. N. 1988. *Hidden arguments: Political ideology and disease prevention policy.* New Brunswick, NJ: Rutgers University Press.

Tessler, R., and Dennis, D. 1989. *A synthesis of NIMH-funded research concerning persons who are homeless and mentally ill.* Washington, DC: National Institute of Mental Health.

Testa, M.F. 1992. Racial and ethnic variation in the early life course of adolescent welfare mothers. In M.K. Rosenheim and M.F. Testa (Eds.), *Early parenthood and coming of age in the 1990s* (pp. 89-112). New Brunswick, NJ: Rutgers University Press.

Testa, M., Astone, N.M., Krogh, M., and Neckerman, K.M. 1993. Employment and marriage among inner-city fathers. In W.J. Wilson (Ed.), *The ghetto underclass* (pp. 96-108). Newbury Park, CA: Sage.

Thomas, G., Farrell, M.P., and Barnes, G.M. 1996. The effects of single-mother families and nonresident fathers on delinquency and substance abuse in black and white adolescents. *Journal of Marriage and the Family*, 58, 884-894.

Thompson, M., Alexander, K., and Entwisle, D. 1988. Household composition, parental expectations, and school achievement. *Social Forces*, 67, 424-451.

Thomson, E., McLanahan, S.S., and Curtin, R.B. 1992. Family structure, gender, and parental socialization. *Journal of Marriage and the Family*, 54, 368-378.

Thornton, A. 1991. Influence of the marital history of parents on the marital and cohabitational experiences of children. *American Journal of Sociology*, 96, 868-894.

Tienda, M., and Stier, H. 1996. Generating labor market inequality: Employment opportunities and the accumulation of disadvantage. *Social Problems*, 43, 147-165.

Tilly, C. 1991. Reasons for the continuing growth of part-time employment. *Monthly Labor Review*, 114, 10-18.

Todd, G. 1993. *The political economy of urban and regional restructuration in Canada: Toronto, Montreal and Vancouver in the global economy, 1970-1990.* Toronto: York University, PhD dissertation, Department of Political Science.

Tonry, M. 1995. *Malign neglect—race, crime, and punishment in America.* New York: Oxford University Press.

Toro, P.A., and Wall, D.D. 1991. Research on homeless persons: Diagnostic comparisons and practice implications. *Professional Psychology: Research and Practice*, 22, 479-488.

Toro, P.A., Bellevia, C.W., Daeschler, C.V., Owens, B.J., Wall, D.D., Passero, J.M., and Thomas, D.M. 1995. Distinguishing homelessness from poverty: A comparative study. *Journal of Consulting and Clinical Psychology*, 63, 280-289.

Townsend, P., and Davidson, N. (Eds.). 1990. *Inequalities in health: The Black report.* London: Penguin.

Tschann, J.M., Kaiser, P., Chesney, M.A., Alkon, A., and Boyce, W.T. 1996. Resilience and vulnerability among preschool children: Family functioning, temperament, and behavioral problems. *Journal of the American Academy of Child and Adolescent Psychiatry*, 35, 184-192.

Tshishimbi, wa B., Glick, P., and Thorbecke, E. 1994. Missed opportunity for adjustment in a rent-seeking society: The case of Zaire. In D.E. Sahn (Ed.), *Adjusting to policy failure in African economies* (pp. 96-130). Ithaca, NY: Cornell University Press.

Tucker, M.B., and Mitchell-Kernan, C. (Eds.). 1995. *The decline in marriage among African Americans.* New York: Russell Sage.

Turner, J.B. 1995. Economic context and the health effects of unemployment. *Journal of Health and Social Behavior*, 36, 213-229.

Turner, R.J., Wheaton, B., and Lloyd, D.A. 1995. The epidemiology of social stress. *American Sociological Review*, 60, 104-125.

Umberson, D. 1992. Relationship between adult children and their parents: Psychological consequences for both generations. *Journal of Marriage and the Family*, 54, 664-674.

Uribe, F.M.T., LeVine, R.A., and LeVine, S.E. 1994. Maternal behavior in a Mexican community: The changing environments of children. In P.G. Greenfield and R.R.

Cocking (Eds.), *Crosscultural roots of minority child development* (pp. 41-54). Hillsdale, NJ: Lawrence Erlbaum.

U.S. Bureau of the Census. 1990a. *Money income and poverty status in the United States.* Current Population Reports, Series P-60, No. 168, 1989. Washington, DC: U.S. Government Printing Office.

U.S. Bureau of the Census. 1990b. *Modified and actual age, sex, race, and Hispanic origin data.* Series CPH-L-74. Washington, DC: U.S. Department of Commerce.

U.S. Bureau of the Census. 1990c. *Supplementary reports, 1990 census of population: Age, sex, race, and Spanish origin of the population by regions, divisions, and states.* Washington, DC: U.S. Government Printing Office.

U.S. Bureau of the Census. 1991. *Money income of households, families, and persons in the United States: 1990.* Current Population Reports, Series P-60, No. 174. Washington, DC: U.S. Government Printing Office.

U.S. Bureau of the Census. 1992a. *Statistical abstract of the United States:1992.* Washington, DC: U.S. Government Printing Office.

U.S. Bureau of the Census. 1992b. *1990 Census of the population*, Part 1. Washington, DC: U.S. Government Printing Office.

U.S. Bureau of the Census. 1993a. *Fertility of American women, June, 1992.* Current Population Reports, Series P-20. Washington, DC: Government Printing Office.

U.S. Bureau of the Census. 1993b. *Poverty in the United States: 1992.* Washington, DC: U.S. Government Printing Office.

U.S. Bureau of the Census. 1993c. *Population projections of the U.S. by age, sex, race, and Hispanic origin data: 1993 to 2050.* Current Population Reports, Series P-25, No. 1104. Washington, DC: U.S. Department of Commerce.

U.S. Bureau of the Census. 1993d. *Statistical abstract of the United States: 1993.* Washington, DC: U.S. Government Printing Office.

U.S. Bureau of the Census. 1994. *Statistical abstract of the United States, 1994.* Washington, DC: U.S. Government Printing Office.

U.S. Bureau of the Census. 1995. *Income, poverty, and valuation of noncash benefits: 1993.* Current Population Reports, Series P-60, No. 188. Washington, DC: U.S. Government Printing Office.

U.S. Bureau of the Census. 1996. *Population projections of the United States by age, sex, race, and Hispanic origin: 1995 to 2050.* Current Population Reports, Series P-25-1130. Washington, DC: U.S. Government Printing Office.

U.S. Conference of Mayors. 1989. *A status report on hunger and homelessness in America's cities—a 27-city survey.* Washington, DC: U.S. Conference of Mayors.

U.S. Congress; Committee on Ways and Means. 1992. *Green Book.* Washington, DC: U.S. Government Printing Office.

U.S. Department of Agriculture. 1990. Nonmetro income growth sluggish. *Economic Research Service Rural Conditions and Trends*, 1, 14-15.

U.S. Department of Health and Human Services. 1995. *Report to Congress on* out-of-wedlock childbearing. DHHS Publ. No. PHS 95-1257. Hyattsville, MD: Public Health Services.

U.S. Department of Justice. 1985. The risk of violent crime. Washington, DC: U.S. Government Printing Office.

U.S. Senate Special Committee on Aging. 1992. Aging America: Trends and projections, 1990-91. Washington, DC: U.S. Department of Health and Human Services.

Uzzell, O., and Peebles-Wilkins, W. 1989. Black spouse abuse: A focus on relational factors and intervention strategies. Western Journal of Black Studies, 13, 10-16.

Vagero, D., and Lundberg, O. 1989. Health inequalities in Britain and Sweden. Lancet, 2, 35-36.

Valdivieso, R., and Nicolau, S. 1994. "Look me in the eye." In R.J. Rossi (Ed.), Schools and students at risk (pp. 90-115). New York: Teachers College Press.

Vanier Institute of the Family. 1994. Profiling Canada's families. Ottawa: VIF.

van IJzendoorn, M.H., et al. 1992. The relative effects of maternal and child problems on the quality of attachment: A meta-analysis of attachment in clinical samples. Child Development, 63, 840-858.

Vega, W.A., and Amaro, H. 1994. Latino outlook: Good health, uncertain prognosis. Annual Review of Public Health, 15, 39-67.

Venezky, R., Kaestle, C., and Sum, A.M. 1987. The subtle danger: Reflections on the literacy abilities of America's young adults. Princeton, NJ: Educational Testing Service.

Vinokur, A.D., Price, R.H., and Caplan, R.D. 1996. Hard times and hurtful partners: How financial strain affects depression and relationship satisfaction of unemployed persons and their spouses. Journal of Personality and Social Psychology, 71, 166-179.

Vogt, R., Cameron, B.J., and Dolan, E.G. 1991. Economics (4th ed.). Toronto: Dryden.

Volpe, R. 1989. Poverty and child abuse: A review of selected literature. Toronto: The Institute for the Prevention of Child Abuse.

Wachs, T.D. 1983. The use and abuse of environment in behavioral genetic research. Child Development, 54, 396-407.

Wachs, T.D. 1987. Specificity and environmental action as manifest in environment correlates of infants' mastery motivation. Developmental Psychology, 23, 782-790.

Wachs, T.D. 1996. Known and potential processes underlying developmental trajectories in childhood and adolescence. Developmental Psychology, 4, 796-801.

Wacquant, L.J.D. 1995. The ghetto, the state, and the new capitalist economy. In P. Kasinitz (Ed.), Metropolis: Center and symbol of our times (pp. 413-449). New York: New York University Press.

Wacquant, L.J.D., and Wilson, W.J. 1989. The cost of racial and class exclusion in the inner city. Annals of the American Academy of Political and Social Science, 501, 8-26.

Wadhera, S., and Strachan, J. 1992. *Teenage pregnancies in Canada, 1975-1989.* Health Reports vol. 3 no. 4. Ottawa: Minister of Industry, Science and Technology.

Wallace, R., and Wallace, D. 1990. Origins of public health collapse in New York City: The dynamics of planned shrinkage, contagious urban decay and social disintegration. *Bulletin of the New York Academy of Medicine,* 66, 391-434.

Waller, J.H. 1971. Achievement and social mobility: Relationships among IQ score, education, and occupation in two generations. *Social Biology,* 18, 252-259.

Wanner, R.A., and McDonald, P.L. 1986. The vertical mosaic in later life: Ethnicity and retirement in Canada. *Journal of Gerontology,* 41, 662-671.

Warr, M. 1993. Age, peers, and delinquency. *Criminology,* 31, 17-40.

Warr, M., and Stafford, M. 1991. The influence of delinquent peers: What they think or what they do? *Criminology,* 29, 851-866.

Warr, P. 1985. Twelve questions about unemployment and health. In B. Roberts, R. Finnegan, and D. Gollie (Eds.), *New approaches to economic life.* Manchester, UK: Manchester University Press.

Warren, J.R. 1996. Educational inequality among white and Mexican-American origin adolescents in the American Southwest: 1990. *Sociology of Education,* 69, 142-158.

Wartella, E. 1995. Media and problem behaviours in young people. In M. Rutter and D.J. Smith (Eds.), *Psychosocial disorders in young people* (pp. 296-323). Chichester: John Wiley and Sons.

Wasserman, G.A., Brunelli, S.A., and Rauh, V.A. 1990. Social supports and living arrangements of adolescent and adult mothers. *Journal of Adolescent Research,* 5, 54-66.

Wasserman, G.A., Rauh, V. A., Brunelli, S.A., Castro, G.M., and Necos, B. 1990. Psychosocial attributes and life experiences of disadvantaged minority mothers: Age and ethnic variations. *Child Development,* 61, 566-580.

Waters, H.F. 1993. Networks under the gun. *Newsweek,* July 12, pp. 64-66.

Weatherall, D. 1992. *The Harveian oration—The role of nature and nurture in common diseases: Garrod's legacy.* London: The Royal College of Physicians.

Werner, E.E. 1990. Predictive factors and individual resilience. In S.J. Meisels and J.P. Shonkoff (Eds.), *Handbook of early childhood education.* Cambridge, UK: Cambridge University Press.

Werner, E., and Smith, R. 1982. *Vulnerable but invincible.* New York: McGraw-Hill.

Werthamer-Larsson, L., Kellam, S.G., and Wheeler, L. 1991. Effect of first-grade classroom environment on shy behavior, aggressive behavior, and concentration problems. *American Journal of Community Psychology,* 19, 585-602.

West, C. 1993. *Race matters.* Boston: Beacon Press.

Wethington, E. 1996. Crime and punishment. In U. Bronfenbrenner et al. (Eds.), *The state of Americans* (pp. 29-50) New York: Free Press.

White, J., Moffitt, T.E. Earls, F., Robins, L.N., and Silva, P.A. 1990. How early can we tell? Preschool predictors of boys' conduct disorder and delinquency. *Criminology*, 28, 507-533.

White, K.R., Taylor, M.J., and Moss, V.D. 1992. Does research support claims about the benefits of involving parents in early intervention programs? *Review of Educational Research*, 62, 91-125.

Whitehead, M. 1990. *Inequalities in health: The health divide*. London: Penguin.

Wilkinson, R.G. 1990. Income distribution and mortality: A "natural" experiment. *Sociology of Health and Illness*, 12, 391-412.

Wilkinson, R.G. 1992. Income distribution and life expectancy. *British Medical Journal*, 304, 165-168.

Williams, D.R. 1990. Socioeconomic differentials in health: A review and redirection. *Social Psychology Quarterly*, 53, 81-99.

Williams, D.R., and Collins, C. 1995. US economic and racial differences in health: Patterns and explanations. *Annual Review of Sociology*, 21 , 349-386.

Wilson, J.B., Ellwood, D.T., and Brooks-Gunn, J. 1995. Welfare-to-work through the eyes of children. In P.L. Chase-Lansdale and J. Brooks-Gunn (Eds.), *Escape from poverty: What makes a difference for children?* (pp. 170-185). Cambridge: Cambridge University Press.

Wilson, J.Q., and Hernnstein, R.J. 1985. *Crime and human nature*. New York: Simon & Schuster.

Wilson, W.J. 1987. *The truly disadvantaged*. Chicago: University of Chicago Press.

Wilson, W.J. 1991a. Studying inner-city school dislocations: The challenge of public agenda research. *American Sociological Review*, 56, 1-14.

Wilson, W.J. 1991b. Public policy research and "the truly disadvantaged." In C. Jencks and P.E. Peterson (Eds.), *The urban underclass*. Washington, DC: The Brookings Institution.

Wilson, W.J. 1996. *When work disappears: The world of the new urban poor*. New York: Knopf.

Winkleby, M., Fortmann, S., and Barrett, D. 1990. Social class disparities in risk factors for disease: Eight-year prevalence patterns by level of education. *Preventive Medicine*, 19, 1-12.

Winkleby, M.A., et al. 1992. Socioeconomic status and health: How education, income, and occupation contribute to risk factors for cardiovascular disease. *American Journal of Public Health*, 82, 816-820.

Wintersberger, H. 1994. Costs and benefits—The economics of childhood. In J. Qvortrup, M. Bardy, G. Sgritta, and H. Wintersberger (Eds.), *Childhood matters: Social theory, practice and politics* (pp. 213-248). Aldershot, UK: Avebury.

Wolfe, B.L. 1995. Economic issues of health care. In B.L. Chase-Lansdale and J. Brooks-Gunn (Eds.), *Escape from poverty: What makes a difference for children?* (pp. 170-185). Cambridge: Cambridge University Press.

Wolfe, B.L., and Hill, S. 1993. The health, earnings capacity, and poverty of single-mother families. In D.B. Papadimitriou and E.N. Wolff (Eds.), *Poverty and prosperity in the USA in the late Twentieth Century* (pp. 89-120). New York: St. Martin's Press.

Wolfgang, M.E., Thornberry, T.P., and Figlio, R.M. 1987. *From boy to man, from delinquency to crime.* Chicago, IL: The University of Chicago Press.

World Bank 1993. *The East Asian miracle economies.* Washington, DC: World Bank.

Wright, J.D. 1989. *Address unknown: The homeless in America.* Hawthorne, NY: Aldine de Gruyter.

Wu, L.L. 1996. Effects of family structure and income on risks of premarital birth. *American Sociological Review*, 61, 386-406.

Yansane, A.Y. 1996. Are alternative development strategies suitable for Africa to remedy its deepening crisis? In A.Y. Yansane (Ed.), *Prospects for recovery and sustainable development in Africa* (pp. 3-33). Westport, CT: Greenwood Press.

Yeo, F.L. 1997. *Inner-city schools, multiculturalism, and teacher education.* New York: Garland.

Zelizer, V.A.R. 1985. *Pricing the priceless child: The changing social value of children.* New York: Basic Books.

Zelkowitz, P., Papageorgigio, A., Zelazo, P.R., and Weiss, M.J.S. 1995. Behavioral adjustment in very low and normal birth weight children. *Journal of Clinical Child Psychology*, 24, 21-30.

Zill, N., and Coiro, M.J. 1992. Assessing the condition of children. *Children and Youth Sciences Review*, 14, 119-136.

Zill, N., and Nord, C.W. 1994. *Running the place: How American families are faring in a changing economy and an individualistic society.* Washington, DC: Child Trends, Inc.

Zill, N., Morrison, D.R., and Coiro, M.J. 1993. Long-term effects of parental divorce on parent-child relationships, adjustment, and achievement in young adulthood. *Journal of Family Psychology*, 7, 91-103.

Zill, N., Moore, K.A., Smith, E.W., Stief, T., and Coiro, M.J. 1995. The life circumstances and development of children in welfare families: A profile based on national survey data. In P.L. Chase-Lansdale and J. Brooks-Gunn (Eds.), *Escape from poverty: What makes a difference for children?* (pp. 11-37). Cambridge: Cambridge University Press.

Zima, B.T., Wells, K.B., Benjamin, B., and Duan, N. 1996. Mental health problems among homeless mothers: Relationship to service use and child mental health problems. *Archives of General Psychiatry*, 53, 332-338.

Zingraff, M.T., Leiter, M.C., Johnsen, M.C., and Myers, K.A. 1994. The mediating effect of good school performance in the maltreatment-delinquency relationship. *Journal of Research in Crime and Delinquency*, 31, 62-91.

Zuckerman, D. 1996. Media violence, gun control, and public policy. *American Journal of Orthopsychiatry*, 66, 378-389.

Author Index

When there are four or more co-authors, only the first co-author is indexed.

Abbott, M., 214
Abell, E., 220
Abrahamse, A. F., 218
Aday, L. A., 71,151
Adler, N. E., 144
Agnew, R., 223
Alba, R. D., 221
Alderson, A. S., 45,213
Alexander, K. L., 80,84,136,215
Alwin, D. F., 104,220
Amaro, H., 141
Amato, P. R., 215,216
Ambert, A. M., 2,104,107,111,114,
        164,177,205,216,219,224
Andersen, H. F., 219,221
Andersen, O., 144
Anderson, K. E., 94,99,215,219
Aneshensel, C. S., 69
Anthony, J. C., 138
Apfel, R. J., 223
Aquilino, W. S., 96
Arber, S., 54
Armey, D., 117
Arnold, M. S., 113,200
Aro, H. M., 49
Aseltine, R. H.,153,163
Asher, S. R., 220
Ashton-Warner, S., 217
Assembly of First Nations, 133
Astone, N. M., 218
Atchley, R. C., 123
Attar, B. K., 223
Avina, J., 39

Baker, D. P., 218
Baker, L., 214
Baker, M., 218
Bane, M. J., 18,46,47,60,225
Bardy, M., 220
Barker, D. J., 223
Barnes, G. M., 99
Barresi, C., 147
Barrett, D., 222
Bassler, O. C., 217
Bassuk, E. L., 152
Baumrind, D., 113
Baydar, N., 48
Beach, C., 214
Becker, G., 218
Beggs, J. J., 130
Bell, C. C., 69
Bell, R. Q., 180
Belsky, J., 219
Bengtson, V. L., 97,125
Benjamin, D., 214
Bennett, N. J., 46,215
Berger, E. H., 79
Bergman, L. R., 225
Bergob, M., 47
Bernhardt, A., 79,87
Berthelot, J. M., 150
Besharov, D. J., 131
Biblarz, T. J.,49
Bickford, A., 201
Billingsley, A., 129
Black, D., 150
Blackburn, C., 145,215,222

Blake, J., 218
Blakeley, E. J., 25,57,60
Blank, R. M., 30
Blau, F. D., 131
Bloom, D. E., 46,215
Bluestone, B., 15,27,60
Bobak, M.,149,158
Bolger, K. E., 220
Boring, C. C., 140
Borjas, G. J., 38
Borkowski, J. G., 218
Bosk, C. L., 41
Bouchard, C., 220
Bould, S., 219
Bound, J., 27,219,221
Bourque, S. L., 113
Bowles, S., 77
Boyd, M., 50
Boyd, R. L., 60,128
Boykin, A. W., 217
Boyle, M., 119
Bradburn, N. M., 154
Brandt, L. J., 99,218
Brantlinger, E. A., 80
Braungart, N. M., 128
Braungart, R. G., 128
Braveman, P., 151
Brenner, M. H., 158
Bridges, E., 78
Briggs, V. M., 39
Brissie, J. S., 217
Bronfenbrenner, U., 182,184,219
Brooks-Gunn, J., 48,49,60,66,95,96,
        203,215,217,220
Brown, G. W., 129,153
Browne, I., 221
Bruce, M. L., 222
Brunelli, S. A., 97
Bumpass, L. L., 46,215,216
Bunker, J. P., 148
Burgoyne, J., 215
Burke, K. C., 153
Burnard, T., 188
Buron, L., 13
Bursik, R. J., 165,216,223

Burton, L. M., 49,97,219
Butler, A. C., 18
Butler, J. S., 60

Cairns, R. B., 224
Caldwell, J. C., 222
Cameron, B. J., 213
Campbell, F. A., 186
Cancian, M., 110
Cancio, A. S., 138
Capaldi, D. M., 96,224
Caplan, R. D., 100
Card, D., 78
Cardozo, B. N., 221
Carey, G., 162
Carini, P., 217
Carstairs, V., 222
Carta, J. J., 79
Caspi, A., 101,180,186,219,223
Catterall, J. S., 53
Cauce, A. M., 113
Cavalli-Sforza, L. L., 224
Ceci, S.J ., 77,85,92,96,171,178,182
Centerwall, B. S., 101,171
Cerny, P. G., 24
Chalmers, D., 223
Chambliss, W. J., 168
Chao, R., 113
Chase-Lansdale, P. L., 215,220
Chavkin, W., 121
Cheal, D., 12,116,123,226
Cherlin, A., 46
Chevan, A., 215
Choi, S. H., 88
Clairmont, D., 64
Clark, W., 52
Clarke, J. N., 148
Clarke, L. L., 148,222
Clingempeel, W. G., 216
Cloward, R., 224
Coe, R. D., 123
Cohen, L., 63
Cohen, S., 222
Coie, J. D., 220

Coiro, M. J., 152,216,220
Coleman, J. S., 64,65,79,82,150,
    167,217
Colin, C., 213
Collins, C., 140,152
Comer, J. P., 81
Comstock, G., 171
Conger, R. D., 100,104,113
Connell, R. W., 84
Connelly, J. P., 217
Contandriopoulos, A. P., 156
Cook, D. A., 113
Cooksey, E. C., 43
Corcoran, M., 17,118,217
Corsaro, W. A., 220
Corse, S. J., 219
Cose, E., 139
Covington, J., 216,223
Cowan, C. P., 219
Cowan, P. A., 219
Craig, P. H., 215
Crain, R. L., 215
Crane, J., 184,217,225
Crnic, K., 219
Crockett, L. J., 96
Crowder, K. D., 225
Crutchfield, R. D., 169
Cruz, J. E., 132
Curtin, R. B., 216

Dale, A., 54
Dandurand, P., 216
Dandurand, R. B., 46
Danziger, S., 29,37,45,92,110,116
Darling, N. A., 112
Dauber, S. L., 80,136
Davey Smith, G., 149,156,158,223
Davidson, N., 146,222,226
Dawson, D. A., 49
Deater-Deckard, K., 113
DeFries, J. C., 177,179
Deniger, M. A., 14,17,18,197
Dennis, D., 217
Denton, N., 60
DeParlee, J., 37

Devereaux, M. S., 47
Devine, J. A., 12,19,37,94,116,131,
    167,193,213,214,224
Diaz, S., 79
DiLeonardi, J. W.,102
DiMaggio, P., 84
Dishion, T. J., 163,220
Dixon, C., 213
Dohrenwend, B. P., 54,222,223
Dolan, E. G., 213
Doris, J., 102
Dornbusch, S. M., 113,163,217,218
Downey, D. B., 92,215
Doyle, D. P., 223
Drakakis-Smith, D., 213
Dreier, P., 24
Dressler, W. W., 131
Driedger, L., 58
Dryfoos, J. G., 218
Dublin, L. I., 188
Dubow, E. F., 118
Dubrow, N., 69, 102
Duncan, C. M., 183
Duncan, G. J., 25,45,60,65,117,
    118,213

Earls, F., 222
Eckenrode, J., 102
Edin, K., 18
Eggebeen, D. J., 19,48,96,116
Eggers, M., 139,222
Ehrenreich, B., 219
Elder, G. H., 100,101,105,180,186,
    219,220,225
Elford, J., 223
Elias, M. J., 80
Eller, T. J., 131
Ellwood, D. T., 18,46,47,203
Elordi, C. A., 113
Elster, A. B., 98,218,219
Engelbert, A., 220
Engerman, S. L., 188,225
Ensminger, M. E., 18,31,52,53,66,
    217,223
Entwisle, D. R., 80,84,136,215

Epstein, J. L., 82
Escalona, S., 96
Escobar, J. I., 222
Evans, R.G., 143,157,158
Evans, S. L., 96
Evans, T. D., 138

Fagan, J., 67,164,166
Farkas, G., 78,136
Farmer, F. L., 148,222
Farmer, M. M., 138
Farrell, M. P., 99
Farrington, D. P., 160,161
Fee, E., 138
Fehrman, P. G., 218
Feldman, N. W., 224
Fennelly, K., 46
Ferguson, R., 78
Fergusson, D. M., 67,223
Fernandez Kelly, M. P., 18,83,94,
    112,137,216
Ferraro, K. F., 138
Ferree, M. M., 203
Ferron, J., 19
Figlio, R. M.,160
Figueredo, A. J., 102
Fine, M., 80,113
Finn, J. D., 218
Finnie, R., 45
Fischer, D. G., 69
Fish, M., 219
Fishman, G., 224
Fitzgerald, H. E., 110,151
Flanagan, C. A., 105
Flora, C. B., 19,216
Florsheim, P., 112
Fogel, R. W., 188,225
Folk, K. F., 97
Forcier, K. I., 153
Ford, E. S., 222
Forste, R., 46
Forthofer, M. S., 153
Fortmann, S., 222
Foster, E. M., 215
Fox, A. J., 222

Frank, J., 158
Franklin, D. L., 47
Fraser, S., 224
Frazier, H. S., 148
Fréchette, M., 161,215
Freeman, H. P., 140
Freeman, R., 170,221
Frenzen, P., 145
Frideres, J. S., 132
Friede, A., 219
Friedman, H. S., 216,224
Fuchs, V. R., 148
Furstenberg, F. F., 2,46,48,49,64
    94-96,107,215,219
Fyfe, A., 9

Gabe, T., 46
Gable, S., 219
Gadsden, V. L., 213
Garasky, S., 44,49
Garbarino, J., 37,63,69,102,106
    171,173
Garcia-Coll, C., 92,138
Garcia, H. A., 92
Gardner, H., 176
Gardner, M., 30
Gariepy, J. L., 224
Garmezy, N., 182,185
Garrett, P., 19,199
Gartley, J., 31,110
Gartner, A., 217
Gates, E. N., 221
Gauthier, P., 215
Ge, X., 180
Geronimus, A. T., 219,221
Gibson, M. A., 84,88
Gilbert, N., 54
Gilbert, S., 52
Gintis, S., 77
Glick, P., 8
Goldenberg, C., 38,79,87,136
Goldsmith, H. H., 180
Goldsmith, W. W., 25,57,60
Gonzalez, N. A., 113
Good, T. L., 217

Gorman-Smith, D., 67,112
Gornick, M. E., 139
Gottfredson, M. R., 167,223
Gottschalk, P., 18,29,45,92,110, 116,214
Gougis, R. A., 86
Graham, J. W., 131
Gramlich, E., 216
Grannis, J. C., 217
Granovetter, M., 221
Grant, J. P., 10
Grasmick, H. G., 165
Grasmick, H. S., 216,223
Green, G., 129
Greenfield, P. M., 195
Greenhalgh, P., 29,92
Groves, W. B., 63,164,223
Guerra, N. G., 223
Gulley, B. L., 223
Gutman, H. G., 129

Hack, M., 151
Hagan, J., 164,168,170,173,224
Hagedorn, J., 224,225
Haggerty, M., 213
Hahn, R. A., 140,222
Haines, D. W., 214
Halfon, N., 119
Halpern, R., 111
Hamilton, V. L., 150,222
Handel, M. H., 223
Handler, J. F., 29,40
Hansen, D. A., 81
Hanson, S. L., 85
Hao, L., 45,46
Harper, L. V., 180
Harrington, A. J., 215
Harris, I. B., 110
Harris, K. M., 11,16
Harris, T. O., 153,222
Harrison, B., 15,27,60
Haskett, M. E., 96
Hauser, R. M., 202
Haveman, R., 13,23,201,205

Hawkins, A. J., 96
Hawton, K., 223
Hayes, C. D., 48
Hayes-Bautista, D., 141
Health, C. W., 140
Heimer, K., 215
Helm, J., 218
Hendersoon, S., 218
Henry, B., 180
Herbener, E. S., 180
Hernandez, D. J., 215
Herrnstein, R., 78,175,223,225
Hertzman, C., 158
Herz, D. E., 30
Hetherington, E. M., 216
Heyns, B., 84,116
Higgins, A., 119
Hilgartner, S., 41
Hill, M. S., 118,218
Hill, P. T., 78
Hill, S., 111,144
Hirschi, T., 167,223
Hirschl, T. A., 213
Hoffer, T., 65,79,217
Hoffman, S., 45,215
Hogan, D. P., 48,66,165
Holden, K. C., 125
Hollingshead, A. B., 222
Holm, M., 10
Holzer, H. J., 110,137,221
Hoover-Dempsey, V., 217
Hooyman, N., 138,147
Horney, J., 170
Horowitz, R., 153
Horwood, L. J., 223
House, J., 100,223
Huber, J., 222,223
Huesmann, L. R., 98
Hughes, M. E., 49
Hunt, M., 67
Huston, A. C., 108

Ippolito, M. F., 118
Isabella, R., 219

Jackson, J. F., 80,217
Jackson, S. A., 119
Jacobson, N., 66,217
Jargowsky, P., 60,225
Jarjoura, G. R., 216
Jarrett, R. L., 114
Jencks, C., 13,65,68,144,168,
    213,223,225
Jenkins, E. J., 69
Jennings, J., 131,141
Jensen, A. R., 77
Jensen, L., 19
Jewell, K. S., 215
Johnson, C., 96,104,113,213
Johnson, G., 27
Johnson, W. R., 136
Johnston, G. M., 213
Jones, D. A., 213
Juhn, C., 214
Julian, T. W., 100

Kaestle, C., 218
Kagan, J., 180,225
Kagan, S., 86
Kahn, H. S., 222
Kahn, J. R., 215
Kalbach, W. E., 221
Karasek, R., 146
Karp, R. J., 220
Karraker, K. H., 96
Kasarda, J. D., 57,60,129,216
Kasinitz, P., 137,165
Katz, L. F., 214
Keith, B., 216
Keith, T. Z., 218
Kellam, S. G., 81,165,223
Kelly, K., 137
Kendler, K. S., 177,181,224
Kerbow, D., 79,83,87,166
Kerig, P. K., 219
Kerr, D., 29,92
Kessler, R. C., 100,150,153,222,223
Ketterlinus, R. D., 98,99,218
Kim, U., 88
Kinard, E. M., 218

King, G., 140
Kingue, M. D., 8
Kitagawa, E. M., 66,165
Kitchen, B., 117,133,168,223
Kiyak, H. A., 138,147
Klebanov, P. K., 60
Klein, T. P., 122
Klerman, L. V., 93,218,220
Knapp, M. S., 78,218
Knickman, J., 120
Kobrin, S., 224
Kochanek, K. D., 138
Kogevinas, M., 146
Kohn, M. L., 84,218
Kolvin, I., 223
Korten, D. C., 10,34,39,214
Koss, M. P., 102
Kostelny, K., 69,102
Kotlowitz, A., 111
Kozol, J., 76,77
Kramer, B. J., 147
Krieger, N., 138,147,221
Krotki, K. J., 127
Krueger, A., 78
Krugman, D., 32
Kupersmidt, J. B., 65,223

Laird, M., 102
Lamb, M. E., 95,98,218,219
Lamberty, J. H., 138
Lamborn, S. D., 113
Lamkin, R. P., 66,217
Land, K., 161
Landale, N. S., 43,46,215
Lareau, A., 82,83,84
Laren, D., 216
Larrivee, D., 29,92
Larson, K. A., 70,80,86,217
Larzelere, R. E., 113
Lash, A. A., 217
Laub, J. H., 111,169,223-225
Lawton, L., 125
Lazure, J., 50
Le Blanc, M., 161,215
Leaf, P. J ., 222

Lee, E. S., 77
Lefley, H. P., 152
Lein, L., 18
Lemann, N., 128
Lenski, G., 213
Leon, D., 222
Leoussi, A., 222
Lerman, R. I., 100
Lester, B. M., 110,117
LeVine, R. A., 195,213
LeVine, S. E., 195
Levitan, S. A., 28,131
Levy, F., 136,225
Lewis, C. E., 223
Lichter, D. T., 43,46,116,213,215
Lieberman, L., 224
Lieberson, S., 39,128
Liebert, R. M., 171
Liem, G. R., 99
Liem, J. H., 99
Lightfoot, S. L., 217
Lillie-Blanton, M., 138
Lim, L. Y., 32
Lind, M., 225
Lindsay, C., 47,215
Lindsey, D., 220
Linhares, E. D., 213
Link, B. G., 71,120
Linn, M. W., 222
Lipsky, D. K., 217
Lloyd, D. A., 216
Lo, O., 215
Lockhead, C., 11,14
Loeber, R., 223,224
Loehlin, J. C., 179
Logan, J. R., 220,221
Lomas, J., 156
London, R. A., 46
Lorion, R., 107
Lotka, A. J., 188
Lowry, R., 150
Lubeck, S., 199
Luckenbill, D. F., 223
Lundberg, O., 144
Luthar, S. S., 225

Lynam, D.R., 161,174,223
Lynskey, M. T., 67,223

MacLeod, D., 218
Magnusson, D., 225
Manlove, J., 215
Manning, W. D., 46
Manor, O., 222
Manson, S. M., 222
Margolin, S., 213
Margolis, P. A., 145
Marks, C., 221
Marmor, T. R., 222
Marmot, M. G., 143,144,146,149,
    156,158,222
Marotto, R. A., 217
Marsden, L., 53
Marshall, I. H., 170
Marsland, D., 222
Martin, S. L., 158
Martin, T. C., 216
Mason, C. A., 113
Massat, C. R., 96
Massey, D., 60,139,201
Masten, A. S., 182,185
Matsueda, R. L., 215
Matthews, K., 222
Maughan, B., 80
Maume, D. J., 138
Maurer, J. D., 138
Maxim, P. S.,221
Maxwell, N., 136
Mayer, S. E., 13,65,68,144,213,216
Maynard, R., 215
McAdoo, H. P., 216,221
McCall, P., 63
McCarthy, B., 164
McCartney, K., 180
McClain, P., 63
McClean, G.E., 177
McClelland, P., 85
McCloskey, L. A., 102
McCord, C., 140
McCord, J., 225

McCormack, T., 155,223
McDonald, P. L., 124
McDonough, P., 144,146
McGrath, E., 152
McGuire, A. M., 224
McKenry, P. C., 100
McLanahan, S., 215,216,218
McLaughlin, D., 125,213
McLeod, J. D., 118,150
McLoyd, V. C., 101,102,105,153,219
McMiller, W. E., 47
McPartland, J. M., 89
Mehan, H., 79,89
Menaghan, E. G., 15,84,203
Mendoza, F. S., 138
Menzies, H., 24
Meyer, D. R., 44
Middle, C., 151
Miles, D. R., 162
Miller, C. K., 46
Miller, J. M., 169
Miller, J. W., 96
Miller, M. K., 148,222
Mincy, R. B., 225
Mines, R., 39
Minty, B., 219
Miranda, L. C., 215
Mishel, L., 12
Mitchell, A., 218,220
Mitchell-Kerman, C., 215
Mitman, A. L., 217
Moffitt, R., 214
Moffitt, T. E., 53,67,114
        160-162,223
Moll, L. C., 79
Molnar, J. M., 122
Montgomery, A. F., 80
Moore, K., 93
Moorman, J., 215
Morgan, S. P., 48,95
Morris, P. A., 49,93,97,110
Morris, R., 222
Morrison, D. R., 216
Morrison, P. A., 218
Moss, V. D., 79

Mosteller, F., 148
Mulinare, J., 140,222
Mulkey, L. M., 215
Muller, C., 79,82,83,166
Mullis, I., 218
Mundy-Castle, A. C., 196
Murnane, R. J., 136,225
Murphy, K., 31,214
Murray, C., 78,175,224,225

Nagin, D. S., 161,162
Neal, D. A., 136
Nelson, J. L., 15,24,26,31,33
Newacheck, P. W., 119
Ng'andu, N., 19
Nguyen, T., 101,186
Nicholas, L. J., 219
Nicolau, S., 61,86
Nielsen, F., 45,213
Nitz, K., 99,218
Noble, D. F., 25
Nord, S., 83,214
Norris, D., 50,58
Norton, A. J., 215

O'Connor, C., 9
O'Connor, T. G., 184
Oden, M. H., 224
Oderkirk, J., 45
Offord, D. B., 119
Ogbu, J. U., 66,75,84,88,89,141,174,
        184,193,221
Ohlin, L., 224
Oldman, D., 218
O'Neill, B. J., 128
O'Neill, J., 136
Orfield, G., 86,218
Ormrod, R., 215
Orok, B., 52
Osgood, D. W., 170
Ouston, J., 80

Padilla, F., 170
Palloni, A., 173
Palosaari, U. K., 49
Pappas, G., 146
Paradise, M. J., 113
Parcel, T. L., 84
Parker, M. B., 93,220
Patterson, G. R., 96,163,219,220,224
Pattinson, G., 219
Payne, S., 111
Peebles-Wilkins, W., 101
Peirce, R. S., 222
Pelton, L., 101,103
Perlman, S. B., 218
Perry, C., 125
Persky, J., 27
Peterson, P., 225
Pettit, G. S., 217
Phelps, J. J., 214
Pierce, B., 214
Pierce, J. L., 218
Pike, A., 175,224
Pillemer, K., 103
Plomin, R., 175,177,179,180,224
Polakow, V., 77
Portes, A., 38,89,90,137,196,218
Powell, B., 92
Power, C., 146,150,222
Pratto, F., 219
Price, R. H., 100
Prilleltensky, I., 226
Pugh, H., 150
Pulkkinen, L., 225

Quinn, J. F., 220
Quinton, D., 67
Qvortrup, J., 32,116,126

Racine, Y., 119
Radwanski, G., 85
Rafferty, Y., 120-122,220
Raftery, A. E., 49
Rainwater, L., 116
Raley, R. K., 46
Ram, B., 58

Ramey, C. T., 85,158,186
Ramey, S. L., 85,158
Rank, M. R., 213
Rasberry, W., 138
Rashid, A., 30,31
Rattner, A., 224
Rauh, V. A., 97
Redlich, F. C., 222
Reed, R. J., 80
Regier, D. A., 152
Reid, C., 163
Reid, J. B., 127,220
Reimer, T. M., 218
Reiss, A. J., 168,224
Reznick, J. S., 180
Rhoades, E., 147
Rhodes, M., 25
Rhodes, R. A., 25
Rice, J., 223
Richards, M. P. W., 215
Richters, J., 91
Ricketts, E. R., 225
Ries, P., 144
Rifkin, J., 28,226
Risman, B. J., 203
Ritter, L. P., 163,217
Rivera-Batiz, F. L., 136
Rivkin, S. G., 75
Roberge, R., 150
Roberts, J., 215
Robins, L. N., 152,161,223
Robins, R. W., 223
Rodgers, H. R., 25,42,43,213
Rodgers, W. L., 117
Rodin, J., 150
Rohe, W. M., 202
Rohner, R. P., 113
Rollins, N., 120,121,122
Romo, F. P., 214
Roosa, M. W., 95
Rose, H., 63
Rose, N., 223
Rosenbaum, J. E., 66
Rosenberg, H. M., 138
Rosenberg, J., 137,165

Rosier, K. B., 220
Ross, C. E., 222,223
Ross, D. P., 11,14
Rossi, P. H., 71
Rossi, R. J., 80
Roth, J., 168
Roth, W. R., 122
Round, J. M., 213
Rowe, D. C., 177,223
Rubin, B. R., 223
Rumbaut, R. G., 89
Rumberger, R. W., 70,80,81,86,217
Rutter, M., 80,173,180-182,184

Saltzman, W., 107
Sameroff, A. J., 118,181
Sampson, R. J., 61,63,64,95,111,
    134,163,164,169,173,215,
    223-225
Sandefur, G., 37,215
Sandfort, J. R., 218
Sandifer, R., 222
Sapolsky, R. M., 222
Saporiti, A., 32,220
Sassen, S., 24,28,34,213
Saucier, J. F., 216
Saudino, K. J., 180
Saugstad, L. F., 153
Sawhill, I. V., 131,213,225
Scarr, S.,81,180,225
Scheper-Hughes, N., 8,10,156
Schiller, B. R., 12,13,29,35,52,92,
    135,214
Schmidt, K., 219
Schoenbach, C., 218
Schooler, C., 218
Schor, E. L., 15,203
Schor, J., 213
Schteingart, J. S., 120
Schuerman, L. A., 224
Schultz, T., 218
Schuster, C. R., 138
Schwab-Stone, M. E., 69
Schwartz, J. E., 216
Schwartz, M., 214

Schwenk, F. N., 124
Sclar, E., 27
Sealand, N., 216
Seifer, R., 118
Seppa, N., 171
Serrill, M. S., 225
Sgritta, G. B., 32,37,116,126,220
Shakoor, B., 223
Shanahan, M. J., 118
Shaper, A. G., 223
Shapiro, L., 78
Shaver, D. M., 217
Shavit, Y., 218
Sheets, R. G., 214
Sheley, J. F., 70,160,224
Sherman, A., 220
Sherman, D., 102
Shields, P. M., 217,218
Shihadeh, E. S., 88
Shillington, E. R., 11,14
Shinn, M., 120-122,220
Shipley, M. J., 223
Sickmund, M., 140
Silva, P. A., 223
Silverstein, M., 125
Simon, D., 8
Simon, J., 12
Simons, L. M., 32
Simons, R. L., 104,113,161
Sklar, H., 219
Skof, K., 58
Skogan, W. G., 26,64,224
Slavin, R. E., 85
Slomczynski, K. M., 218
Slusarcick, A. L., 31,52,53
Smeeding, T., 25,116,213,220
Smith, A. P., 222
Smith, D. R., 216
Smith, G. D., 222
Smith, J., 45,220
Smith, M. D., 224
Smith, R., 225
Smith, S. E., 47
SmithBattle, L., 48
Smock, P., 45

Snidman, N., 180
Snyder, H. N., 140
Solon, G., 51
Sorlie, P. D., 138
South, S. J., 43,100,226
Spiegelman, M., 188
Spitze, G., 100,220
Sprafkin, J., 171
Squires, T. S., 140
Srole, L., 222
Sroufe, L. A., 181
St. Peter, R. F. 119
Stafford. M., 223
Starrels, M. E., 219
Statistics Canada, 52,59,122,133,
        145,151,152,154,213-215,
        222
Steelman, L. C., 92
Steffensmeier, D. J., 88
Stegman, M., 202
Stein, S., 222
Steinberg, L., 65,89,112,113,217
Sternberg, K. J., 102,112
Stevens, J. A., 222
Stevenson, D. R., 218
Stevenson, H. W., 83
Stier, H., 137
Stigler, J. W., 83
Stoddart, G. L., 157
Stokes, R., 215
Stokols, D., 145
Stollard, K., 219
Stouthamer-Loeber, M., 223
Strachan, J., 47
Strasburger, V., 171
Straub, L. A., 145
Straus, M. A., 112
Strawn, J., 37,116
Strobel, F. R., 26,192
Strobino, D. M., 219
Stull, D., 147
Suarez-Orozco, M. M., 88
Sucoff, C. A., 69
Sudarkasa, N., 215
Sui-Chu, E. H., 78,128

Sullivan, M., 99,134,165
Sum, A. M., 218
Swadener, B. B., 80,90,200
Sweet, J. A., 46,216

Taeuber, C., 124
Takeuchi, D. T., 222
Taylor, M. J., 79
Taylor, R., 216,223
Terman, L. M., 224
Tesh, S. N., 222
Tessler, R., 217
Testa, M., 43,47,48
Teti, D. M., 95
Teutsch, S. M., 140,222
Theorell, T., 146
Thomas, G., 99
Thompson, M., 215
Thompson, W. M., 220
Thomson, E., 216
Thorbecke, E., 8
Thornberry, T. P., 160
Thornton, A., 215
Tienda, M., 137
Tigges, L., 129
Tilly, C., 15,28
Todd, G., 24
Tolan, P. H., 67,112,223
Tonry, M., 167-169,224
Toro, P. A., 70,71,220
Townsend, P., 146,222,225
Trejo, S. J., 38
Tremblay, R. E., 225
Trickett, P. K., 219
Tschann, J. M., 185,223
Tshishimbi, wa B., 8
Tucker, M. B., 215
Turnbull, B. J., 78
Turner, J. B., 100,222,223
Turner, R. J., 216
Tyrell, D. A., 222

Umberson, D., 125
Uribe, F. M., 195

U.S. Bureau of the Census, 29,43,54, 86,116,123,125,132,213-215, 220,221
Uzzell, O., 101

Vagero, D., 144
Valdivieso, R., 61,86
Van Ijzendoorn, M. H.,95
Vaughan, L., 95
Vega, W. A., 141
Venezky, R., 218
Vinokur, A. D., 100
Vogt, R., 213
Volpe, R., 101

Wachs, T. D., 175,186,222
Wacquant, L. J., 35,60,63,88,134
Wadhera, S., 47
Waite, L. J., 218
Wall, D. D., 220
Wallace, D., 216
Wallace, R., 216
Waller, J. H., 223
Walzer, N., 145
Wanner, R .A., 124
Warr, M., 223
Warr, P., 223
Warren, J. R., 86
Wartella, E., 224
Wasserman, G. A., 97,196
Waters, H. F., 172
Weatherall, D., 224
Weimann, G., 224
Weinberg, D., 37
Weintraub, S., 91
Weiss, C. C., 96
Weiss, H. B., 218
Weitzman, B. C., 120
Welch, F., 31
Werner, E., 182,185
Werthamer-Larsson, L., 223
West, C., 167
West, D. J., 162
Wethington, E.,160,168,174,205
Wheaton, B., 216

Wheeler, L., 223
Whincup, P., 223
White, H. R., 223
White, J., 161
White, K. R., 79
Whitehead, M., 145,146
Wiewel, W., 27
Wilkinson, R. G., 144,222
Willett, J. B., 225
Williams, D., 140,152,156
Williamson, D. F., 222
Willms, J. D., 78,218
Wilson, J. B., 203
Wilson, J. Q., 223
Wilson, L., 153
Wilson, W. J., 61,65,88,93,128,129, 134,135,138,164,166,167, 215,223
Winkleby, M. A., 222
Wintersberger, H., 214
Wise, A. W., 78
Wolfe, B., 23,111,119,144,201,205
Wolfgang, M. E., 160
Wolfson, M., 150
Wright, J. D., 12,13,19,37,70,71,94, 116,131,160,167,193,213, 214,217
Wu, C., 222
Wu, L. L., 49,215

Yansane, A. Y., 8
Yelaja, S. A., 128
Yeo, F. L., 86
Yeung, W. J., 117

Zamsky, E. J., 215
Zelizer, V. A. R., 32
Zelkowitz, P., 219
Zill, N., 83,216,220
Zima, B. T., 121
Zingraff, M. T., 223
Zucker, R. A., 151
Zuckerman, B., 110
Zuckerman, D., 171
Zuo, J., 216

Subject Index

Abilities, 176,182,184
Abuse
    child, 101,102
    of parents, 103,104
    spousal, 100-102
Actualization
    of abilities, 176,184,185
    of negative traits, 176,184,185
Adolescent mothers, 18,47,93-98,
        204,218,219
Africa, 7-10
African American(s), 88,125,127,
        131,163,167,168,187-189,
        225
    child poverty, 46,47,116,131
    childrearing practices, 95,105,113
    families, 43,46,93,97,101,125
    health, 138-141,146
    and jobs, 27,93,129,136
    middle class, 60,128,129
    migration to the north, 60,61,128
    and neighborhoods, 59,60,63-64,
        138,165,195,196,221
    poverty, 20,46-48,93,123,134,
        165,216,220
    and schools, 77,78,86,87,123,136
    unemployment, 93,129
Assets, 51,131
Assimilation, 89,196
Assortative mating, 30,31,207

Behavior genetics, 175-178
Behavioral problems, 119,161
Birth weight, 96,119,121,151
Blacks. See African American(s)

Canada and the United States, 6,
        11,12,24,35,58,59,221
Capital, 82
    human, 82,83,150,167
    social, 64,82,83,104,150,167
Causality, 1,142
Chain of events, 152,180-182
Child, children
    development, 93-100,118-120,182
    health, 121,158
    homeless, 120-122,164
    mortality, 10,119,140,147,148,222
    neglect, 102,103
    poverty, 37,47-51,68,115-120
    at risk, 95,182
    and schools, 122
    social construct, 116
Childrearing (parenting) practices,
        112-114,177,179,224
Class. See Social class
Community(ies), 152
    functional, 65,79,217
Competitiveness, 25,39,40
Computers, computerization, 24,
        191,196
Conduct disorders. See Behavioral
        problems
Context, 1,95
Contraception, 92,94
Corporations, 24,33,34,40,191,
        192,214
Cross-pressure, 67,208
Culture of poverty. See Subculture
        of poverty

Debt
    national, 36
    personal, 14,46

Delinquency, 98,159
  as a cause of poverty, 53,54,159
  development of, 67,160-162,
    173,174
  as a result of poverty, 159,164-174
Depression, 108,152,153,210,212
Discrimination, 127,130,135-138,
  167,201
Disorganization. *See* Social
  disorganization
Divorce, 42
  and poverty, 45,46,124
Downward mobility. *See* Social
  mobility
Dropout (school), 35,51-53,170,
  202,214
Drug trade, 67,166,168

Education, 40,76,77,83,84,94,
  122,136. *See also* Schools
Educational requirements, 31-32
Elderly poverty, 109,122-125
  minority, 123
  women, 109,124,125
Ethnic cultures, 194-197

Families, family, 106,214
  single-parent,14,64,93,100,163
  two-parent,14,64
  two-wage earner, 30,31
Family size, 28,91-93
Fathers, single, 99,100,116
Fertility, 10
Financial sector, finances, 24,33,34,
  191
Free trade agreements, 23,24,35

Gap (between classes, rich and poor),
  8, 14-16,33,117,143-145,
  148,191,194
GDP, 204

Genes and environment, 155,158,
  175,186
Genetic inferiority, 175,186-189
Genetic potential, 176,182
Genotype-environment correlations,
  177-180,207,210,211
Globalization of the economy, 10,
  23-25,192
GNP, 8,209
Guns, 70

Health, 146,158,222
  differentials by SES, 124,143-154
  elderly, 124,158
  minority, 138,139,140
  women, 124,125
Health care, 62,63
Hispanic, 60,80,127,131
  health, 138,140,141
  immigration, 127
  poverty, 60,116,131
Home ownership, 51,202,215,
  216,226
Homelessness, 70,71
Housing, 149,156,182,201,202

Illness, 54,146
Immigrant(s), immigration, 38,39,61,
  127,132,141,195
Income, 145,213
  differences, 136,137,144
  distribution, 43,51,52,123,144
Industries and industrialization,
  25-27,156
Inner-city
  concentration of poverty, 57,61,
    134,193
  crime in, 61,70
Intergenerational transmission, 95-97,
  118,155,183,187,189,200
IQ, 77,78,84,154-156,176,
  185,187,224

Jobs
  creation, 28,29,197
  entry-level, 26
  in inner cities, 24,26,32,33,60,61
  loss, 25-27,60,61
  low-paid, 27-30,31,203
  low-skilled, 30
  part-time, 28,29
  relocation, 32,33,60,214

Life expectancy, 140,141,146-150

Manufacturing jobs, 25-27,31,197
  loss of, 26-27,60
Marital conflict, 100,101
Maternal employment, 17,18,30,
  108,203
Media, 166,171-173,184,205,224
Medical care, 139,146-149,156-158,
  203
Mental illness, 54,152-154
Meritocracy, 196-198
Mexican Americans, 43,60,86-88,
  116,132,140,141
Middle class, 12,82-85,103,111,218
Minorities, 130,168
  education, 85-87
  segregation, 60,61,129,130
  voluntary and involuntary, 87-90
Mobility. *See* Social mobility
Monitoring. *See* Supervision (of
  children)
Mothers, 16,107,110,112,114,115,
  219,220. *See also* Adolescent
  mothers; Single mothers

Natives, 58,88,123,127,132,147,221
Neighborhoods
  and child outcomes, 65,66,111
  and crime, 61,63,67,103
  dangerous, 103,166

Neighborhoods *(continued)*
  disadvantaged (poor), 53,57-73,94,
    100-102,130,134,165,186,
    201-204,217
  disorganization of, 61,63,106,
    163,169
  and family relations, 64,65,102,
    105,111,166
  middle-class, 65,66,71,72,217
  segregation, 134,135,166-169

Parents, parental, parenting, 172,207,
  224
  authoritative, 65,104,112
  authority, 114,115,220
  blaming of, 111
  burden, 103,104,108,111
  competence, 96,103
  expectations, 52,83,84,96
  investment, 107
  resources, 82-85,155
  skills, 104-107,165
  supervision, 83,102-104,163,166
Peers, peer group, 98,100,217,220
  influence of, 68,69,94,104,165
  minority children and, 89,90
  peers' parents, 104,217
Personality, 178,179
Poverty, 13,130
  adaptations to, 94,95,199,218
  causes of, 1,2,23,49,54,55
  concentration of, 129,193,201-204
  consequences, 1,2,155,176,179,
    183,186
  cutoffs, 12,122,215
  discourse on, 39,191,200,201
  employed poor, 13,14,191
  mobility in and out, 16-18,183
  personal causes, 41-55
  rural, 19,20
  systemic causes, 23-40,142,191,
    194,211
Profit, emphasis on, 33,34,192
Puerto Rican(s), 60,61,132

Racial inequality, 130-133,165,167
Racism, 128-130
Resilience, 150,181
Resources, parental, 82-85,97
Rich (the), 14-16,33,199-201
Rural, 145,148
    poverty, 9,19,20,57,75,216,220

Schools, 165,196,218
    disadvantaged, 75-78,202
    families and, 75,78,81,82
    and minorities, 85-87
    parents and, 78,79,82-85
    personnel, 77,78
    and poor children, 77,80,81
    in poor neighborhoods, 31,70,
        75-90
    segregation, 86,87
    successful, 81
Segregation, 58,61,86,87,133-135,
        166-169,193,194,216
Service sector, 27,28,211
Single fathers. See Fathers, single
Single mothers, 91,129. See also
        Adolescent mothers
    child outcomes, 111,215
    child poverty, 95-97,215
    divorced, 42
    employment, 29
    neighborhoods, 63,111,114
    never-married, 42,46,47,48
    poverty, 29,43-45,105,111,115
Single parenting, 42-50
Skills, 50,174
    work-related, 135,136,196-198,
        221
Social assistance. See Welfare
Social class, 58,211
    differences by, 80,83-85,143-156,
        182
Social control, 64,164-166
Social disorganization, 61,63,106,
        163,169,171
Social mobility, downward, 49,150,
        208

Social pathologies, 198-200
Socialization (of children/
        adolescents) 194
    collective, 66,217
    in poor neighborhoods, 65-68
Socioeconomic status. See Social
        class
Stigma, 17,89,111
Stress, stressors, 105,145,149,150,
        181,186
Subculture of poverty, 193-197,225
Supervision (of children), 83,102,
        103,104,163,166
    collective, 69,103
    and neighborhoods, 68,69

Technology, technologization, 19,
        191,196-198
Television, 166,184,229
Temperament, 81,82,101,165,185

Unemployment, 35,61,105,144,153,
        154,169,191,222

Victimization, 63,64
Violence, 69,160,166,168,171,184

Welfare, 11,41,47,99,117
    low payments, 36,37,203
    mobility out of, 16-18,48,131
Women, 143. See also Adolescent
        mothers; Single mothers
    earnings, 28,29,110
    elderly, 109,124,125
    health, 111
Work, 16,135-138,197
Work habits, 83,185

Youth unemployment, 26,35,36

T - #0490 - 101024 - C0 - 212/152/17 - PB - 9780789002327 - Gloss Lamination